THIRD EDITION

Fundamentals of MENTAL HEALTH NURSING

Kathy Neeb, RN, BA
Case Manager for Workers Compensation
HealthPartners
Minneapolis, MN

F. A. DAVIS COMPANY ■ Philadelphia

F. A. Davis Company
1915 Arch Street
Philadelphia, PA 19103
www.fadavis.com

Printed in the United States of America

Last digit indicates print number: 10 9 8 7 6 5 4 3 2

Acquisitions Editor: Lisa M. Deitch
Developmental Editor: Alan Sorkowitz
Art Manager: Carolyn O'Brien

As new scientific information becomes available through basic and clinical research, recommended treatments and drug therapies undergo changes. The author(s) and publisher have done everything possible to make this book accurate, up to date, and in accord with accepted standards at the time of publication. The author(s), editors, and publisher are not responsible for errors or omissions or for consequences from application of the book, and make no warranty, expressed or implied, in regard to the contents of the book. Any practice described in this book should be applied by the reader in accordance with professional standards of care used in regard to the unique circumstances that may apply in each situation. The reader is advised always to check product information (package inserts) for changes and new information regarding dose and contraindications before administering any drug. Caution is especially urged when using new or infrequently ordered drugs.

Library of Congress Cataloging-in-Publication Data
Neeb, Kathy
    Fundamentals of mental health nursing / Kathy Neeb—3rd ed.
        p.   cm.
    Includes bibliographical references and index.
    ISBN 10: 0-8036-1401-2   ISBN 13: 978-0-8036-1401-7
1. Psychiatric nursing.   2. Practical nursing.
    [DNLM: 1. Mental Disorders—nursing.   2. Nursing, Practical.   3. Psychiatric
Nursing—methods. WY 160 N373f 2006] I. Title.
    RC440.N415 2006
    616.89′0231—dc22   2005014728

This book is dedicated to the special people in my life:

- **To the many friends, colleagues, and especially the patients who have graciously shared their stories and their journeys with me as I have walked through my journey:**
  Thank you. I am eternally indebted to you all.

- **To my wonderful family:**
  I love you all very much!

Preface

For years now, my students in practical nursing have labored through textbooks of mental health nursing. The information in these textbooks, although interesting and accurate, has gone far beyond the scope of practice for the practical/vocational nurse.

Many students at this level of preparation do not have the opportunity for clinical experience in a mental health setting, and, in fact, many are not employed in "psych units." Much of what the LPN/LVN experiences of mental health problems is actually learned on medical-surgical clinical rotations.

It is therefore one goal of this text to provide basic information pertaining to areas of mental health that can be recognized more easily and used more accurately by the nurse in a medical-surgical venue.

Psychology is the study of the mind. It has many subdivisions and specialty areas. More than 50 theories pertain to personality development and therapy. The brain is an amazing organ; its effects on health and illness are infinite. It is important for nurses to recognize the mind-body connection that exists in each person. There are as many variables in diagnosing and treating mental illnesses as there are patients who have them.

As recently as May 2004, the World Health Organization released a study showing that rates of mental illness, especially depression, anxiety, eating disorders, and substance abuse are higher in the United States than any other country in the world. Ukraine ranked second. Clearly, the need for nurses worldwide to have education and clinical training in caring for people who have mental disorders, is of paramount importance.

This text attempts to point out some of the common correlations between physical and psychological illness and healing. Many chapters include case studies. These are fictional, and any association with a specific individual is purely coincidental. By working through these materials, students will have the opportunity to simulate the patient-care situations they will encounter in clinical practice.

A second goal of this text is to present the concept of the unlimited possibilities in the world of psychology. This is a "soft" science with many theories and few absolute answers. The possibilities are endless. It is important to expand your scope of thinking and be open to the many ideas and potentials that are present when you begin to work with individuals and their minds and bodies. You will begin to learn to think in concepts and abstracts and to ask, "What if . . .?"

I have chosen to "personalize" much of the text for two reasons. First of all, I want the book to emulate a conversation or a comfortable lecture/discussion format. Second, I want to prepare you as students to realize that you ARE (or soon will be) the nurse! Very soon, the situations and actions presented here will be yours to experience in your nursing practice; by personalizing the text and critical thinking questions, I hope that each of you will put yourself in the position of "virtual nurse!"

Fundamentals of Mental Health Nursing, Edition 3, offers students and instructors some new features. In addition to a new four-color format, it has added graphics in the form of photos, tables, and other drawings to help create impact of certain topics. I hope visual learners will find that especially helpful.

I have chosen to expand this edition by adding two new chapters. Editions 1 and 2 purposely did not include the special population of children and adolescents. Many instructors asked us to incorporate some of that information. In response to those requests, I am pleased to offer a chapter focusing on some of the childhood and adolescent disorders you may commonly encounter in your nursing life. The other new chapter expands on what was previously an appendix. As our population changes and becomes ever more diverse, so health care needs to be able to diversify to meet the needs of the people of those cultures and belief systems. Therefore, a full chapter has been dedicated to exploring some of the alternative modalities being introduced into mainstream nursing practice.

Throughout the text, you will find several new and updated case studies. I have added questions in the new NCLEX testing formats to assist in preparing for licensure examination. For instructors, I have included an expanded PowerPoint presentation and test bank to the Instructor's Resource Disk for the book.

I hope you find this text as much of a joy to use as it was for me to write. In the big picture, this is just a "day trip" into the great journey of psychology. It is a difficult, challenging, and very exciting excursion. I wish each of you a pleasant journey!

For the instructor, this book is accompanied by a comprehensive instructor's guide, an extensive Cybertest computerized test bank, and PowerPoint presentations for most chapters.

Kathy Neeb

Contributors

Robin A. Spidle, RN, PhD
Payson, Arizona

Brenda Agee, RN, MSN
Nursing Instructor
Delaware Technical and Community College
Georgetown, Delaware

Consultants to the Third Edition

Sue Garland, RN, MSN, ARNP
Division Chair, Allied Health and Related
    Technologies
Practical Nursing Program Coordinator
Big Sandy Community and Technical College
Paintsville, Kentucky

Debra Hodge
Licensed Practical Nursing
West Virginia Academy of Careers and
    Technology
Beckley, West Virginia

Maureen L. McGary, RN, MSN, NP-C
Former Program Head, Practical Nursing
Virginia Western Community College
Wirtz, Virginia

Consultants to Previous Editions

Ethel Avery, RN, MSN, EdS
Instructor
H. Councill Trenholm State Technical College
Montgomery, Alabama

Sharon M. Erbe, RN, BSN, MSN(c)
Nursing Coordinator
WSWHE BOCES
Hudson Falls, New York

Gloria Ferritto, RN, BSN, PHN
Assistant Director, Vocational Nursing Program
Maric College
Vista, California

Frances Francis, RN, ADN, BS
Practical Nursing Instructor
Hazard Regional Technology Center
Hazard, Kentucky

Nancy T. Hatfield, RN, BSN, MA
Instructor, Practical Nursing Program
Career Enrichment Center
Albuquerque Public Schools
Albuquerque, New Mexico

Christine D. Herdlick, RN, BA
Nursing Instructor
Marshalltown Community College
Marshalltown, Iowa

Phyllis Lilly, RN, BSN
Instructor
Isabella Graham Hart School of Practical
    Nursing
Rochester General Hospital
Rochester, New York

**Betty Richardson, RN, PhD, LPC,
LMFT, CS, CNAA**
Instructor, Practical Nursing Program
Austin Community College
Austin, Texas

Judy Stauder, RN, MSN
Coordinator
Practical Nursing Program of Canton City
    Schools
Canton, Ohio

Table of Contents

1

Foundations for Mental Health Nursing

1

History of Mental Health Nursing

Learning Objectives ▪ ▪ ▪

1. Identify the major contributors to the field of mental health nursing.
2. Know the basic tenets or theories of the contributors to mental health nursing.
3. Define three types of treatment facilities.
4. Identify three breakthroughs that advanced the field of mental health nursing.
5. Identify the major laws and provisions of each that influenced mental health nursing.

Key Terms ▪ ▪ ▪

- American Nurses Association
- Asylum
- Deinstitutionalization
- Free-standing treatment centers
- Hospital
- National League for Nursing
- Nurse Practice Act
- Psychotropic
- Standards of care

▪ THE TRAILBLAZERS

For centuries, nurses have been many things to many people. We have nurses to thank for cooking, cleaning, and ministering to those who fought our battles.

Long before we knew what aerobic or anaerobic microorganisms were, nurses knew when to open or close the windows. Nurses helped women give birth to their young and nursed the babies when mothers were unable to or when mothers died during or shortly after giving birth. The first flight attendants were nurses. For centuries, nurses have gone about the business of caring for people, but they haven't always done that quietly. Who were the nurses who took the risks? Who were the ones who spoke out on behalf of the patient and the profession? In times when nursing was considered only "women's work," and when women were not politically active, the major trailblazers were female.

FLORENCE NIGHTINGALE

Florence Nightingale (1820–1910) has been called the founder of nursing. Her story and her contributions are numerous enough to fill many volumes. She was born of wealth and was highly educated. When she was very young, she realized she wanted to be a nurse, which did not please her parents. Conditions in hospitals were poor, and her parents wanted her to pursue a life as wife, mother, and society woman.

Florence worked hard to educate herself in the art and science of nursing. Her mission to help the British soldiers in the Crimean War earned her respect in the world as a nurse and administrator (Fig. 1-1). This was no easy task because many of the soldiers at Scutari resented her intelligence and did what they could to undermine her work.

It is due to her observations and diligence that the relationship between sanitary conditions and healing became known and accepted. Within 6 months of her arrival in Scutari, the mortality rate dropped from 42.7 percent to 2.2 percent (Donahue, 1985, p. 244). She insisted on proper lighting, diet, cleanliness, and recreation. She understood even then that the mind and body worked together, that cleanliness, the predecessor to our clean and sterile techniques of today, was a major barrier to infection, and that it promoted healing. She carefully observed and documented changes in the conditions of the soldiers, which led to her adulation as "The Lady with the Lamp" (from the poem "Santa Filomena" by H. W. Longfellow).

Above all, she was a crusader for the improvement of care and conditions in the military and civilian hospitals in Britain. Among her books are *Notes on Hospitals* (1859), which deals with the relationship of sanitary techniques to medical facilities; *Notes on Nursing* (1859), which was the most respected nursing textbook of the day; and *Notes on Matters Affecting the Health, Efficiency and Hospital Administration of the British Army* (1857) (Donahue, 1985, p. 248).

The first formal nurses' training program, the Nightingale School for Nurses, opened in 1860. The goals of the school were to train nurses to work in hospitals, to work with the poor, and to teach. This meant that students cared for people in their homes, an idea that is still gaining in popularity and professional opportunity for nurses. Florence Nightingale died at the age of 90. What a role model!

DOROTHEA DIX

Dorothea Dix (1802–1887) (Fig. 1-2) was not actually a nurse, but rather a schoolteacher. She believed that people did not need to live

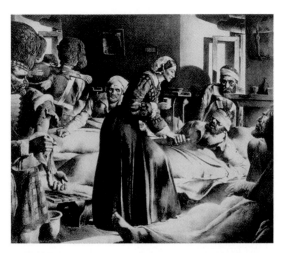

FIGURE 1-1. Florence Nightingale at work during the Crimean War.

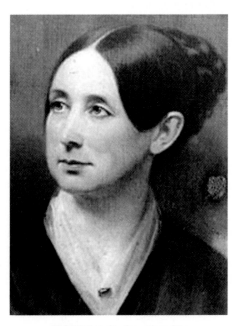

FIGURE 1-2. Dorothea Dix

in suffering and that society at large had a responsibility to aid those less fortunate. Her primary focus was the care of prisoners and the mentally ill. She not only lobbied in both the United States and Canada for the improvement of **standards of care** for the mentally ill, but she went one step further and suggested that the governments take an active role in providing help with finances, food, shelter, and other areas of need. She learned that many criminals were also mentally ill, a theory that is borne out in continuing studies today. Because of the efforts of Dorothea Dix, 32 states developed asylums or "psychiatric hospitals" to care for the mentally ill. There is a monument to her and her efforts on the Women's Heritage Trail in Boston.

LINDA RICHARDS

While Dorothea Dix was working for political help in the field of mental health, a nurse named Linda Richards (1841–1930) (Fig. 1-3) was pushing to upgrade nursing education.

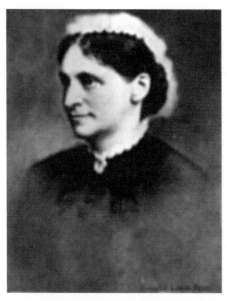

Linda Richards
America's First Trained Nurse
Born in Potsdam, 1841

FIGURE 1-3. Linda Richards

She was the first American-trained nurse, and in 1882 she opened the Boston City Hospital Training School for Nurses to teach the specialty of caring for the mentally ill. By 1890, more than 30 asylums in this country had developed schools for nurses. Linda Richards was among the first nurses to teach and work seriously with planning and developing nursing care for patients. In cooperation with the **American Nurses Association** (ANA) and the **National League for Nursing,** she was instrumental in developing textbooks specifically for nurses that had stated objectives for outcomes of nursing education and patient care.

HARRIET BAILEY

The first textbook focusing on psychiatric nursing was written in 1920 by Harriet Bailey.

EFFIE JANE TAYLOR

Ms. Taylor initiated the first psychiatric program of study for nurses in the year 1913. She is also well known for her development and implementation of patient-centered care. Patient-centered care with an emphasis on the emotional and intellectual life of the patient was also stressed by Ms. Taylor.

MARY MAHONEY

Mary Mahoney (1845–1926) (Fig. 1-4) is considered to be America's first African-American professional nurse. Her contributions lay primarily in home care and in the promotion of the acceptance of African-Americans in the field of nursing. An award in her name is presented annually at the ANA convention to a person who has worked to promote equal opportunity for minorities in nursing. During her career it was necessary to open separate schools of nursing for African-American students because they were banned from the white schools. Two of these schools of note were Spelman

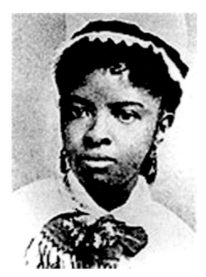

FIGURE 1-4. Mary Mahoney

Seminary, in Atlanta, and Tuskegee Institute, in Alabama.

HILDEGARD PEPLAU

Dr. Hildegard Peplau (1909–1999) (Fig. 1-5) was a nurse ahead of her time. She believed that nursing is multifaceted and that the nurse must be a tool to educate and promote wellness, as well as a person who delivers care to the ill. In her book, *Interpersonal Relations in Nursing* (1952),

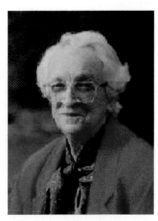

FIGURE 1-5. Hildegard Peplau. (Photo copyright Letitia A. Peplau. Reprinted with permission.)

Dr. Peplau brought together some interpersonal theories from psychiatry and melded them with theories of nursing and communication. She believed that the nurse works in society—not merely in a hospital or clinic—and that we need to use every opportunity to educate the public and follow role models in physical and mental health. Peplau saw the nurse as

1. *Resource person.* Provides information.
2. *Counselor.* Helps patients to explore their thoughts and feelings.
3. *Surrogate.* By role playing or other means helps the patient to explore and identify feelings from the past.
4. *Technical support.* Coordinates professional services (Peplau, 1952).

In addition to this, she believed in building a collaborative therapeutic relationship between the nurse and the patient. In her book she cites four stages of this relationship (Peplau, 1952):

1. *Orientation.* Patient feels a need and a will to seek out help.
2. *Identification.* Expectations and perceptions about the nurse-patient relationship are identified.
3. *Exploration.* Patient will begin to show motivation in the problem-solving process, but some testing behaviors may be seen; patient may have a need to "test" the nurse's commitment to his/her individual situation.
4. *Resolution.* Focus is on the patient's developing self-responsibility and showing personal growth.

In 1954, the first graduate-level nursing program was developed by Dr. Peplau at Rutgers University to provide training for clinical nurse specialists for psychiatric nursing.

HATTIE BESSENT

In the early 1980s, the National Institute for Mental Health granted money to be used for the education and research of minority nurses who were choosing to upgrade to Masters and Physicianate levels of practice. Hattie Bessent is credited with the development and directorship of that program.

■ THE FACILITIES

People who have mental illnesses are everywhere; popular statistics say that about one in every three Americans will experience some form of mental illness at some point in life. The "trailblazers" realized that mental illness was different from medical-surgical disorders. They understood that each person's mind was truly unique and that therefore nurses needed information and training specific to those illnesses. To help meet those needs, actions were taken to improve the quality of care for those patients. This was not enough, however, and it became evident that persons with mental disorders were often better served through care in special facilities.

ASYLUMS

These special facilities were called **asylums,** which Webster Online, in part, defines as "1: a place of refuge 2: protection given to esp. criminals and debtors 3: an institution for the care of the needy or sick and esp. of the insane" (Merriam-Webster, 1994). Patients were often treated less than humanely. Custodial care was provided, but patients were often heavily medicated. Nutritional and physical care was minimal, and often these patients were volunteered for various forms of experimentation and research.

HOSPITALS

As treatment facilities evolved, the term *asylum* and the connotations associated with it became unpopular. Until the Community Mental Health Act of 1963 was passed, much housing of this clientele was handled by the individual state hospital system. Today, such a facility is called a **hospital** or treatment center or is known by a specific name, such as the Betty Ford Center.

Hospitals handle patients with psychological needs according to the size of the hospital and its resources. To comply with regulations surrounding mental health issues, smaller communities may see these patients in the emergency room and then refer them to other clinics or hospitals. Communities large enough to support such programs may provide in-house treatment as well as outpatient treatment and aftercare. Metropolitan areas commonly provide treatment via several options, including hospitals and free-standing treatment centers.

FREE-STANDING FACILITIES

Free-standing treatment centers may be called detoxification (detox) centers, crisis centers, or by similar terms. They provide care ranging from crisis-only to more traditional 21-day stays. This, too, depends largely on the size and needs of the individual community. More discussion on the types of treatment facilities occurs in the section on The Laws.

■ THE BREAKTHROUGHS

It was not until 1937 that formal clinical rotations in mental health began for nurses. Today, these rotations are required for students in professional and registered nursing programs, but students in practical or vocational nursing are usually exposed to mental health theory or very short observational experiences. In 1955, theory relating to mental health nursing became a requirement for licensure for all nurses.

Throughout the 1800s and early 1900s, progress was made in developing humane, effective treatment of mental illnesses. With the best knowledge available to them as a profession, nurses were forward thinkers in providing specialized care to people unfortunate enough to have illnesses that were somehow different from the tuberculosis, smallpox, and influenza that filled hospitals. There was one major difference, however: Medicines existed to help in treating those diseases. At that time, no one had been able to find pharmacologic help for people with emotional, behavioral, or physical brain disorders. Then came the 1950s.

PSYCHOTROPIC MEDICATIONS

Chemists were experimenting with combinations of chemicals and their effects on people. In 1955, a group of **psychotropic** medications called phenothiazines was discovered to have the effect of calming and tranquilizing people. What a world of possibility this opened for people living with and caring for mental disorders! Suddenly it was possible to control behavior to a degree, and patients were able to function more independently. Other forms of therapy became more effective because patients were able to focus differently. Some improved so dramatically that it was no longer necessary for them to remain hospitalized and dependent on others. Between the mid-1950s and the mid-1970s, the number of patients hospitalized with mental illnesses in the United States was cut approximately in half, mainly because of the use of psychotropic drugs.

DEINSTITUTIONALIZATION

The use of phenothiazines became so effective that state hospitals and other facilities dedicated to the care and treatment of people with mental illness saw a large decline in population. It became costly to run these large buildings and continue to employ staff. The combination of these effects, as well as new laws pertaining to the care of the mentally ill, resulted in a movement called **deinstitutionalization.** People who had formerly required long hospital stays were now able to leave the institutions and return to their communities and their homes. Deinstitutionalization was and still is a controversial issue, but it was a huge step in returning a sense of worth, ability, and independence to those who had been dependent on others for their care for so long.

NURSING ORGANIZATIONS AND RECOMMENDATIONS

A natural progression from the breakthroughs that were happening in nursing was the development of organizations for nurses. The American Nurses Association (ANA) is recognized as an organization for professional nurses (registered nurses, or RNs). One of its goals is to promote standardization of nursing practice in the United States. It also promotes the certification of nurses who meet specific criteria. The concept of psychiatric nurse specialists, clinicians, or advanced practice nurses is a result of the work of the ANA. The American Psychiatric Nurses Association provides leadership in recommending standards of care for nurses who care for people with mental illness. This organization invites nurses who are RN-prepared. Further information can be obtained at their Web site, www.apna.org.

The National League for Nursing evolved from the National League for Nursing Education and became known as the NLN in 1952. Its focus is on nursing education, and the NLN is the accrediting agency for many schools of nursing across the United States.

Every state has adopted its own code or set of rules by which all nurses are expected to perform. This is called the **Nurse Practice Act** and is based on federal guidelines that have been adapted to the needs of the individual state. The Nurse Practice Act is discussed in more detail in Chapter 3.

Sigma Theta Tau is an honor society for nurses who have shown special talents in research or leadership. Again, it is open to baccalaureate-degree nursing students, graduate students in nursing, and leaders in the nursing community.

Specific to the licensed practical/vocational nurse are two organizations. One is the National Federation of Licensed Practical Nurses, Inc. (NFLPN), welcoming licensed practical nurses and licensed vocational nurses and practical/vocational nursing students in the United States. The organization consists of licensed practical nurses, licensed vocational nurses, and practical/vocational nursing students. In September 1991, a new category of affiliate membership was established to allow those who have an interest in the work of NFLPN but who are neither LPNs nor PN students to join. The NFLPN has a published set of Nursing Practice Standards for the LPN/LVN. They can be found on the Web site www.nflpn.org.

The other organization is the National Association for Practical Nurse Education & Service, Inc. (NAPNES). The organization was founded by practical nurse educators in 1941 and identifies as the world's oldest nursing organization dedicated exclusively to the promotion of quality nursing service through the practice of licensed practical nurses (LPN) and licensed vocational nurses (LVN). NAPNES promotes multidisciplinary organization of individuals, facilities, and schools that advocate the professional practice and practical and vocational nursing. Visit the NAPNES Web site at www.napnes.org to read the NAPNES position paper, dated 7/18/2004, titled, "Supply, Demand and Use of Licensed Practical Nurses."

The National Coalition of Ethnic Minority Nurse Associations (NCEMNA) is made up of five national ethnic nurse associations: Asian American/Pacific Islander Nurses Association, Inc. (AAPINA), National Alaska Native American Indian Nurses Association, Inc. (NANAINA), National Association of Hispanic Nurses, Inc. (NAHN), National Black Nurses Association, Inc. (NBNA), and Philippine Nurses Association of America, Inc. (PNAA). Goals include advocating for equity and justice in nursing and health-care for ethnic minority populations and endorsement of best practice models for nursing practice, education, and research for minority populations. More information can be located at their Web site, www.ncemna.org.

The American Assembly for Men in Nursing (AAMN) provides a framework for nurses, as a group, to meet to discuss and influence factors that affect men as nurses. Among its objectives is to encourage men of all ages to become nurses and join together with all nurses in strengthening and humanizing health care. The organization also supports men who are nurses to grow professionally and demonstrate the increasing contributions being made by men in the nursing profession. As do the other professional organizations, AAMN advocates for continued research, education, and dissemination of information about men's health issues, men in nursing, and nursing knowledge at the local and national levels.

Appendix C of this text provides more contact information for these and other agencies designed to promote and assist nurses, particularly at the LPN and LVN level of preparation.

■ THE LAWS

Many changes and advancements were being made at this time in medicine and nursing in general. The area of mental health was a particular challenge. There were ethical considerations that had not surfaced in earlier years. Psychotropic and psychoactive medications were benefiting many patients but had their own problems as well; side effects were not always pleasant. More drugs were being developed, and more questions arose: How much is too much to give people? Do we keep them completely sedated? People were asking which was worse: the illness or the medication? People are still asking that question.

Nonetheless, it was necessary to begin regulating the health-care industry a bit more. A series of laws governing various aspects of care for persons with mental illnesses were published. The laws have changed somewhat and have been renamed in some cases, but the collective intention is to provide funding, treatment, and ethical care for this segment of society.

HILL-BURTON ACT

In the 1930s, the Hill-Burton Act was the first major law to address mental illness. It provided money to build psychiatric units in hospitals.

NATIONAL MENTAL HEALTH ACT OF 1946

The National Mental Health Act of 1946 was part of the result of the first Congress to be held after World War II. It provided money for nursing and several other disciplines for training and research in areas pertaining to improving treatment for the mentally ill. The National Institute of Mental Health (NIMH) was established as part of the National Mental Health Act of 1946.

THE COMMUNITY MENTAL HEALTH CENTERS ACT OF 1963

The Community Mental Health Centers Act resulted from President John F. Kennedy's concern for the treatment of the mentally ill. Its main purpose was to provide a full set of services to the people living in a particular community. These services were to include inpatient care, outpatient care, emergency care, and education. This was to be a national effort, funded federally at first. The goal was for the center to generate enough services so that, eventually, the community could support it financially.

In 1981, the bill was amended in Congress. Called the Omnibus Budget Reconciliation Act (OBRA), it allows money to be allocated differently. There is currently less money available in the federal budget, and that money can be withheld at any time. Unfortunately, with the turmoil in the insurance and health-care delivery systems today, mental health benefits are often among the first services to be cut back or eliminated.

PATIENT BILL OF RIGHTS

In 1980, the image of the patient was changing. The Civil Rights Movement of the 1960s was giving way to the provision of rights for all groups of people. Patients were beginning to be identified as "clients" who purchased services from health-care providers. Persons of very young or very old age or persons with certain physical, intellectual, or communication difficulties became politically recognized as "vulnerable." The outcome was the development of the Patient Bill of Rights, which is discussed in more detail in Chapter 3.

Key Concepts ▪ ▪ ▪

1. Mental health nursing has a long and rich history. It has evolved from very rudimentary skills before the time of Florence Nightingale to the specialty area of nursing that we see today.
2. Patients with mental illness are treated in many different types of facilities, depending on the diagnosis and the availability of care in the particular community.
3. The 1950s were important years to all of the mental health industry. The first psychotropic medications were developed, making it possible for people to return to their homes and communities (deinstitutionalization). These medications also allowed other treatment forms to be used more effectively.

4. Nurses at all levels of preparation are integral parts of the mental health treatment team. Our observations, documentation, and interpersonal skills make us effective tools in patient care.

5. A series of laws over the past 50 years have provided for money, education, research, and improvements in the care of the mentally ill. Financial difficulties in the insurance and health-care industry contribute to cutbacks in money and services for care and treatment of the mentally ill.

REFERENCES

Donahue, MP (1985). *Nursing, the Finest Art.* St. Louis: CV Mosby.

Webster Online (2004). **www.merriam-webster. com**

Peplau, HE (1952). *Interpersonal Relations in Nursing.* New York: GP Putnam's Sons.

CRITICAL THINKING EXERCISES ■ ■ ■

1. The "trailblazers" were risk takers. One of the professional responsibilities of nursing is to try to give something back to our profession. How will you, as an individual, become a trailblazer? What direction should nursing as a whole take to strengthen our profession? What criteria should be important when deciding what level of preparation in nursing should allow the nurse to be a specialist in mental health?

2. The laws have said that people who have mental illnesses should be treated using the least restrictive alternative. Deinstitutionalization allows these people to live among us in the community. Consider the following scenario: Your city has just purchased the house next door to you, and the plan is to develop this into a halfway house for women who have been child abusers. You are the parent of a 3-year-old and you are also a mental health nurse. What would you do? What are your thoughts about this situation? What are your feelings about this situation?

3. Your employer has announced that your company is changing its medical insurance policy. The company will be providing you with a set amount of money to spend on insurance benefits. The three insurance services you have to choose from offer either family coverage or mental health services. You are a single parent with two preschoolers. You also have a diagnosis of bipolar depression for which you need medications, therapy, and periodic hospitalization. What will you choose?

TEST QUESTIONS ■ ■ ■

MULTIPLE CHOICE QUESTIONS

1. The main goal of deinstitutionalization was to:
   A. Let all mentally ill people care for themselves.
   B. Return as many people as possible to a "normal" life.
   C. Keep all mentally ill people in locked wards.
   D. Close all community hospitals.

2. A major breakthrough of the 1950s that assisted in the deinstitutionalization movement was:
   A. The Community Mental Health Centers Act
   B. The Nurse Practice Act
   C. The development of psychotropic medications
   D. Electroshock therapy

3. The set of regulations that dictates the scope of nursing practice is called:
   A. National League for Nursing
   B. American Nurses Association
   C. Patient Bill of Rights
   D. Nurse Practice Act

4. As a result of deinstitutionalization and changes in the health-care delivery system, nurses can expect to care for people with mental health issues in which of the following settings?
   A. Psychiatric hospitals only
   B. Outpatient settings only
   C. Medical-surgical hospital settings
   D. All of the above

2

Basics of Communication

Learning Objectives ■ ■ ■

1. Identify three components needed to communicate.
2. Differentiate between effective and ineffective communication.
3. Identify six types of communication.
4. Identify five challenges to communication.
5. Identify common blocks to therapeutic communication.
6. Identify common techniques of therapeutic communication.
7. Identify five adaptive communication techniques.
8. Define key terms.

Key Terms ■ ■ ■

- Aggressive
- Aphasia
- Assertive
- Block
- Communication
- Dysphasia
- Hearing impaired
- Ineffective
- Laryngectomy
- Message
- Neurolinguistic programming
- Nonverbal
- Receiver
- Sender
- Therapeutic
- Verbal
- Visually impaired

Human beings communicate. Everything we do or say has a message and a meaning. Sometimes, the words and the actions send different meanings to different people. For example: Sally and Jim meet for report in the morning. Sally's eyes are red and swollen, and she is unusually quiet. Jim asks her if something is wrong, and she responds, "No, everything is just fine." Jim has observed some changes in Sally's behavior and appearance. Sally has verbally com-municated that nothing is wrong. What is really being communicated here?

People of different cultures communicate differently. Men and women communicate differently. **Hearing-impaired** people communicate differently from people who are not hearing impaired. People in the medical professions communicate differently from people in business professions. We communicate all the time in everything we do. **Communication** is an ongoing process.

■ COMMUNICATION THEORY

SENDER, RECEIVER, AND INTERPRETATION OF MESSAGE

One of the challenging parts of communicating with others is that the process requires three parts: a **sender** (Sally), a **message,** and a **receiver** (Jim). That means the sender is really only partially responsible for the communication. Sally cannot totally control Jim's interpretation of her message. As it turns out, Sally is a victim of severe allergies. She was visiting her friend who has cats. Sally is very allergic to them, and the redness and swelling were symptoms of her allergic response. She simply didn't wish to burden Jim with her problem during report, so she opted to respond by telling him everything was "just fine."

What did you decide was being communicated in the example just given? On what did you base your decision? What "spoke" louder to you: Sally's words or her actions and appearance? What is the danger in making this assumption about Sally's message?

It is very important for the sender and receiver to double-check the message. In nursing, this is even more necessary, because we use our own professional "language"; when dealing with the health and safety of our patients, we need to be very sure that there are not "mixed" or "missed" messages.

■ TYPES OF COMMUNICATION

VERBAL AND WRITTEN COMMUNICATION

Verbal communication is the process of exchanging information by the spoken or written word. It is, therefore, the objective part of the process. In the example given earlier, Sally's reply that "everything is just fine" is an example of verbal communication. The expertise a nurse develops in the areas of written and verbal communication is largely responsible for the credibility of that nurse.

NONVERBAL COMMUNICATION

Nonverbal communication is more subtle. It consists of our actions, our tone of voice, the way we use our body, our facial expressions, and so forth. It is the subjective part of the process. Nonverbal communication is estimated to be 70 percent of the message we send (Fig. 2-1). The old saying is true: A picture is worth a thousand words!

A note of caution: Be careful with "slang" word and hand gestures. Have you ever heard the expression, "S/he talks with her/his hands"? Many people use hand gestures when speaking. Making the "OK" sign with one's fingers is normally a sign of encouragement, agreement, or congratulations. For people of certain cultures, however, it is a vulgarity. An example from this author's teaching experience is the word "gals." For people of my generation, being part of the "guys" or the "gals" was a good thing. It demonstrated acceptance and belonging to one's social group. In a discussion class on the very topic of words and gestures and what they mean, one African-American female student spoke up. She shared with the class that "gals" in her world was a demeaning term relating to the degrading role of the African-American woman in history. To say the least, I was dumbfounded. Who knew? It was I who learned the lesson that day. Moral of the story: Be ready to learn from each other every day. Be prepared to make known those terms or gestures that are uncomfortable for yourself and your patients. Make a conscious effort not to use those words when in the company of those they may offend. (See Box 2-1.)

AGGRESSIVE AND ASSERTIVE COMMUNICATION

The terms *aggressive* and *assertive* are sometimes used interchangeably in American culture, but they have very different meanings.

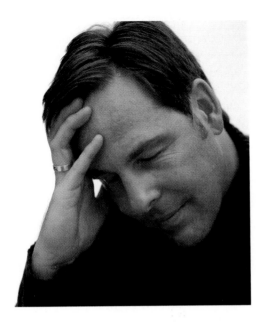
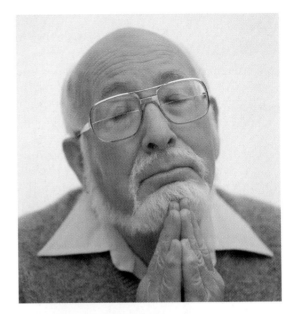
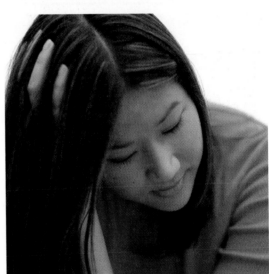

FIGURE 2-1. Nonverbal communication is subjective, but it represents 70 percent of the message we send to others. It includes the way we use our body, our facial expressions, and so forth. What do the following photographs represent to you?

Aggressive Communication

Aggressive communication is communication that is not self-responsible. Aggressive statements most often begin with the word *you*. Aggressive communication, like aggressive behavior, is meant to harm another person. It is a form of the defense mechanism projection, or blaming, and it attempts to put the responsibility for the interaction on the other person.

EXAMPLE

"You make me so angry when you don't help with the housework!"

Assertive Communication

Assertive communication, on the other hand, is self-responsible. Assertive statements begin with the word *I*. They deal with thoughts and feelings and they deal with honesty.

BOX 2-1	*Examples of Communication with Cultural Implications*

Words that are seemingly harmless to some people can be very hurtful to others. We don't usually know that until we take the time to ask! These are examples of communication that may have different cultural implications. How many more can your class identify?

- Eye contact with strangers or those in perceived positions of power or respect is not considered appropriate among some populations.
- Hand gestures may communicate different meanings to different groups of people.
- Slang terms may be inappropriate, offensive or may exclude people who do not understand the meaning of the word.
- Gender-reference terms such as "you guys" when the group is mixed or not male.
- Terms such as "master" and "slave" frequently used in computer-related issues may offend African-American people and others.
- African-American women displayed in subservient roles.
- Distortion or omission of important developments in the lives of African-Americans.
- Pictures, photographs that do not portray accurate skin tones, hair texture, and physical features of certain ethnic groups.

EXAMPLE

"I feel angry when you don't help with the housework!"

Assertive behavior and communication are also techniques of personal empowerment. People *choose* to think or feel a certain way; others do not have the power to make us think or feel anything we do not choose to think or feel. To be able to say "I think" or "I feel" keeps us in control of our emotions, yet it allows honest, open expression of the feelings we have as a result of someone else's behavior. Still, the feelings and thoughts belong to the person choosing them, not to anyone else.

SOCIAL COMMUNICATION

People usually alter their style of communicating according to who is receiving the message. For example, teenagers usually communicate with their peer group in a different manner from the way they communicate with their parents. So, too, do nurses communicate differently with their patients than they do with their friends or family.

Social communication is the day-to-day interaction we have with personal acquaintances. We may use "slang" or "street language," and we may be less literal and purposeful in our social interactions. Quite simply, social interaction has a different purpose than a nurse's professional communication.

THERAPEUTIC COMMUNICATION

Therapeutic communication is a language of its own. It requires testing out new methods of communicating and new ways of listening. Therapeutic communication is purposeful: We are trying to determine the patient's needs. Sometimes, for various reasons, the patient is not comfortable sharing his or her needs and concerns. At those times, it is up to the nurse to try to uncover the problem by using two tools: techniques of therapeutic communication and "active" or "purposeful" listening (or "listening between the lines"). The techniques and blocks to them will be discussed at the end of this chapter.

NEUROLINGUISTIC PROGRAMMING

Neurolinguistic programming (NLP) is a form of communication developed primarily by Milton Erickson, a hypnotherapist; John Grinder, a psychologist and linguistics professor; and Richard Bandler, a mathematician and editor (Grinder & Bandler, 1981). It is a way of learning to frame statements and questions while attempting effective communication. One of the theory's tenets, not unlike other communication theories, is that humans cannot fail to communicate. The theory builds on the idea that humans tend to communicate in basically three ways: hearing, seeing, and tactile experience. Choice of wording can make a difference in how the words a nurse says to a patient are actually "heard" by that patient. Remember: Communication must have a sender and a receiver. NLP is one method being taught to health care providers to assist in the successful completion of the communication loop.

It is important to note that this is not hypnosis; it is a form of communication. NLP can be used in conjunction with hypnosis and other treatment modalities. In most states, hypnosis can only be performed legally by professionals specially trained and licensed to do so.

Further explanation and some simple examples of NLP phrasing are provided in Chapter 9, on Alternative Modalities.

■ CHALLENGES TO COMMUNICATION

Communicating is something that humans often take for granted—until they no longer can do it! Who hasn't had the experience of trying to answer the telephone during a nasty bout with laryngitis? Have you ever tried to sign a check while your arm was in a cast? Do you remember trying to read the traffic signs after your last eye examination? These are uncomfortable situations, but for the most part, they are temporary. What about your patients and coworkers for whom this situation is permanent?

PEOPLE WHO ARE HEARING IMPAIRED

It is important for the nurse to be very patient when communicating with people who are hearing impaired. Be aware that the hearing-impaired person's frustration is even greater than your own in trying to communicate. Try to establish a trusting, team-approach relationship with your hearing-impaired patients. Let them know you will try whatever it takes for you to be able to understand each other. Find out what has worked for that person in the past and remember to maintain an appropriate sense of humor while you build this new skill.

Not all hearing-impaired people use sign language. Lip reading may be inaccurate and could lead to incorrect communication. Sometimes writing a note is the most effective way to communicate with a person who is deaf or hard of hearing.

PEOPLE WHO ARE VISUALLY IMPAIRED

The nonverbal part of communication is the challenge with this group of people. Nursing is a highly affective art, so that certain nonverbal cues, such as our tone of voice, body position, and facial expressions, "speak" most strongly to our patients. How does a sightless person or someone who is severely impaired visually interpret these nonverbal cues?

Nurses must learn to become detail-oriented storytellers. It is important to learn to describe to **visually impaired** patients what the call signal sounds like, what the people in the hall are laughing at, why the voices suddenly switch to a whisper when another person enters the room, and who has just entered. Think about a time when you walked into the lunchroom after everyone else was at lunch, and as you walked in everyone quit speaking. What was your first response? How did that feel? Sightless people can't see a wave of the hand or see when you leave or enter a room; these events must be verbalized.

Patient teaching takes on a new dimension because it involves physically moving, touching, or verbally explaining in much more detail than usual. Learning to eat can be difficult for a newly sightless person. Usually, the teaching involves relating the food position to the numbers on a clock face. Sightless patients need to rely on their other senses to compensate for the eyes they can't use.

Sometimes individuals have more than one need to be considered when you are communicating with them. For example, some people are both hearing impaired and visually impaired. When communicating with these individuals, a nurse needs to be creative. Investigate methods that have worked for this person in the past and explore methods such as a conversation board or printing the message on the person's palm.

PEOPLE WHO HAVE LARYNGECTOMIES

Under some circumstances, people have to live with partial or total removal of their larynx ("voice box"). Imagine what it would be like to be able to speak one day and have no voice at all the next! The larynx is one of those body parts that is very much taken for granted. How do you answer the phone? Order a pizza? Call for help? Cheer on the home team?

PEOPLE WITH LANGUAGE DIFFERENCES

Ours is a global society. Look at the students in the room with you. Listen to their speech. Even though English is the predominant language in the United States, it may not be the primary language for many of the people you will be working with and caring for. You may find yourself in an area where you are the one who does not speak the primary language. How will you communicate? How will you ensure safe care of your patients? If Dr. XYZ gives a verbal order, how will you know you have heard it correctly? What about those people who say they are speaking English, but you or their patients are not able to understand them? It can be very embarrassing and potentially insulting for all parties involved. Techniques for ensuring understanding are discussed at the end of this chapter.

PEOPLE WHO HAVE APHASIC/DYSPHASIC DISORDERS

People whose speech is difficult or who have no speech present other challenges. The amount of speech a patient possesses is related to many things, such as age, cause of difficulty, and severity of involvement. There are different types of **aphasia** (Table 2–1).

It will be up to the physician and the speech therapist to determine the cause and extent of involvement, but the nurse will be part of the plan of treatment. This will be a very individualized type of communication skill. Patients may know what you want when you ask for the comb; they may think they are handing you the comb, but you

TABLE 2-1	*Types of Aphasia*
TYPE OF APHASIA	**DESCRIPTION**
EXPRESSIVE	Difficulty expressing himself or herself in written or verbal forms of communication
RECEPTIVE	Difficulty interpreting or understanding written or verbal forms of communication
GLOBAL	Combination of receptive and expressive forms of aphasia

actually get the coffee cup. Someone may try to read aloud a passage from a book, but what comes out of the patient's mouth may be a long line of obscenities! The person would be very embarrassed if he or she knew what was said. The nurse must be very understanding and willing to try over and over to have correct communication with persons with various forms of aphasia. We must remember, too, that any "nasty words" are not to be taken personally; chances are very good that those "nasty words" were really a sincere attempt by the patient to say, "Thank you, Nurse!"

■ THERAPEUTIC COMMUNICATION

It is possible to hold a helping, therapeutic conversation with most people, but it takes some practice. These "techniques" need to be practiced in much the same way that one learns any other language: by hearing them, practicing them, and making them part of your professional (and social) vocabulary.

There is another old saying that "the road to defeat is paved with good intentions." Sometimes, our good intentions as nurses get us in trouble with our communication skills. We unintentionally set ourselves up for **ineffective** communication. The following is a list of ways nurses "block," or impede, helpful interactions with patients:

1. *False Reassurance/Social Clichés.* These are phrases we use in an effort to sound supportive. In social communication, they sound friendly, but in a therapeutic relationship they invalidate the patient's concerns.
2. *Minimizing/Belittling.* These, too, are used socially to try to relieve the tensions of others. There is a security in numbers, and to share that many people are experiencing the same thing as the individual is somehow supposed to make the problem seem lighter. In therapeutic use, the implications are different.

3. *"Why?"* This simple little word needs to be virtually eliminated in therapeutic interactions. "Why" connotes disapproval, displeasure. "Why ask why?" is a good question for the health-care provider to remember. The patient often doesn't know "why" and can end up feeling responsible for providing an answer anyway. The nurse often needs to know "why," but there are other ways to ask that are less stress-producing to the patient.
4. *Advising.* Alcoholics Anonymous sometimes uses the statement, "Don't 'should' on yourself." Nurses must not "should" on their patients, either! This sets the stage for expectations that the patient may not be able to meet. It also sets up, in the patient's mind, some sort of value system that puts the nurse's value as the "right" one. It can sound very judgmental.
5. *Agreeing or Disagreeing.* Socially, we agree or disagree for several reasons. Sometimes we are just expressing our opinion. Sometimes we are trying to make a favorable impression. Therapeutically, it is wise to avoid statements that express your own opinions or values.
6. *Closed-Ended Questions.* These are forms of questions that make it possible for a one-word "Yes" or "No" answer. They discourage the patient from giving full answers to your questions. Closed-ended questions are those that start with phrases such as "Can you ... ," "Will you ... ," "Are they ... ," and "May I .... " It doesn't help to add a *please*, either, as in "Please, may I ask you a question?" or "Will you please take out the trash?" This courtesy still leaves the possibility for the receiver to say "Yes" or "No." The *please* makes it sound more polite in social venues, but the same questions can be made assertive and therapeutic by stating or asking for what we want ("I need to ask you a question" or "Please take out the trash").

The general rule for making an open-ended question from a closed-ended question is to simply drop off the first two words.

EXAMPLE

Closed: "Will you help me, please?"
Open: "Help me, please."

This can also be accomplished by adding words like *how* and *what* to the beginning of the question.

EXAMPLE

Closed: "Can I help you?"
Open: "How can I help you?" OR "What can I do to help you?"

7. *Providing the Answer with the Question.* This is a technique that television interviewers use frequently. You may have heard the expression, "They put words into my mouth." Perhaps you have experienced someone doing that to you. It assumes an answer. For instance, a question that answers itself is, "Didn't you really know that the committee would reject the proposal?" A better way to ask a question that you really want answered from the interviewee's perspective is to change the question to "What were your thoughts about how the committee might react?"

8. *Changing the Subject.* Nurses do this inadvertently sometimes. When schedules get busy and patients all need our attention at the same time, our own agenda takes over and we start to see to our own needs. It is very easy to give a quick "Um-hum" in answer to a patient's question and then proceed with our own information getting and giving. Unfortunately, that may send the message to the patient that the nurse doesn't care or that this problem is not worthy of a nurse's time. This patient may be reluctant to offer more information to that nurse in the future.

Changing the subject may also reflect the nurse's comfort (or discomfort) level with the subject. If the nurse just experienced the death of a loved one from a heart attack, for example, it may be very uncomfortable to answer a patient's questions about recovery and prognosis following his or her bypass surgery. The nurse may answer quickly and move on to a more comfortable topic, like "Well, your physician has advanced your diet; that's good news!"

9. *Approving or Disapproving.* This is similar in many ways to minimizing or agreeing. The patient perceives a value system that puts the nurse in the position of the expert, and, in many ways, we are. That puts a big responsibility on our shoulders, however, and that responsibility includes being supportive without being judgmental or portraying our personal idea of what is right or wrong, good or bad.

The nurse is in a partnership of sorts with the patient. We collaborate with the patient to determine the best way to help the patient help himself or herself. If we can look at the relationship with that attitude, there is no "right" or "wrong," because each person is just a little different. No two patients are the same, so what is helpful to each one is "right" for that patient.

Table 2–2 gives some help in identifying the blocks and the effect they may have on the patient.

TECHNIQUES OF THERAPEUTIC/HELPING COMMUNICATION

Hildegard Peplau envisioned the nurse as a "tool" for ensuring positive interpersonal relationships with patients. Nurses are with the patient for approximately 8 hours daily. Compare that with the amount of time a physician is able to spend with the patient and it is easy to see how the nurse becomes the therapeutic tool that helps the patient help himself or herself. Our patients develop

TABLE 2-2 ■	*Blocks to Therapeutic (Helping) Communication*	
TYPE	**EXAMPLE**	**EFFECT ON PATIENT**
FALSE REASSURANCE/ SOCIAL CLICHÉS	"Don't worry! Everything will be just fine!"	1. Tells patient his or her concerns are not valid 2. May jeopardize patient's trust in nurse
MINIMIZING BELITTLING	"We all have felt that way sometimes."	Implies that the patient's feelings are not special
THE WORD "WHY"	"Why did you refuse your breakfast?"	1. Patient feels obligated to answer something he or she may not wish to answer or may not be able to answer 2. Probes in an abrasive way
ADVISING	1. "You should eat more." 2. "If I were you, I'd take those pills, so I'd feel better." 3. "You ought to try a hobby."	1. Places a value on the action 2. Gives idea that the nurse's values are the "right" ones 3. Jeopardizes nurse's credibility if the "should" doesn't work for the patient
AGREEING OR DISAGREEING	1. "You're wrong about that." 2. "I think you're right!"	1. Places a value of "right" or "wrong" on the action 2. Can be argumentative 3. Patient may feel reluctant to change his or her mind, because the nurse has expressed a value
CLOSED-ENDED QUESTIONS	1. "Can you tell me how you feel?" 2. "Do you smoke?" 3. "Can I ask you a few questions?"	1. Allows a "Yes" or "No" answer 2. Discourages further exploration of the topic 3. Discourages patient from giving information
PROVIDING THE ANSWER WITH THE QUESTION	1. "Are you feeling afraid?" 2. "Didn't the food taste good?" 3. "Do you miss your mom/dad?"	1. Combines a closed-ended question with a solution 2. Discourages patient from providing own answers
CHANGING THE SUBJECT	1. "Did your doctor say anything about discharging you today?" while the patient is asking about another topic.	1. Discounts the importance of the patient's need to explore personal thoughts and feelings 2. May be a reflection of the nurse's own "*un*comfort" level with this topic
APPROVING/ DISAPPROVING	1. "That's the way to think about it! Good for you!" 2. "That's not a good idea."	1. Can sound judgmental 2. Can set the patient up for failure if the approval or disapproval doesn't help; can lower nurse's credibility

a different kind of rapport with us because they learn to trust us. Although our technical skills are very important and must never be allowed to get rusty, it is the appropriate use of our verbal and nonverbal communication skills that cements the relationship with our patients and that ultimately promotes their healing.

The previous section pointed out some of the bad habits of conversation. It is now time to learn new habits. These will feel awkward at first, but with practice and trust, they will help improve the quality of your interactions not only with your patients, but in most interpersonal communication as well. They are little "tricks of the trade" that may be as little as a one-word change in the way a sentence or request is presented, but they get a lot of mileage in the way people respond.

Remember: These communication methods will not all work for all people in all circumstances, but if you use them faithfully you will see improvements in the way you relate to your patients and in the way they respond to you.

1. *Reflecting, Repeating, Parroting.* This technique seems to be the easiest to learn and therefore is used the most often. Parrots are often trained to repeat words or phrases. "Polly want a cracker?" is heard over and over again when people try to get a parrot to speak to them.

   Reflecting, repeating, and parroting refer to this technique because that is what the nurse does: He or she picks a word or phrase that seems to be a key word or idea in what the patient is trying to communicate. It sometimes involves a degree of guessing on the part of the nurse to check out the perceived message. For instance, if the patient says to you, "I want to get out of here; everyone is against me," you have several options for checking the main concern of the patient. The nurse will repeat a word or phrase of the patient's statement to reflect, or

parrot, whatever is perceived to be the main concern. The nurse could say "Everyone?" or "Against you?" to try to encourage the patient to expand on these ideas. *Caution:* Because this technique might seem obvious to the patient, use parroting sparingly. It will not take the patient too many times of hearing his or her words repeated before perhaps suggesting that the nurse look into having a good audiometric examination!

2. *Clarifying Terms.* We live and work in a very global society. There are many different people with whom nurses interact as patients and coworkers. We use words in different ways, sometimes. The Americanized vocabulary pronounces many words the same but spells them differently.

EXAMPLE

There, their, they're OR one, won

English is a very complex language to learn. Some people use terms very literally. Nursing is a profession that is filled with inference and nuance; it is highly affective. Because of that, it is very important to clarify terms with patients and other workers. Nurses must be sure that the terms they choose are correct and mean the same thing to all parties involved in the interaction. The technique is easy to learn: Simply ask. "When you say 'I can't do that,' what do you mean?" is one way of clarifying a statement. The patient may mean "I am not physically able" or "I am not morally able" or "I do not know how to do that" or any number of things that the word *can't* may mean. If we don't try to clarify that simple word, we could infer incorrectly the patient's level of ability or cooperation.

3. *Open-Ended Questions.* These are the essence of successful nurse-patient communication. They are also among the hardest techniques to learn,

because we are constantly bombarded with incorrect usage in social interaction and in the world of talk shows and news reporters.

One of the goals of helping communication is to get the patient to participate, so it is important to present questions in a way that will encourage the patient to provide information without the nurse's sounding persistent or intrusive. Such a perception by the patient will be a major interference in future attempts at communication.

In some instances, "yes" or "no" may be all the nurse needs to know or all that the patient is capable of responding at the time. In those instances, closed-ended questions may be used until the patient is able to provide more information. Otherwise, open-ended questions are the more correct form and will get more productive results.

EXAMPLE

"Ms. Green, are you in pain?" could win the nurse several different answers.

Depending on the patient's culture or her religious preference, or both, "pain" may or may not be acceptable. She may answer "yes" or "no" on the basis of those beliefs. If Ms. Green has a chemical dependency that has not been shared with you, she may say "yes" to get the benefit of the pain medication. Pain is a very individual experience. What one person considers to be extreme pain, another might brush off as a minor irritation. The closed-ended nature of this question doesn't require the patient to provide useful, measurable information that allows the nurse to be helpful or therapeutic. A more helpful form of this question would be in an open-ended format, such as, "Ms. Green, on a scale of 0 to 5, how do you rate your pain?" or "Ms. Green, please tell me about

your pain; where is it and how severe is it right now?"

4. *Asking for What You Need or Want.* This relates to the discussion on assertive versus aggressive communication. Nurses can ask for what is needed and wanted from patients and coworkers and still maintain a pleasant, professional tone of voice. This technique requires the user to start the sentence with the words "I want" or "I need." Taking the direct approach with people is usually the safest way to be sure that the receiver gets the message the sender intended to send.

EXAMPLE

"I want to switch shifts with Mary next Tuesday, please." OR "Mr. Baker, I need to change your dressing. When would you prefer: now or after your walk?"

These two examples show ways to be assertive, direct, and self-responsible while still maintaining politeness and allowing the patient to have some control over his or her care.

5. *Identifying Thoughts and Feelings.* This is another difficult technique to master. Because words conveying thoughts and feelings are used incorrectly more frequently than they are used correctly in our society, it is hard to reinforce the proper technique. The rule is simple: A feeling is an emotion. A "feeling statement" must identify an emotion that you are experiencing or are trying to explore with a patient. For example, "I feel proud that I earned this promotion" or "I feel frightened to walk alone at night."

A thought is an opinion, idea, or fact that one wishes to express. "I think I deserve this promotion" and "I think security needs to be improved in the parking area" are examples of "thinking statements."

"I feel security needs to be improved in the parking area" and "I feel the patient needs a different pain medication" are incorrect uses of the word "feel." There is no emotion identified in these statements. "Feeling" is certainly implied, but implied thoughts and feelings need to be clarified to avoid mistaken conclusions. In both of these statements "feel" should be replaced with "think" for correct usage.

Using words pertaining to thought and feeling correctly will minimize the amount of time the nurse must spend clarifying and will maximize the quality of the interaction. In the mental health specialty, it becomes even more important for the nurse to use such terms appropriately to help the patient identify and label his or her emotions and thoughts to facilitate therapy.

6. *Using Empathy.* Empathy is also tied into feelings. There is a big difference between sympathy and empathy. Sympathy is used socially when people wish to share emotional experiences. It is not a therapeutic technique because it involves experiencing the emotion. Empathy involves identifying emotions without experiencing the emotion. Nurses need to use empathy with patients. We need to be able to identify the emotion and relate to it while keeping the focus on the patient's needs. We need to be able to help the patients deal with their feelings and still maintain professional control of the situation; we need to remain the helper.

Sympathy often allows both persons to become emotionally invested in the moment. The focus is shared by both people. In therapeutic relationships, the focus must remain on the client.

Consider the following situation: You notice a patient in the lounge. She is crying. You want to help, so you approach her, sit down, and offer your assistance. She explains to you that she just found out that her pet died.

The pet had been her "family" since her divorce. They had been through many experiences together. The pet had always been there for her and now the pet had died while she was in the hospital and couldn't be there. Your response options are:

Sympathy: Remembering your own favorite pet who died, you say "I know just how you feel; my pet died suddenly, too" and begin crying as well.

OR

Empathy: Remembering your pet who died, you allow yourself to feel that pain, and then say, "I am so sorry. It must be very painful to lose something you feel so close to. I'd like to hear about your pet when you think you'd like to talk about it."

Socially, chances are that we might take the "sympathy" option, which would be appropriate with people who are not patients. Our patients need us to be sensitive but still be the helper. The "empathy" option is more appropriate in most therapeutic situations.

7. *Silence.* Silence serves many functions in communication, yet many people are very uncomfortable with it. American society seems to value conversation. People use vocabulary and the ability to talk about a variety of topics as a measure of intelligence and social grace. Watch what happens at a social gathering or in the break room when a short silence occurs. Often, people fidget nervously or make "small talk" just to break the silence.

Silence, as a therapeutic technique of communication, serves two main purposes: First, it allows the nurse and the patient a short time to collect their thoughts, and, second, it shows patience and acceptance on the part of the nurse. Sitting quietly for a period of time, usually 2 to 3 minutes, and maintaining an open body posture send the message that you are willing to wait if the patient has more to say or that you accept the fact that the interaction may be over for the present. Silence can be just as powerful and effective as any verbal interaction.

Caution: Do not allow the silence to go on too long. If nothing has been said by either party within 2 to 3 minutes, it is wise to suggest to the patient that it might be time for a rest. Then take your cues from the patient's response. Perhaps the conversation will begin again, or maybe the patient will be grateful for your suggestion to rest. Either way, you can let the person know that you are there if he or she wants to talk again at another time.

8. *Giving Information.* This is very different from the communication block of giving advice. Giving information relates to the helping relationship because it involves a form of teaching.

As mentioned earlier, physicians are usually with their patients for very short periods of time, whereas nurses are usually with the same patients for an 8-hour shift. It is very natural for nurses and patients to have more quality time for talking. This is one reason patient teaching is becoming a bigger part of a nurse's responsibility in all levels of nursing.

Nurses provide information in all phases of hospitalization, from preoperative teaching to discharge planning. It involves using pamphlets, videos, resource manuals, or other resource persons.

Caution: Most state Nurse Practice Acts still place the stipulation that the nurse may not legally give information to the patient before the physician has given the initial information. This means that nurses may not give lab reports, read diagnostic information, talk about possible treatments, and so forth until these have first been discussed between physician and patient. How do we know this has occurred? We use therapeutic techniques that allow us to ask questions that get us results.

EXAMPLE

"Mrs. Brown, I'd be happy to discuss your surgery with you. What did your physician explain already?"

Using this combination of offering assistance and asking an open-ended question serves three purposes: You've maintained rapport, you've gotten Mrs. Brown to tell you her level of prior knowledge, and you have let her know that you presume she has had a conversation with the physician. What if Mrs. Brown hesitates or tells you outright that the physician hasn't been in yet? You pull out the techniques of stating your needs and using empathy, and you tell her very honestly, "Mrs. Brown, I can sense your frustration, but I cannot legally (or ethically) give you that information until you and your physician have discussed it first. I'll be happy to call your physician to let her know that you wish to see her as soon as possible. After you have talked, I'll be happy to answer any questions you may have."

9. *Using General Leads.* This is a method of encouraging the person to continue speaking. It lets the speaker know that you are listening and interested in hearing more. The technique is fairly simple: It involves verbal and usually nonverbal communication. Examples of general leads are saying "Yes?" while maybe raising the eyes, "Go on ..." while maintaining eye contact and possibly nodding the head in an affirmative motion or maybe just saying "... and then?" if the person pauses in the middle of a statement or concern.

10. *Stating Implied Thoughts and Feelings.* This takes a combination of skills. It requires using some guessing (like you did in reflecting), using empathy, and making an observation about a behavior or condition you see in the patient.

This technique is helpful in initiating conversation that might be difficult to start with other techniques. It is hard to deny that something is not right when someone identifies a specific behavior or action that supports the suggestion that something is different about the patient. Nurses are assessing their patient's physical and emotional states all the time.

When a patient is reluctant to share this situation, the nurse can preface the question with an observation and then follow with an educated guess at the emotion that is being experienced.

EXAMPLE

A nurse observes a patient, Mr. Trent, and his wife. They usually have a lively, pleasant visit, but today all is quiet and tense. Few words are spoken. When Mrs. Trent leaves, the nurse decides to try to state an implied feeling by saying, "Mr. Trent, I just saw your wife leave. The two of you were unusually quiet today. I get the feeling that you are unhappy or uncomfortable with something. I'd like to help if I can."

Because the nurse has identified a change in behavior pattern, it is difficult for Mr. Trent to deny there is a "problem." The nurse has chosen to use a generic form of emotional response to see which way Mr. Trent will take the conversation. Offering assistance lets Mr. Trent know that the nurse does care about his feelings.

Table 2–3 helps define the techniques for helping communication skills and the effects they may have on nurse-patient relationships.

TABLE 2-3	*Techniques for Therapeutic (Helping) Communication*	
TECHNIQUE	**EXAMPLE**	**EFFECT ON PATIENT**
REFLECTING/ REPEATING/ PARROTING	Patient: "I'm so tired of all of this." Nurse: "Tired?"	1. Encourages exploring meaning of the statement 2. *Caution: Use sparingly;* can be irritating if overused
CLARIFYING TERMS	"When you say 'tired,' do you mean it in a physical way or an emotional way?"	1. Encourages patient to restate the comment 2. Improves chances that the message sent is the message received
OPEN-ENDED QUESTIONS	1. "How are you feeling today?" 2. "What can I do to help, Mr. Jones?"	1. Discourages "Yes"/"No" answers 2. Encourages patient to express self in his or her own terms
ASKING FOR WHAT YOU WANT OR NEED	1. "Mrs. Smith, I need to ask you a few questions, please." 2. "Mr. Harris, I would like next Tuesday off, please."	1. States purpose for the interaction 2. Keeps speaker assertive and self-responsible
IDENTIFYING THOUGHTS AND FEELINGS	1. "I feel angry when you are not honest with me." 2. "I think honesty is important in all relationships."	1. Helps the patient to identify and label thoughts and emotions 2. May give insight to underlying concerns or complications of healing

(continued)

TECHNIQUE	EXAMPLE	EFFECT ON PATIENT
USING EMPATHY	1. "It must feel very demeaning when others are dishonest." 2. "I feel very sorry that you are in such pain."	1. Acknowledges patient's feelings 2. Keeps nurse in position of control and helpfulness
SILENCE		1. Shows that nurse is comfortable with what patient says and is willing to hear more 2. Allows nurse and patient to collect their thoughts
GIVING INFORMATION	1. "Ms. Harris, I'd be glad to explain this diagnosis to you. Tell me what the doctor has said, and I'll clarify it for you any way I can."	1. Increases rapport 2. Eases patient's anxiety 3. Honestly confirms that the physician has given prior information 4. Suggests collaboration
USING GENERAL LEADS	1. "Yes?" 2. "Go on ..." 3. "And then?"	1. Tells patient nurse is listening 2. Encourages patient to elaborate
STATING IMPLIED THOUGHTS AND FEELINGS	1. "Ms. Johnson, you're not smiling today like you usually do. I sense something is bothering you. How can I help?"	1. Lets the patient know you are paying attention to him or her 2. Identifies a specific behavior or change in behavior, which lowers chance of denying it. 3. Patient hears that the nurse cares and wishes to help

■ ADAPTIVE COMMUNICATION TECHNIQUES

Some populations of people, such as those mentioned in the previous section, require special considerations when you are communicating with them. These are some ways of facilitating communication with people who live with certain disabilities or who have varied degrees of ability.

PEOPLE WHO ARE HEARING IMPAIRED

When communicating with your patient who is hearing impaired, it is important to know the extent of the impairment. Does the person speech-read? Is he or she reliant on a hearing aid? What is the emotional attitude of the patient?

Communicating can be very frustrating for hearing-impaired patients as well as for the nurse. There are several methods of signing. Hearing-impaired patients often use sign language, but most "hearing" people do not know sign language. Sometimes paper and pencil writing is effective, but it is slow. Speech reading is helpful to some hearing-impaired people, but it is not always accurate. Because many words that look the same are in fact very different in meaning, and because not all speaking people say words the same way (because of dialect or different primary language from that of the hearing-impaired person), speech reading can be misleading at best.

PEOPLE WHO ARE VISUALLY IMPAIRED

Adaptive devices such as books on tape, braille-prepared computers, and seeing-eye dogs can be extremely helpful. The type of adaptive device depends on the type and severity of the impairment.

Caution: Visually impaired people are not necessarily hearing impaired, too! It is usually not necessary to talk slower or louder to a person with a visual impairment.

PEOPLE WHO HAVE LARYNGECTOMIES

Technology has developed several different aids that amplify the vibrations of speech. For some patients with **laryngectomies,** placing this amplifier over the area of the larynx and talking will produce a buzzing sound that replicates their former voice. It is a monotone sound, but it greatly improves the ability of these patients to communicate in a more natural manner. Not everyone can use these devices, however. Some people need to rely on communication boards and pictures to communicate (Fig. 2-2). Some people make use of new computer-assisted devices. The patient will be in close contact with a speech therapist. Nurses need to be involved with the therapist as well, so that the patient has continuity of therapy and good evaluation of the ability to use the devices. The goal is to restore the person to his or her surgical maximal ability of speech. It can be a frightening and frustrating time for the patient and the health-care team, but the rewards are great when speech, at whatever level, begins to return.

PEOPLE WITH LANGUAGE DIFFERENCES

Honesty is the best policy here. This discussion comes up in several sections of this text, but it is much better to apologize and admit when you are not receiving the sender's message. Serious mistakes can be made when one assumes the meaning of the message. It is also important to remember that communicating is often a highly cultural activity; people are not always com-

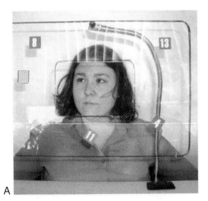
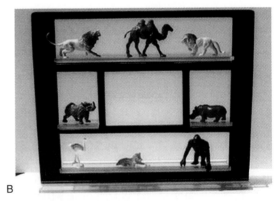

A   B

FIGURE 2-2. Communication boards for persons with severe physical disabilities and communication disabilities. A, The Eye-Talk Communicator, model 3700, is equipped with a self-contained, height-adjustable stand. This clear board enables the user to communicate using an eye gaze while still being able to see the person being communicated with and the surroundings. B, The 3-D Eye-Talk!, model 3705, like the Eye-Talk Communicator, enables the user to communicate using an eye gaze while still being able to see the surroundings as well as the person being communicated with. The 3-D Eye-Talk! features a self-contained stand with three shelves and a clear board. Small objects can be placed on the shelves, permitting the user to communicate using actual items, instead of pictures or symbols. (Photos courtesy of Enabling Devices, Hastings-On-Hudson, NY.)

fortable asking for correction or clarification from someone of a different gender, age, or social or professional status. Using assertive, honest communication skills will usually get positive results. Remember: When not positive about the meaning of a message, ask!

PEOPLE WHO HAVE APHASIC/ DYSPHASIC DISORDERS

This is another area that offers many options for adaptive techniques. Nurses must be aware of the type and degree of aphasia/**dysphasia** for each patient. The physician and speech pathologist or therapist are excellent resource people to help in deciding what type of adaptive technique will be the most effective. Your documentation of the responses of your patient to the various techniques will also help in these decisions.

Techniques range from changing the rate or pitch of our speech to actually using objects, pictures, spelling boards, or computerized equipment if the patient has access to it (Fig. 2-3). Nurses need to be cautioned, however. Do not answer for the patient. Finishing sentences or trying to play guessing games with people who have these types of disorders is usually not in the best interest of the patient. It usually takes a longer time for these patients to process the information and get the answer out. Be patient. When you see that the patient is getting frustrated or is truly unable to respond properly, it may be because the words you used were unfamiliar or maybe too much time has passed and the patient has forgotten the question. Gentle hints or rephrasing your question may be enough to help the patient. It may be just one little word that makes the difference between the patient's being successful or not.

Communication in all forms is essential to the work of a nurse. Taking the time to learn and use these techniques can make your relationships with patients and coworkers very pleasant and rewarding.

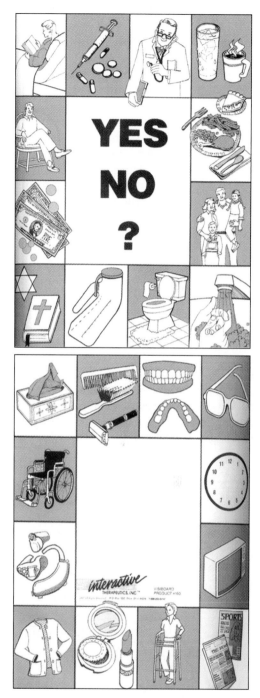

FIGURE 2-3. Picture board for patients with aphasia. (Courtesy Visiboard, ©1987, Interactive Therapies, Inc., Stow, Ohio. Reprinted with permission.)

Key Concepts ▪ ▪ ■

1. Humans cannot NOT communicate. Interpersonal communication is a complex process.
2. Therapeutic or helping communication is a language that is learned and shared by nurses. It is a purposeful skill that requires practice.
3. People communicate verbally and nonverbally. Nonverbal communication sends a stronger message than verbal communication.
4. Communication can be assertive or aggressive. Assertive statements are the more helpful of the two; they start with the word "I." Aggressive statements are designed to place responsibility on another person. They start with the word "you."
5. Nurses need to be aware of what blocks therapeutic communication and the techniques to use to encourage effective, helping communication with patients.
6. Special techniques are used when communicating with populations who have special communication needs.

REFERENCES

Grinder, J. and Bandler, R. *Trance Formations—Neuro-Linguistic Programming and the Structure of Hypnosis*, Real People Press, Moab, Utah, 1981.

Special Mention: Deirdre Michael, MA, CCC/SLP, University of Minnesota Hospitals, for her thoughts concerning people with conditions affecting their capacity for verbal communication.

CRITICAL THINKING EXERCISES ■ ■ ■

1. Write one feeling statement and one thinking statement for each of the following situations:
   A. A coworker who is a BSN is routinely coming late to work and overstaying breaks, causing patients to have unsafe care and you to have extra work. You speak to your nurse manager, who appears to ignore your concerns, so you approach the coworker.
   B. Your patient is suddenly uncooperative and verbally abusive to you. To the best of your knowledge, you have done nothing to deserve this kind of behavior and you attempt to discuss this with the patient.
   C. You are a person who speaks differently than your coworkers. You overhear your patient and another nurse talking. You hear the statement, "I don't care to work with that person, either. That's the worst accent I have ever heard." You guess they are talking about you.

2. With two of the above situations what communication techniques will you use to try to improve the situation?

3. Turn the following aggressive statements into assertive statements.
   A. "You make me so angry when you stop at the bar before you come home."
   B. "You always take the 'easy' assignment and that's not fair."
   C. "Mark always gets the days off he asks for; why can't I?"

TEST QUESTIONS ■ ■ ■

MULTIPLE CHOICE QUESTIONS

1. Which of the following is an example of a therapeutic, open-ended question?
   A. "Why did you do that, Mrs. Jones?"
   B. "How can I help you, Mr. Thompson?"
   C. "Can I help you, Ms. Greene?"
   D. "Please, can I ask you a question, Mark?"

2. The purpose of "therapeutic communication" is to:
   A. Develop a friendly, social relationship with the patient.
   B. Develop a parental, authoritarian relationship with the patient.
   C. Develop a helping, purposeful relationship with the patient.
   D. Develop a cool, businesslike relationship with the patient.

3. You observe a patient in the family lounge. She appears to be talking to herself. You want to find out what is wrong. Your best approach to her might be:
   A. "Who are you talking to?"
   B. "Please stop talking. You are disturbing the other people."
   C. "I saw your lips moving. Can you tell me what you are talking about?"
   D. "Why are you talking to yourself?"

4. Your patient asks you the results of his blood tests. You respond:
   A. "They are all negative."
   B. "Why do you want to know?"
   C. "I think you should wait until your physician comes in."
   D. "I am not able to tell you right now, but I will call your physician and have her stop in to explain them to you."

5. Your patient is a single parent who has just been diagnosed with terminal cancer. She is concerned about returning to work and asks many questions. Finally, the patient says, "What do you think I should do?" You say:
   A. "I think you should just stay busy."
   B. "I wouldn't worry about it."
   C. "What are your thoughts about returning to work?"
   D. "Oh, you'll be just fine. There are lots of people worse off than you."

6. Your patient has refused all of your attempts to care for him. You say:
   A. "I'd like to help you; what can I do?"
   B. "Why don't you like me?"
   C. "What is the matter with you?"
   D. "You must do this; physician's orders!"

7. Your patient is Jewish and refuses to eat non-Kosher food. You say:
   A. "I will ask the dietitian to come and talk with you."
   B. "The dietitian will come to see you."
   C. "It's the best we can do. You need to eat."
   D. "You're right. The hospital food does leave much to be desired!"

8. Your patient is commenting that the physician has not been in to visit for two days. You say:
   A. "I hate it when that happens!"
   B. "What do you need to know?"
   C. "Well, he is very busy!"
   D. "You feel ignored by your physician?"

9. Your patient, who is usually very talkative, does not respond to you when you enter the room. You say:
   A. "Ms. Smith, you are so quiet this afternoon. Is something bothering you?"
   B. "Ms. Smith, is something bothering you?"
   C. "Can I help you?"
   D. "Why are you so quiet this afternoon?"

10. Ms. Smith responds to your question (see #9), "I feel like nobody cares." You respond:
    A. "Why do you say that?"
    B. "Like nobody cares? Please try to describe the emotion you are truly 'feeling.'"
    C. "Ms. Smith, you're wrong about that. Of course we care."
    D. "Ms. Smith, maybe the doctor can change the dosage of your medication. You'll feel better."

11. An example of a therapeutic response conveying support or encouragement is:
    A. "That must feel very discouraging."
    B. "Maybe you shouldn't worry quite so much."
    C. "Why do you say that?"
    D. "Nobody would deliberately try to hurt you."

12. "I feel like the patient's family does not understand the situation" is an example of what kind of statement? _____. Briefly explain your answer. _____

13. In a therapeutic or helping communication, which of the following communication techniques would be the most appropriate?

SELECT ALL THE ANSWER CHOICES THAT APPLY

A. Silence

B. Open-ended questions

C. Closed-ended questions

D. Asking "why?"

E. Sharing observations

F. Giving advice

G. General leads

MATCHING QUESTIONS

Directions

Match the "block" or "technique" on the left with the best statement on the right.

COLUMN A	COLUMN B
1. General Lead	A. "You said you aren't hungry . . . ?"
2. Agreeing	B. "It will be just fine!"
3. Share Observations	C. "You should take a long trip!"
4. Giving Advice	D. "Go on . . ."
5. Reflecting	E. "You are crying. What is wrong?"
6. Giving Information	F. Allow, but do not focus on this.
7. Belittling Feelings	G. "We all feel pain sometimes."
8. Ensuring Understanding	H. "I'm not sure I understand . . ."
9. Reassuring Clichés	I. "I'll bring you some information on that."
10. Crying	J. "Your physician is very competent!"
	K. "You're right; we are short-staffed!"

CONVERSATIONAL PRACTICE

Directions

Read the following situation. There are five therapeutic verbal or nonverbal techniques and five blocks. On your answer sheet, identify the techniques that are therapeutic on spaces 1 through 5 and the blocks on spaces 6 through 10. If the technique or block is a group of words, write the exact words. If the technique is nonverbal behavior, identify the behavior. (The 10 verbal or nonverbal items are identified by an asterisk [*] and are in bold print.)

Situation

You are the staffing nurse for your facility. One nurse is frequently late for work. You have the following conversation with that nurse:

You: "Hello, Marie. Thank you for stopping in. ***I need to talk to you about your attendance."**

Marie: ***"Why? *Is something wrong?"**

You:	*"I see by your time card that you have been late for work four times this month.** That is significant and I am concerned. *Can you tell me what the problem is?"**
Marie:	"No. I don't have a problem." *(Marie starts to cry.)**
You:	*(Silence for a short time) *"Marie, you really should start exercising.** It takes away stress."
Marie:	"I didn't say anything about stress—it's none of your business, anyway!"
You:	*"You're wrong, Marie.** I have two options today: I can put you on probation, or I can work out a plan with you to improve your attendance. Which would you prefer?"
Marie:	"I didn't think it was a big deal to be a few minutes late. *I guess I'd like to improve my attendance."**
You:	"I'm glad! Here are some bus schedules to look at. Let's start there." (And you continue to work with Marie.)

THERAPEUTIC/HELPING

1. _____

2. _____

3. _____

4. _____

5. _____

NONTHERAPEUTIC/BLOCKS

6. _____

7. _____

8. _____

9. _____

10. _____

CHAPTER

3

Ethics and Law

Learning Objectives ■ ■ ■

1. Define professionalism.
2. Identify the standards of nursing practice.
3. State an understanding of the Nurse Practice Act.
4. State the importance of honesty and accuracy in verbal reporting and written documentation.
5. State the importance of confidentiality.
6. Define HIPAA and its role in heath care delivery.
7. Define JCAHO and its role in health care delivery.
8. Identify responsibility to self, patients, and coworkers.
9. Explain the Good Samaritan Act.
10. Explain involuntary commitment.
11. Explain voluntary commitment.
12. Identify patients' rights and nursing considerations for them.
13. Define patient advocacy.
14. Identify community resources in general, as well as those in your community.

Key Terms ■ ■ ■

- Advocacy
- Commitment
- Confidentiality
- Culture
- Culture of nurses
- Ethics
- Patient Bill of Rights
- Professional
- Proxemics
- Responsibility
- Standards of care

■ PROFESSIONALISM

Professional is a word with many different meanings. Merriam-Webster Online defines *professional* as an adjective meaning "(1) characterized by or conforming to the technical or ethical standards of a profession." It may be a term that requires a nurse to rely on the therapeutic communication skill of clarifying.

Nursing is a profession. Nurses care for patients and perform designated services for a salary. As a profession, however, the different levels of nursing disagree as to who is a "professional nurse." We all receive pay for our work, yet it is commonly accepted that only registered nurses (RNs) are considered professional nurses; the licensed practical nurse (LPN) or licensed vocational nurse (LVN) is considered a nonprofessional. In areas with union representation in nursing, the two levels usually belong to separate organizations. Some nursing groups believe that only RNs who are baccalaureate-prepared and beyond are considered professional.

Regardless of your beliefs in this discussion, *all* nurses are expected to behave in a professional manner; that is to say, we are to perform at the highest level of preparation we have achieved. We are to abide by the federal, state, and local guidelines that are set down for us. Sometimes this code of behavior is called **ethics**, which is a combination of professional expectations that borders on legal issues. Ethics are born more out of patients' expectations from nurses than out of actual legal boundaries. Ethical nurses have a high sense of professional pride and honor. Their conduct is of the highest quality they can give to their profession.

Nurses must be aware of their state's Nurse Practice Act and perform within its parameters. A nurse's personal problems are to be handled outside of the work environment. We are expected to be respectful of the beliefs of our patients and coworkers and not to force our personal beliefs on others at work. We are expected to perform honestly. We are expected to report any infractions we notice in other nurses. In short, we are expected to behave and perform in a manner that promotes the pride and reputation of the nursing profession, not as a detriment to that profession.

STANDARDS OF CARE

In 1941, the National Association for Practical Nurse Educators and Service developed a code of ethics for the LPN. Nineteen states are active in this organization.

The National Federation of Licensed Practical Nurses (NFLPN) has also adopted a code of ethics for the LPN/LVN. In 1965, the International Council of Nurses produced the first code of ethics for nurses as a whole.

The American Nurses Association (ANA) has written guidelines for minimum **standards of care** that nurses at each level of preparation are expected to perform. These were originally written in 1973 and have been updated most recently in 2001. The ANA also writes standards for some specialty areas within nursing. There is a set of Standards of Psychiatric-Mental Health Clinical Nursing Practice, last updated in 2000. These standards can be accessed at the ANA Web site www.nursingworld.org/ethics/code/protected_nwcoe303.htm. The purpose of the ANA is to promote high standards of practice, improve working conditions for nurses, and promote the general well-being of nurses. Each state has some autonomy in the interpretation and implementation of the guidelines of all the groups mentioned earlier.

NURSE PRACTICE ACT

The Nurse Practice Act dictates the acceptable scope of nursing practice for the different levels of nursing. When a nurse is questioning whether or not to perform a certain skill or perhaps is accused of wrongdoing, it is typically the Nurse Practice Act that is consulted to find out if that nurse is performing at the accepted level of preparation. For example, if your state does not allow the LPN/LVN to supervise patient care, yet an LPN or LVN is the only licensed staff on duty on the night shift, the Nurse Practice Act for your state may have been ignored, and that nurse could be held liable for damages in a court of law. This can be an ethical dilemma as well. It may be the interpretation of the facility that it is permissible to allow that LPN/LVN to function as supervisor if an RN is on call. This may or may not be the interpretation of the particular state. A phone call to the Board of Nursing will give the answer. Any nurse has the right and responsibility to make that phone call.

ACCURACY

The ultimate goal of the helping person in health care is to "do no harm." Safety for our patients and ourselves must be in our thoughts at all times as we progress through our professional lives.

A nurse's best defense is the quality of verbal and written communication. In her book, *Legal, Ethical, and Political Issues in Nursing*, Tonia Aiken indicates that spelling errors are crucial in liability cases, as they reflect on a nurse's general ability to care for patients. Legally, the general assumption is "if it is not charted, it has not been done." Some situations can impede our efforts at accuracy in charting. First of all, nurses are busy. Patient care is the primary focus of our workday. Many times, it seems that the 8-hour day is over before it starts! Charting may be scaled down to a minimum, especially if the employer does not pay for overtime.

Some facilities use a form of charting that may be called "charting by exception." This type of documentation is based on flow-sheet charting. Normal values, the guidelines for which are established at the facility, are written on the chart form, and the nurse uses a series of check marks and arrows to indicate that certain assessments have been made. The nurse then initials the check marks and arrows and uses a full signature at the bottom of the page. Only situations outside of the established normal parameters are mentioned in some sort of nurse's note. Although this type of charting saves time, it is sometimes challenged legally because it is not always enough documentation.

Sometimes the nurse is deficient in reading, writing, and spelling skills. Not only might this be a source of extreme embarrassment to the nurse, but also it is unacceptable as professional, safe nursing practice. It is important to note as well that this is a much more common problem in the United States than one might think and that it is not just people from other countries who experience this difficulty!

No matter what the situation, it is imperative that the nurse takes as much time as necessary to carry out complete, accurate documentation on each patient. Your competency to practice nursing can be questioned if for some reason your documentation is subpoenaed in a court case and your spelling and grammar are of poor quality according to American standards.

All agencies have an established method for verbal reporting. It may be a taped shift report, a grand rounds type of report, or a one-on-one report with the patient's care plan. Again, it is important to prepare to spend as much time as needed to get the message from your day's work to the receiver for the oncoming shift. Be thorough but as concise as possible. It is usually standard procedure to discuss vital signs, physical assessments, any visits from physicians or visitors, new orders, responses to medications and treatments, and any change in condition. An area that is sometimes forgotten is the mental, emotional, and behavioral status of the patient. We know that physical healing is to a large extent a result of attitude and emotional condition; therefore, be sure to include the patient's psychological status in your verbal report. Always check with the incoming nurse to be sure that there are no further questions and be sure to inform that nurse of anything you may not have completed.

HONESTY

It may seem insulting to discuss honesty and integrity with nursing students. Honesty, or "veracity" as it is also called, is after all, one of qualities of professionalism, isn't it? The discussion is necessary, though, because honesty means different things to different people. It may mean "surviving" or "helping someone less able than myself" or "telling the physician what he or she wants to hear." Honesty is a concept that can be highly cultural.

Honesty can also mean the difference between keeping and losing your nursing license. Sadly, nurses are a group of people with a high percentage of chemical dependency. Inappropriate use and misuse of mind-altering chemicals such as alcohol or prescription and nonprescription drugs can render a nurse legally unsafe. Continuing to practice nursing while using these chemicals displays unprofessional behavior and poor judgment. A nurse in this situation who is fearful of losing a license or unable to seek help may consider inaccurate charting, omission of certain charting, or blatant lying about a situation as a way to remain employed. The patient's safety is not the nurse's primary concern when this happens.

The professional choice is always to tell the truth. It may be painful, frightening, or embarrassing to admit personal conflicts or errors or omissions in patient care, but you will avoid further potential harm to your patient as well as to your professional reputation by admitting to mistakes and taking the appropriate corrective measures. Nurses are human. Despite our best efforts and multiple medication checks, we make mistakes occasionally. Recognizing them, admitting them, and taking corrective measures to ensure the patient's safety are the signs of sound judgment and professional nursing behavior.

CULTURE OF NURSES

A commonly accepted definition of **culture** includes nonphysical traits, rituals, values, and traditions that are handed down from generation to generation. Nursing is an occupation that passes down its professional values, rituals, and traditions from generation of nurse to generation of nurse (Fig. 3-1). The affective, or attitudinal, components of nursing are behaviors that nurses typically learn from role modeling other nurses. It is this concept that spawned the term *culture of nurses* (Neeb, 1994).

As mentioned earlier, we exist in a global community. We are nurses who have been born and raised in many different places. We have different ideas about politics and social issues. However, when we come

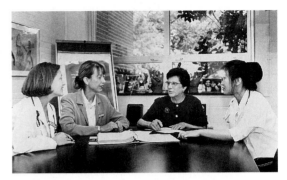

FIGURE 3-1. The culture of nursing. Through role modeling, professional values, rituals, and traditions are passed from one generation of nurses to the next. (From Sorrell, J.M. and Redmond, G.M., *Community-Based Nursing Practice: Learning Through Students' Stories.* F.A. Davis Company, Philadelphia, 2002, p. 358. Reprinted with permission.)

together as a profession, we meld these ideas into behaviors that are consistent in order to provide our patients with the best possible care. We may need to give up some personal ideas while working, to make the whole of nursing greater than the sum of its parts. This means that skills such as spelling and grammar that may be "correct" or actually considered unimportant in personal situations will not be acceptable for practicing nursing in the United States (Aiken, 1994). This is not an issue of labeling a nurse's personal or cultural belief system as right, wrong, good, or bad. Rather, it means that we must remember the components of professionalism and our basic tenets of communication.

Another component is highly cultural, and that is a field of study called **proxemics.** Proxemics concerns space, time, and waiting, which are all influenced by one's culture. If you have ever traveled between the northern tier and the southern tier of the United States, you may have noticed a cultural difference in time and waiting. People in the northern states tend to be much more rushed. They may watch the clock in restaurants, in classrooms, and while on hold on the telephone. In the southern states, life is a bit slower-paced. That burger doesn't need to be there in 2 minutes; people just sit to wait, and they relax. This is not an issue of right or wrong, good or bad. It is an issue of differences in the way people are acculturated.

For nurses from countries in which timeliness is not an issue, punching a time clock or serving a medication within the allotted amount of time may not be a priority. As nurses know, however, this sort of timeliness is a very important part of our nursing culture. A patient who is in pain and asks for a pain medication expects the nurse to be on time with it. If the nurse replies, "I'll be there in a minute," the patient might hear the word "minute" and take it quite literally. After all, the patient is the one in need. It may actually have taken you 15 minutes to return with the medication, and in that time you may have answered two more call signals, helped someone to the bathroom, and taken a physician's order, but that patient who is waiting for you knows only that you haven't returned yet. Depending on that patient's culture, the call signal may have been on immediately after 1 minute passed or the patient may feel it is grossly disrespectful to ask again and thus suffer silently.

Space and distance also constitute a big part of nursing culture. Nurses must touch patients in order to do their jobs. We make full body assessments, catheterize, give suppositories, and perform prenatal and postnatal checks. Male and female nurses work on male and female patients. In a way, we become desensitized to these functions, as they become a routine part of our jobs. Some patients are very timid and modest. In their culture, strangers may not touch strangers in certain ways, and these individuals may prefer to have family members perform those tasks. Some nurses feel uncomfortable waking postoperative patients for their routine vital signs check because in their culture, it is not proper to awaken sick people; it is proper to let them sleep and not disturb them. Proxemics is a very complex field of study; this has only touched on some basics. It is important for nurses to understand, however, that the concepts of space,

time, and waiting are highly cultural in their interpretation.

Nurses must work together for the betterment of patient care. When in doubt, ask. Learn from each other. There is no better way for personal and professional enrichment.

■ CONFIDENTIALITY

Confidentiality is so important that it is singled out as one of the federal and state patient rights. *Confidential* means **1:** marked by intimacy or willingness to confide **2:** private, secret (*confidential* information) **3:** entrusted with confidences **4:** containing information whose unauthorized disclosure could be prejudicial to the national interest (Merriam-Webster Online).

Remember how you felt when you told your best friend your deepest secret only to hear that secret had been repeated to someone else? That was a break in confidentiality. In a manner of speaking, your patient's diagnosis and plan of care are a secret to everyone but the patient and the health-care team; this information is very private and must be kept that way. But what happens when the patient shares something with you that must be passed on?

The Doctrine of Privileged Information is a bond between patient and physician. Under this doctrine, the physician has the right to refuse to answer certain questions (e.g., in a court of law) and can cite "privileged physician-patient information." Nurses are usually not included in this relationship. If information is requested of us, we are bound to answer as truthfully as we can. So, how does one maintain honesty and confidentiality at the same time? First and foremost, communicate honestly to the patient that you cannot make promises. When you sense that the patient is telling you information that is potentially legally sensitive, it is a good idea to tell the patient right away that you as a nurse are not protected by the Doctrine of Privileged

Information. The patient should be told that you would be happy to call the physician, but if the person still chooses to share this information with you, a good technique is to let the patient know that you may need to tell the information to a supervisor or others involved in the patient's treatment. The legal case of Tarasoff vs. Regents of the University of California in 1976 is the standard for this law. It also protects intended victims of patients who may be hospitalized or incarcerated. Let the patient know that only those parts of the conversation that are directly related to his or her care will be shared but that if information is requested by a legal representative, you will be required to answer.

Temptations are great, especially for the student nurse. It is fun and exciting to learn new information and to see your skills making a difference in someone's recovery. It is easy to start chatting about your experiences to another student or to a staff nurse, but be careful. The person nearby (e.g., in the elevator with you) may be a friend or family member. Unless specifically indicated by the patient, these people do not ordinarily have rights to information about the patient. There are many horror stories about innocent conversations that were overheard by the "wrong" people, which resulted in negative consequences to the patient and/or the nurse involved.

Whoever said hospitals were quiet places probably never worked in a hospital. Nurses and physicians are often talking continuously, and usually not quietly. "Dr. X is on the phone about Mrs. D's bowel surgery," calls the unit coordinator to the nurse across the hall. "Is Mr. B's insulin up yet?" asks the nursing assistant from the kitchenette. "Nurse Y needs to know."

Sound familiar? How many other patients or people passing through the area heard those interchanges? How would the patient feel if he or she knew that personal information had been handled so thoughtlessly? Remember that patients could interpret the message differently than the nurse might. These breaches of confidentiality happen all the time, but that does not make them acceptable. Take the extra couple of steps it requires to give or receive information quietly to the appropriate people (Fig. 3-2).

Charts, too, can be culprits of confidentiality. How many eyes may have seen that chart you accidentally left open when you went to answer that last call signal? What about your report sheet? Some nurses call these sheets their "brains." Be sure to keep yours with you at all times! A story about a "brain" that was found on the floor was told by a nurse who was studying to be a lawyer. The report sheet had fallen from a nurse's pocket and had been picked up by a family member. This person could have brought the paper to the desk immediately and the story would have ended there, but that was not the case. At the end of the shift, the family member brought the "brain" to the nurse in charge. None of the items on the list had been carried out, according to the family

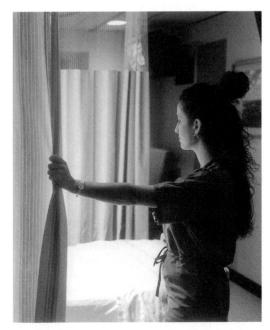

FIGURE 3-2. Maintaining privacy is a patient right and conveys caring to the patient. (From Williams, L.S. and Hopper, P.D., *Understanding Medical Surgical Nursing*, 2nd ed., F.A. Davis Company, Philadelphia, 2003, p. 13. Reprinted with permission.)

member who had been there the greater part of the day. Unfortunately for the nurse, the tasks had been charted as being completed. This display of unprofessional and irresponsible behavior was one thing; the family member maintained, however, that anyone could have picked up that piece of paper and learned many personal things about the patient. The family member sued for breach of confidentiality and won the suit. Granted, this is a drastic example of what can happen, and laws regarding these situations may vary from state to state. The moral of the story: Be careful with patient information of any kind and always maintain honesty in documentation. In these days of computerized, paperless documentation we are just as vulnerable to breeches of confidentiality. Two regulatory agencies intimately involved in documentation and privacy issues are the Health Insurance Portability and Accountability Act of 1996 (HIPAA) and the Joint Commission on the Accreditation of Healthcare Organizations (JCAHO).

HIPAA was developed by the Department of Health and Human Services to provide national standards pertaining to the electronic transmission and communication of medical information between patients, providers, employers, and insurers. HIPAA allows more control on the part of the patient as to what part of their information is disclosed. It addresses the security and privacy involved with medical records and how that information is identified and passed between care providers. For example, Social Security numbers, not long ago routinely used as a patient identifier, are either not used or used in some manner that is difficult to track, such as a partial number or a backward number. HIPAA became effective in April of 2003. Some areas of health care, such as Workers Compensation are either exempt from HIPAA rules or are slightly less stringent in the passing of information.

In June of 2004, the U.S. Department of Health and Human Services Substance Abuse and Mental Health Services Administration Center for Substance Abuse Treatment published a 25-page document entitled "The Confidentiality of Alcohol and Drug Abuse Patient Records Regulation and the HIPAA Privacy Rule: Implications for Alcohol and Substance Abuse Programs." Whew! The document can be located at www.samhsa.gov. It carefully details what can and cannot be disclosed and strongly emphasizes the patient's rights (discussed later in this chapter) and the necessity for the patient's signed informed consent (discussed in the Crisis Intervention section in the Treating Mental Health Alterations chapter).

JCAHO is the leading, national accrediting body of health-care organizations. Earning accreditation by the Joint Commission, once only achievable by hospitals, indicates commitment to quality on a daily basis within the entire facility. Two other goals of a JCAHO accreditation are reducing the risk of undesirable patient outcomes and encouraging continuous improvement. Long-term care facilities and clinics, including specialty clinics associated with mental heath issues, are becoming accredited to provide quality geriatric, mental health, and substance abuse treatment to children, adolescents, and adults. Accredited facilities and clinics have demonstrated compliance with the highest standards of clinical care and administrative quality.

Also in 2004, came the publication of the "2004 National Patient Safety Goals." Sentinel events, patient identifiers, and a list of "dangerous abbreviations" are among the regulations that will be surveyed on unannounced visits, typically with state and/or JCAHO surveys. Frequently asked questions (FAQs) about the safety goals can be found on the Joint Commission Web site at www.jcaho.org.

■ RESPONSIBILITY

Responsibility, or accountability, is a key concept at all levels of nursing practice; however, these words do not necessarily mean independence. Responsibility to the professional RN can mean different things than it does for the LPN/LVN. Nurses are expected to know their scope of practice for their state. Responsibility means performing to the best of your ability within the boundaries of that scope of practice. Sometimes this means knowing when to say "No." Sometimes it means calling the state governing agency to ask specific questions.

Responsible behavior for a nurse also means keeping our personal lives in a manageable state. "Nurse, heal thyself" is not an unrealistic statement to think about. We need to be physically and emotionally prepared to be helpful to our patients, and we cannot do that if we neglect our own personal health. How prepared do you feel to perform clinically after a week of studying for exams? Would you want to be cared for by a nurse who is not eating well or sleeping well? Chances are, you would answer a resounding "No!" to that last question. Yet how many times do we go to work or school when we are exhausted or feeling ill? "I'm fine. I just need a cup of coffee. It's just a little cold." A good rule of thumb is to follow the recommendations in our personal lives that we would give to our patients.

Being accountable or responsible in nursing means being able to work independently and honestly within that scope of practice. It means knowing when to ask for help or to find a reference to refresh your memory or look up that medication you are not familiar with. It means doing everything you possibly can to ensure that you are providing the safest, most accurate care to your patients.

It is the responsibility of the nurse to communicate with patients and coworkers. We must be alert to changes in the patient's condition, both physically and psychologically. The actions we perform, the observations we make, and the documentation we complete are the most effective ways to be helpful and to ensure continuity of care for those patients.

We also have a responsibility to those we work with. Agencies have different ways of organizing the way we perform our jobs;

some practice "team" nursing and some assign primary-care patients for whom the nurse is responsible for managing care during the entire hospitalization. Some facilities use a "buddy" system to ensure help for lifting and to cover the patient load during breaks or meetings. Regardless of the system used, each nurse is in some way interdependent with the other staff members.

You depend on the other staff members to come to work. What happens when you must work one or two people short? Who really suffers as a result? How do you feel when your "buddy" or helper overstays a break or mealtime? What is your response to that? What has happened to the amount of time your patients may have needed? What about your ability to perform safely when you are filling in for someone who is not there?

Many times, the response is some form of anger or resentment. Now that you are familiar with the techniques of healthy communication, you will be able to confront these behaviors more assertively. The responsibility we need for each other professionally may be different from the kind we have for our patients, but it is every bit as important, for it ultimately affects the quality of care we are able to give.

■ ABIDING BY THE CURRENT LAWS

GOOD SAMARITAN ACTS

Good Samaritan acts offer immunity for citizens who stop to help someone in need of medical help. Nurses, physicians, and other medically trained personnel may not always be protected by Good Samaritan laws. The Good Samaritan law came out of tort law. Tort means a "a wrongful act other than a breach of contract for which relief may be obtained in the form of damages or an injunction" (Merriam-Webster Online). The Good Samaritan law varies from state to state, so it is important to understand the implication of this law in your state. The basis for all Good Samaritan laws, however, is that a third party cannot be charged with negligence unless help is given recklessly or if that person makes the situation significantly worse, according to the guidelines for that particular state.

INVOLUNTARY COMMITMENT

Each state has its own regulations about people who need to be hospitalized against their will. This action is reserved for people exhibiting behavior that makes them potentially dangerous to themselves or to others. The average length of time for involuntary **commitment** is approximately 72 hours but could be more or less than that, depending on your state law. During this time, the person is observed and examined by the medical and nursing staff. The patient has full ability to exercise his or her rights under the **Patient Bill of Rights** in that state. At the end of the legal "hold," the patient either chooses to leave or to stay for further treatment. Most of the time, the person realizes a need for help and stays.

Sometimes it is the professional opinion of the treatment team that the person remains a threat to self or the community but that the patient cannot make the appropriate decision. This then becomes an issue of proving incompetence and becomes part of the legal system.

VOLUNTARY COMMITMENT

Most patients who are hospitalized for some type of mental illness are there voluntarily; that is to say, at some point they realized they needed help. It does not mean they will be happy to be there, of course. There remains a stigma in the United States about being hospitalized for problems relating to a person's emotions or behavior. Many times, society assumes that these disorders are weaknesses in character rather than illnesses. It can be very embarrassing to be labeled "mentally ill"; this diagnosis can follow a person for life and has affected patients' personal and professional relationships. It is no wonder that sometimes people allow themselves to be hospitalized for a mental illness only as a last resort. Patients who agree to voluntary treatment are legally allowed to sign themselves out; this is often discouraged by the treatment staff except under certain situations, and it is possible for the staff to institute an involuntary commitment for this patient if they consider the person to be potentially dangerous. Voluntary and involuntary commitment is discussed again in Chapter 8.

Nurses must be very aware of all laws and circumstances affecting the commitment. We must maintain the physical and emotional safety of the patient during the time of hospitalization. Confidentiality is crucial. Educating the public will be helpful in continuing to eliminate the negative implications of issues surrounding mental illness.

■ PATIENT'S RIGHTS

In the 1960s, again during the leadership of President John F. Kennedy, civil rights became a burning issue. Gaining rights for oppressed people of many backgrounds was actively sought by groups such as the American Civil Liberties Union (ACLU). It was largely due to the efforts of this group that civil rights were addressed for people in prisons and for those warehoused in institutions for the mentally ill.

By the 1980s, knowledge of a document called the Patient Bill of Rights became a requirement for people receiving care in a facility, as well as for the health-care workers providing that care. These requirements vary from state to state but are based on federal guidelines and are supported in most states. Agencies in states subscribing to a Patient Bill of Rights are to have the rights listed and displayed in a prominent place in the facility. Patients are to be informed of the implications of their rights and are to be given a copy of the Bill of Rights upon admission to the health-care facility. Table 3-1 lists the most frequently adopted patient rights.

TABLE 3-1	*Most Frequently Adopted Patient Rights*	
PATIENT RIGHT	**DESCRIPTION**	**NURSING CONSIDERATIONS**
1. Treatment in the least restrictive alternative	Patients are not to be held in any stricter conditions than their behavior or diagnosis warrants.	Patients are not to be hospitalized if they can be treated as outpatients or are not to be kept in lockup if not dangerous, and so on. Check the agency protocol and physician's orders for the individual patient. You must still maintain safety for the patient and others.
2. Freedom from restraints and seclusion	The patient is isolated either socially or by being placed in solitary lockup. Restraining can be with either physical or chemical restraints. Many areas require specific diagnosis-related restraint orders.	Be aware of the individual's diagnosis and correlating orders. ■ Make accurate observations and documentation about the patient's physical and behavioral response to restraint. ■ One guideline is to check circulatory function every half hour and to exercise and reposition the patient in restraint at least every 2 hours.
3. Give or refuse consent for medications (including electroconvulsive therapy and psychosurgery)	All patients have the right to say yes or no to treatments that affect them. This must be *informed* consent, meaning the patient fully understands the treatment, potential outcomes, and potential effects of refusal.	Nurses can reinforce the physician's explanation of treatment. Examine the patient's understanding; if there is little or no understanding of treatment, the nurse needs to have the physician return and explain again to the patient and significant others.
4. Possess and have access to personal belongings	Anything of a personal nature that the patient wishes to remain with him or her must be given to the patient.	Carefully document any teaching about safety of personal items. If your local laws allow, have the patient sign a waiver of responsibility for personal items.
5. Daily exercise	Patient needs some form of physical activity at least once daily.	Exercise is according to patient's ability and activity order. Exercise can range from passive range of motion (PROM) to the most strenuous activity the patient can safely perform.
6. Visitors	Patient can visit with anyone he or she chooses.	Determine at time of intake who will be visiting regularly. In cases of family concern over certain people the patient may wish to visit, safety must be a key issue. At times, nurses may need to monitor visits and visitors. Carefully document the patient's emotional and physical outcome of visits. *(continued)*

PATIENT RIGHT	DESCRIPTION	NURSING CONSIDERATIONS
7. Writing materials	Paper, pencils, pens, and so forth must be available to patients.	Unless contraindicated for safety reasons, nurses can assist in ensuring that these items are available at all times. If safety is an issue (e.g., stabbing self or others with a sharp object), this condition needs to be noted in charting.
8. Uncensored mail	Mail must not be opened before the patient receives it.	If patient is unable to physically open the mail or if there is concern that cognitively the patient will lose a check, for example, the nurse or another agent of the facility may witness the opening of the mail. Arrangements can be made with a family member or guardian to sign checks or see to the patient's affairs if the patient is unable to do so.
9. Courts and attorneys	Legal access remains intact for anyone who is hospitalized, whether voluntarily or involuntarily.	Patients can call an attorney at any time. Nurses and agency representatives may be asked to help them. In cases when this seems inappropriate, patient, staff, and family can discuss alternatives in a family conference. Any outcomes need to be incorporated into the care plan and documented.
10. Employment compensation	Wages are not to be withheld during hospitalization.	Under certain legal conditions, compensation may be withheld for reasons other than a stay in a health-care facility. This would be confidential information but must be incorporated into the care plan and documentation.
11. Confidentiality (records, treatment, and so on)	Information about the patient is to be kept secure and private.	Discussion of the patient's condition must take place only in designated places and with designated persons. ■ Many states have cautioned nurses against giving *any* information regarding the patient over the telephone. In some states, a nurse can be in jeopardy of losing a license for releasing information over the phone. ■ Be careful of the wording in your charting. ■ Release information only to those people who are specifically required or legally entitled to have it.

(continued)

TABLE 3-1 ■	*Most Frequently Adopted Patient Rights (Continued)*	
PATIENT RIGHT	**DESCRIPTION**	**NURSING CONSIDERATIONS**
12. Be informed of these rights	Patients must have full understanding of their civil rights while under facility care.	The nurse or the facility representative will explain in detail the meaning of these rights for the patient. Depending on your local law and agency policy, the patient may be asked to sign a document stating that these rights have been explained. Usually, a copy is then kept with the patient record and the patient keeps a personal copy.

In addition to these most frequently adopted patient rights, some states are adopting a set of patient rights for psychiatric patients. These rights may include the right to

- Marry or divorce
- Sue or be sued
- Be actively involved in his or her care
- Be employed if possible
- Retain licenses (driver's license, license to practice one's profession)

It is important that nurses and other health-care professionals educate patients who may have a mental illness diagnosed. In December of 1999, the Hazelden Foundation, an internationally known center for treating chemical dependency, surveyed 1500 adults across the United States. Sixty percent of those responding indicated that they believe alcoholism is an illness, but 47 percent of all respondents stated that, given a choice between two equally qualified individuals, one chemically dependent and one not chemically dependent, they would hire the person who was not chemically dependent. That is a strong bias against people with a mental illness.

patients' needs. These individuals are either volunteers within the community or paid workers from an agency whose job is to ensure that patients, especially those considered vulnerable, are being treated in a safe, legal manner.

Everyone is responsible for reporting abuse and neglect of those who are considered vulnerable. Nurses and health-care workers have a moral, legal, and ethical responsibility to report known or suspected abuse of people who cannot care for themselves. Part of our scope of practice is to be a voice, or an advocate, for the patients under our care. This is the meaning of patient **advocacy.**

Sometimes the nurse is just not sure if abuse is occurring. It is usually better to err on the side of safety for your patient and to report your concern to your supervisor. In most areas, it is acceptable to contact the investigating agency directly. Regardless of the procedure you choose to report your concerns, always check your agency's policy and procedure for such reporting and for the documentation that is required.

■ PATIENT ADVOCACY

With the emergence of the Patient Bill of Rights, patient advocates and patient ombudsmen became visible to speak out for

■ COMMUNITY RESOURCES

According to the provisions of the Community Mental Health Centers Act, every community offers some form of help to people in need. This help can be in the form of hospital emergency rooms, shelters, crisis centers, or social service offices. Most communities have a list available just for the asking. Clinics and hospitals provide lists to people who are at risk or who ask for the resources. Depending on the facility's policies, the nurse may be able to help patients choose a community resource to access after discharge. Be sure to provide information on fees for the services provided by the individual agencies. They vary greatly in relation to offered services, fees, and acceptable insurance. Some are free, whereas some provide assistance on a "sliding scale" or according to ability to pay.

If a patient is reluctant to discuss community resources at the time of discharge, the nurse can suggest that, if the time comes, the patient can look in the yellow pages of the local phone book. The nurse can also inform the patient that it is always acceptable to call the hospital to request a list. Shelters for battered persons usually are *not* advertised; these are kept confidential to maintain safety for the people who need them.

Key Concepts ■ ■ ■

1. It is the nurse's responsibility to know the code of ethics and standards of nursing practice for the state in which he or she is practicing. They will vary from state to state.
2. Collaborative practice means working together with all levels of nursing and all ancillary disciplines to provide the best possible care for the patient.
3. Honesty in nursing practice and excellence in verbal and written communication are crucial to the care of the patient and to the credibility of the nurse. Legally, you will be judged by correct spelling and grammar (American format) in a court case. Your competency can be questioned if your spelling and grammar are poor.
4. Cultural considerations such as space, time, waiting, language, and touch (to name a few) are important parts of the nurse-patient relationship. They are also important in the culture of nursing. What we may believe or have been brought up to believe personally may be different from the standards that are part of the culture of nurses. The patient's well-being and wishes, the state Nurse Practice Act, and agency policy dictate how we can care for the patient in a safe and respectful manner.

CASE STUDY 1 ■ ■ ■

Nurse P, LPN, had worked for Agency X, a nursing home in a small midwestern community, for 10 years. Over the years, Nurse P gained the trust and respect of everyone she worked with or cared for on the job. Nurse P's reputation was very good in the community as well. On one particular day, Nurse P was asked by a patient to "Go to my purse and get my glasses, would you please?"

This apparently had happened many times before, so Nurse P sensed no reason for concern. Several hours later, a family member noticed that the patient was missing an amount of cash and a wedding ring, which the patient kept in the purse "for safe-keeping." The patient recalled asking Nurse P to retrieve the glasses from the purse. Other patients and staff had also seen Nurse P in the patient's purse. The case went to small claims court. Nurse P was found guilty and was made to pay restitution. In addition, Nurse P's license to practice nursing in that state was revoked.

1. What could Nurse P have done to avoid this situation?

2. What are your thoughts about this situation? For the patient? For Nurse P? For the "fairness" of the situation?

3. What are your feelings about this situation?

4. What are Nurse P's chances of becoming licensed again? In her state? In another state? What would the situation be if this were your state?

CASE STUDY 2   ■ ■ ■

You have been working as a nurse in the ob-gyn department of a major clinic in your town. Ms. PG has been scheduled for a visit with the doctor. From her chart, you learn her home pregnancy test was positive—twice! She is unmarried and wants to abort this fetus. She has a history of petty larceny and drunk, disorderly conduct. After the examination, you search for the chart to complete your documentation only to be told the doctor has taken the chart, and others, home with him. He does this quite often, you learn.

1. What is your agency policy regarding location of the patient's medical record? Who has access to it, whether by paper or electronically?

2. What law(s) may regulate the decision to allow patient records in a personal vehicle, residence, or anywhere off premises?

3. What is your ethical responsibility in this case?

REFERENCES

Aiken, T.D. with Catalano, J.T. (1994). *Legal, Ethical, and Political Issues in Nursing.* FA Davis, Philadelphia.

American Nurses Association (2001). *American Nurses Association Code of Ethics for Nurses with Interpretive Statements.* American Nurses Publishing, Washington, D.C.

Fossett, B. and Nadler-Moodie, M. (2004). *Psychiatric Principles and Applications for*

General Patient Care, 4th ed. Western Schools, Brockton, MA.

Merriam-Webster Online (2004). Merriam Webster, Incorporated. www.m-w.com

National Federation of Licensed Practical Nurses. *Nursing Practice and Standards.* National Federation of Licensed Practical Nurses, Raleigh, NC.

Neeb, K. (1994, October). The culture of nurses. *Nursingworld Journal, 20,* 1.

CRITICAL THINKING EXERCISES ■ ■ ■

1. You are an LPN or an LVN on the surgical unit of your county hospital. In shift report, you are told that you will be getting a new postoperative patient within the hour. When the patient arrives, a police officer is in attendance. The officer tells you that this person is a suspect in a homicide. The officer instructs you to report anything the patient says to you. When you begin your postoperative vital signs, the patient says, "Nurse, I shot the guy and he deserved it. I'll do it again if I have to. I can tell you, because you can't tell anyone!" How will you handle this situation?

2. You have just started working on the medical unit in your hospital. You have been assigned a female patient called "Ms. X." You are curious about the fact that Ms. X is not using her real name. While reading her chart, you learn she is in an abusive relationship. You see the warning that "Ms. X's husband is not allowed in the unit at any time." When you go to meet her, you are shocked; Ms. X is your next-door neighbor. What do you do? What do you say to her husband? What do you say when your family asks you "What happened?"

3. You are working the 0700 to 1500 shift. Your station uses the "buddy system" for patient care. You and your buddy have had a very busy morning. You are the "new" nurse and are still learning, but your "buddy" has been away from the floor for a very long time. You have performed much care for your buddy's patients. When you go to chart your care, the charts are already signed off by your buddy. What course(s) of action would be best? What might be the outcomes of your actions for yourself? For your patients? For your buddy?

4. You are the nurse who is supervising care on the 2100 to 0700 shift. Another nurse who works this shift routinely has poor-quality charting. Nothing is hidden or omitted from the chart, but it contains many misspelled words and many grammatical errors. You decide to "keep the peace" and say nothing because you get along well with this nurse and the patients all like the individual. Patient X falls out of bed on your shift, and the family sues for negligence. The other nurse is found incompetent by virtue of written documentation that the lawyers cannot decipher. To your dismay, you are also implicated as the supervising nurse on that shift because you did nothing to improve the quality of this nurse's writing skills. What do you feel right now? What might this mean for you? What will your defense be to the court? How will you handle this differently in the future?

Return to Case Study 2 above. It was on a Friday that Ms. PG's chart left the office. The doctor's plan was to enter his notes on the weekend and he needed the lab reports in order to do so and develop his plan of care. Unfortunately, the doctor's car was hit by another vehicle that ran a red light. The doctor is in critical condition and the vehicle was totaled. The records were located, but they are strewn about the car and the immediate area. It is not certain if the entire chart is intact or if some is missing. On her next visit, Ms. PG mentions that she has been getting phone calls from attorneys and pro-life groups offering their assistance. She is unsure how they got her phone number. What would HIPAA law likely dictate in this situation? Should Ms. PG be told that her chart was affected when the doctor's vehicle was hit? What are your clinic policies and procedures for handling this situation? Who should approach the doctor? What is in your medical record that you would not want others to have access to?

Community Resources Worksheet

Directions: Contact a community agency in your community. Explain that you are a student nurse and that you are trying to determine the resources available in your community.

Your name: _____

1. Name of agency:

2. Who are the target groups for this agency?
   a. Gender?
   b. Age?
   c. Specific problem such as chemical abuse, ageism, and so forth?

3. How do people access this agency?

4. What are the fees for services here?

5. What types of insurance does the agency accept?

6. What services does the agency provide?

7. What hours is the agency open?

8. Do people need appointments to come here?

9. Do you keep records? How do you maintain confidentiality?

10. Other questions you may wish to ask.

11. STUDENTS: What is your impression of this agency? Would you feel comfortable coming here or referring a patient here? Why or why not?

TEST QUESTIONS ■ ■ ■

MULTIPLE CHOICE QUESTIONS

1. The code of behavior that combines professional expectations that border on legal issues is called:
   A. Commitment
   B. Ethics
   C. Nurse Practice Act
   D. Patient Bill of Rights

2. The document that defines the scope of nursing practice in each state is called:
   A. Commitment
   B. Ethics
   C. Nurse Practice Act
   D. Patient Bill of Rights

3. The set of rules designed to protect patients and others who are described as "vulnerable" is called:
   A. Doctrine of Privileged Information
   B. Collaborative practice
   C. Nurse Practice Act
   D. Patient Bill of Rights

4. Sandra is an RN who is working with you. Sandra is from the local pool/registry and you are the staff LPN or LVN at the facility. You see Sandra charting her medications and treatments before she administers them. Choose the best therapeutic communication technique to use when approaching Sandra.
   A. "Why are you doing that?"
   B. "I am concerned about the legality and safety of charting before giving medications, Sandra."
   C. "You know it is wrong to chart before giving the medications."
   D. "You really shouldn't do that, Sandra."

5. A few hours later, Sandra gets sick and goes home. You know that she charted before giving her medications, and you saw her passing some medications. You are not sure who got their medications and who did not. Mrs. G, a patient who is alert and oriented and a reliable historian for herself, sees you and says, "That new nurse forgot my medication this morning. It's my heart medication and I need it. Would you get it for me?" You see the medication has been charted already. Your next action would be:
   A. Refuse the patient, telling her, "You're mistaken, Mrs. G. That medication is signed for, so you must have gotten it."
   B. Give Mrs. G her heart medication and assume she is right.
   C. Call the physician.
   D. Inform your supervisor of the entire situation.

6. The Health Insurance Portability and Accountability Act:
   A. Requires patients to be treated in designated regional treatment centers.
   B. Approves of patient records being transported in personal vehicles by medical staff.
   C. Allows patients to have some say in what medical information can be divulged and to whom.
   D. Prohibits all transmission of medical records electronically.

7. Mr. Ouch has just had bilateral total knee replacement. He is in your transitional care unit. He repeatedly calls out in pain, disturbing the other residents, yet he refuses to take the prescribed pain medication, stating "You're all just trying to knock me out." You:
   A. Shut his door, leaving him alone with some privacy until he settles.
   B. Offer another pain relief technique, realizing he has the right to refuse medication.
   C. Have additional staff come to the room to assist while you administer a prescribed injection.
   D. Inform him his behavior is not appropriate and is disruptive to others and that he needs to stop calling out.

MATCHING QUESTIONS
Directions
Match the ethical or legal concept on the left with its definition or application on the right. There is one "best" answer for each concept. There is one answer that matches none of the concepts.

ETHICAL OR LEGAL CONCEPT

1. _____Involuntary Commitment
2. _____Good Samaritan Act
3. _____Patient Advocacy
4. _____Ethics
5. _____HIPAA
6. _____JCAHO
7. _____Nurse Practice Act
8. _____Patient's Bill of Rights

DEFINITION OR APPLICATION

A. Result of work by American Civil Liberties Union
B. Provides immunity for speaking out for patients' needs
C. Dictates the acceptable scope of nursing practice
D. Leading national accrediting body of healthcare organizations
E. Legal medical "hold," averages 72 hours
F. Characterized by or conforming to the technical or ethical standards of a profession
G. Addresses the security and privacy involved with medical records and how information is identified and passed between care providers
H. Speak out for patients' needs
I. Combination of professional expectations that borders on legal issues

4

Developmental Psychology Throughout the Life Span

Learning Objectives ■ ■ ■

1. Identify major theories of personality development from newborn through adult development.
2. Identify developmental tasks from prenatal development through death, according to the major theorists.
3. Identify possible outcomes of ineffective development, according to the major theorists.
4. Identify the five stages of grief/death according to Kübler-Ross.

Key Terms ■ ■ ■

- Accommodation
- Assimilation
- Autonomy
- Behavioral
- Cognitive
- Ego
- Elisabeth Kübler-Ross
- Erik Erikson
- Id
- Jean Piaget
- Lawrence Kohlberg
- Lunar month
- Maslow's Hierarchy of Needs
- Menarche
- Psychoanalytic/Psychosexual
- Puberty
- Sigmund Freud
- Superego
- Unconscious

The study of developmental psychology encompasses the study of human growth and development, which is a specialty subdivision of psychology. This text covers only the very basics of human development. A sample of the main theorists in the field of child development is presented, along with others whose theories are applied more in the areas of adult personality development. For the separate developmental age groups, a chart is shown delineating the general physical and behavioral traits that are commonly seen in these age groups. The characteristics may cover beliefs from several of the individual theorists you will study.

Remember, these are only theories. Many scientific studies have been performed in the specific disciplines; however, it has yet to be proved that any one is true for *everyone* in *every* instance. Each person is unique. Individuals are subjected to different factors such as genetics and environment, which may affect development. Each person develops at his or her own pace. While reading and learning about these theories, compare them with your personal experiences and observations, as well as with the patient assessments you will be performing. Some theorists may have more validity to you than others.

■ DEVELOPMENTAL THEORISTS: NEWBORN TO ADOLESCENCE

SIGMUND FREUD (1856–1939)

The theories of **Sigmund Freud** (Fig. 4-1) are considered controversial in today's world. Sigmund Freud was an Austrian neu-

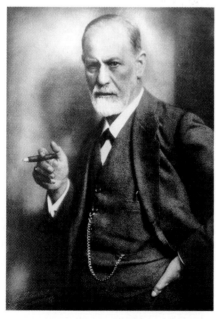

FIGURE 4-1. Sigmund Freud

rologist. He believed, after observing behaviors of children, that the personality was fully developed by age 12. He said that the personality must develop in a certain way and at strictly defined ages and that failure to progress in this manner would certainly lead to dysfunction. Bear in mind that the life span of young Western Europeans during these years was much shorter than it is today, so that 12 years of age seemed much older than it does by today's standards.

One of Freud's main tenets, or beliefs, is that behaviors resulting from ineffective personality development are **unconscious**. He believed that ineffective personality development was in some way related to the relationship of the child to the parent and that it was related to what he called **psychosexual** development.

Freud's theories have validity for some people today, but others denounce them as ridiculous. At no time will you be expected to "convert" to any of the theories discussed in this text; it is, however, necessary to have a working knowledge of the main theories of personality development. Freud is of particular interest because, in addition to his highly debated ideas, he was the first to also offer a reasonably organized method of treatment. Because he was the first publicized theorist, all other theories have evolved as a result of his. Whether you respect his ideas or not, Sigmund Freud's beliefs surface in almost every topic covered in this text. All other theorists compare their theories with Freud's, either in agreement or in opposition.

Table 4-1 shows Freud's psychosexual or **psychoanalytic** stages of development. Included in the table are some of the expected behaviors Freud thought one might witness as the child passes through these ages. The last column lists some behaviors that have been suggested as outcomes of failure to progress through his idea of proper personality development. Discussion of Freud and his theories continues later in this chapter.

TABLE 4-1	*Freud's Stages of Development (Psychoanalytic or Psychosexual Stages)*		
STAGE OF DEVELOPMENT	**APPROXIMATE AGES**	**TASKS/ CHARACTERISTICS**	**EXAMPLES OF UNSUCCESSFUL TASK COMPLETION**
ORAL	Birth–18 months	Use mouth and tongue to deal with anxiety (e.g., sucking, feeding)	Smoking, alcoholism, obesity, nail biting, drug addiction, difficulty trusting
ANAL	18 months–3 years	Muscle control in bladder, rectum, anus provides sensual pleasure and parent pleasing; toilet training can be a crisis	Constipation, perfectionism, obsessive-compulsive disorder
PHALLIC	3–6 years	■ Learn sexual identity and awareness of genital area as source of pleasure; conflict ends as child represses urge and identifies with same-sex parent ■ Electra Complex: "Penis envy"—Daughter wants father for herself; discovers boys are different from her ■ Oedipus Complex: Son wants mother to himself; father is a rival	Homosexuality, transsexuality, sexual identity problems in general, difficulty accepting authority
LATENCY	6–12 years	Quiet stage in sexual development; learns to socialize	Inability to conceptualize; lack of motivation in school or job
GENITAL	12 years–adulthood	Sexual maturity and satisfactory relationships with the opposite sex	Frigidity, impotence, premature ejaculation, serial marriages, unsatisfactory relationships

ERIK ERIKSON (1902–1994)

Erik Erikson (Fig. 4-2) was a psychoanalyst who was a follower of Freud. Erikson took Freud's main concepts and expanded them to include nonphysical criteria. Erikson understood that people are individuals and that no matter how young the person, everyone is different. Erikson's observations indicated a variable that was different from the psychosexual and age-specific theory offered by Freud. That variable is what we now call an emotional component. Table 4-2 shows Erikson's eight stages of development. Frequently, his stages are identified by the words highlighted in the column headed Developmental Tasks. Your instructor may choose to have you learn them by stage or by the developmental task, or both. Note that the developmental tasks are always

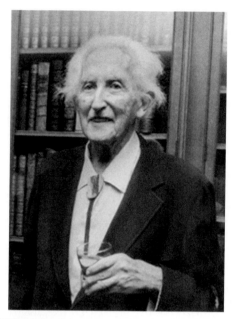

FIGURE 4-2. Erik Erikson (Courtesy of Harvard Gazette, Cambridge, MA.)

listed as contradictions of each other. This is one way that Erikson indicated his ideas about emotional fluctuation in people.

JEAN PIAGET (1896–1980)

Jean Piaget (Fig. 4-3) was a Swiss psychologist with a completely different outlook on development from his colleagues Freud and Erikson. Piaget's theory is called cognitive development. *Cognitive* means the ability to reason, make judgments, and learn. Piaget believed that development was not as much a part of chronologic age as of experiential age. We as nurses are obviously interested in humans; Piaget was so sure of his ideas that he said they were applicable to any living organism; the catch is to make the observations and comparisons about the cognitive process according to the expected ability for that organism. Piaget believed that intelligence consists of coping with the environment (Dennis & Hassol, 1983). He believed that a person must complete each stage of development before he or she can progress to the next stage. Table 4-3 shows the four stages of Piaget's theory of development.

LAWRENCE KOHLBERG (1927–1987)

The last of the theorists we will discuss for this age of development is **Lawrence Kohlberg** (Fig. 4-4). Kohlberg was a believer in Piaget's theories, but he perceived that very young people have the ability to understand and judge right and wrong. Kohlberg's theory is therefore called the development of moral judgment. *Caution:* Morality, the ideas that people consider to be "right" and "wrong," is highly cultural. Nurses are usually guided away from putting a moral value on their patients and their patients' beliefs.

Kohlberg was for many years a professor at Harvard University. He developed and published his theory of moral development in 1958 as his doctoral thesis. It was based on some of the ideas of Jean Piaget. His true interest was in the mechanisms people use to justify their decisions. Although he was interested in the morality of his subjects, he was especially interested in how they supported their decisions. He studied only male subjects ranging in age from 10 to 16 years. Kohlberg's theory is expressed in three levels. Each level has two sections. Table 4-4 shows these stages.

Kohlberg believed that these stages build on the learning achieved from the stage before it. Therefore, the stages must be experienced in the exact order, and one is not to backtrack, or revert to a previous stage. Part of his belief was that moral development can be promoted via formal education. In fact, there is a mild resurgence of Kohlberg's theory emerging in some classroom environments today. Kohlberg's theory has been criticized on the grounds that it is sexist and culturally biased. It indicates that some cultures and peoples never progress to the highest level and suggests that behaviors that are acceptable in some cultures are "wrong." Kohlberg's theory also does not consider the emotional responses that daily problems and stressors can produce. Psychologist Carol Gilligan published a book in 1982 indicating that boys and girls and men and

TABLE 4-2	Erikson's Eight Stages of Development			
STAGE	APPROXIMATE AGES	DEVELOPMENTAL TASKS	EXAMPLES	EXAMPLES OF UNSUCCESSFUL TASK COMPLETION
SENSORY	Birth–18 months	Trust vs. mistrust	Nurturing people build trust in the newborn.	Suspiciousness, trouble with personal relationships
MUSCULAR	1–3 years	Autonomy vs. shame and doubt	"No!"—Toddler learns environment can be manipulated.	Low self-esteem, dependency (on substances or people)
LOCOMOTOR	3–6 years	Initiative vs. guilt	Child learns assertiveness can manipulate environment—disapproval leads to guilt in the toddler.	Passive personality, strong feelings of guilt
LATENCY	6–12 years	Industry vs. inferiority	Creativity or shyness develops.	Unmotivated, unreliable
ADOLESCENCE	12–20 years	Identity vs. role confusion	Individual integrates life experiences or becomes confused.	Rebellion, substance abuse, difficulty keeping personal relationships; may regress to child-play behaviors
YOUNG ADULT	18–25 years	Intimacy vs. isolation	Main concern is developing intimate relationship with another.	Emotional immaturity; may deny need for personal relationships
ADULTHOOD	21–45 years	Generativity vs. stagnation	Focus is on establishing family and guiding the next generation.	Inability to show concern for anyone but self
MATURITY	45 years–death	Integrity vs. despair	Individual accepts own life as fulfilling; if not, he or she becomes fearful of death.	Has difficulty dealing with issues of aging and death; may have feelings of hopelessness

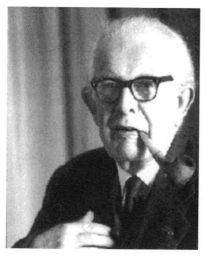

FIGURE 4-3. Jean Piaget (Courtesy of allpsych.com)

women are all able to feel compassion and morality but that the genders process their morality from different perspectives, a variable that was not considered in Kohlberg's study.

■ DEVELOPMENTAL THEORISTS: ADOLESCENCE TO ADULTHOOD

SIGMUND FREUD (1856–1939)

In addition to his five psychosexual stages of development, Sigmund Freud had a model for the components of personality. He said

TABLE 4-3	*Developmental Theory of Jean Piaget*	
STAGE	**APPROXIMATE AGE**	**EXPECTED ABILITY**
SENSORIMOTOR	Birth–2 years	■ Uses senses to learn about self ■ Schemata develop, which are plans or ways of learning to assimilate and accommodate. They include the behaviors of looking, hearing, and sucking.
PREOPERATIONAL	2–7 or 8 years	2–4 years: ■ Thinks in mental images ■ Symbolic play ■ Develops own languages 4–7 or 8 years: ■ Egocentrism—sees only own point of view but *cannot* do this until age 7 or 8. With age, this ability develops.
CONCRETE OPERATIONAL	8–12 years	■ Ability for logical thought increases. ■ Moral judgment begins to develop. ■ Numbers and spatial ability become more logical.
FORMAL OPERATIONS	12 years–adult	■ Develops adult logic. ■ Able to reason things out. ■ Able to form conclusions. ■ Able to plan for future. ■ Able to think in concepts or abstracts.

that the personality consists of three parts: the **id**, the **ego**, and the **superego**. Remember as you study this information that Freud believed that *all* the components of our behavior are set in the unconscious. The behaviors may appear to be very purposeful and deliberate, but in Freud's theories, they are supposedly responses to situations of which we are not aware.

Id is the part of our personality that is concerned with the gratification of self. You may have heard the terms "pleasure principle" or "if it feels good, do it!" These are attitudes that arose from people who believe that we have underdeveloped ids, and these individuals promote the idea that people need to allow the id to take care of "me, myself, and I."

Ego, in Freud's world, had a different connotation from the modern-day common use of the word. Ego, as Freud taught, is the

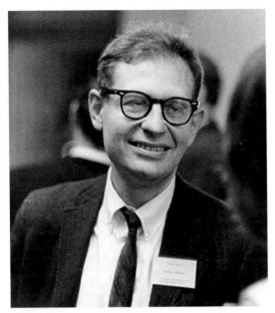

FIGURE 4-4. Lawrence Kohlberg (Courtesy of Harvard Graduate School of Education, Cambridge, MA.)

TABLE 4-4 ■ *Lawrence Kohlberg's Theory of Development of Moral Reasoning*			
STAGE	**"RIGHT" BEHAVIORS**	**WHY WE SHOULD DO "RIGHT"**	**WHAT IF WE DO NOT DO "RIGHT"**
LEVEL I: PRECONVENTIONAL			
1. Punishment and obedience orientation	*Do not do it* if it will result in punishment.	To avoid punishment and to see what one can "get away with"	I will be punished and I do not like that.
2. Concerned with having own needs met	It is "right" if I (or if *we*) get something I want out of it.	To help me get my needs and wants fulfilled	I will lose recognition for the importance of "others."
LEVEL II: CONVENTIONAL			
3. "Good boy, good girl" orientation	"Good" means living up to what is expected of us.	Self and others think we are "good."	Avoiding "blame" is more ethical than getting a "reward."
4. "Law and order"	"Right" means obeying the laws and rules.	It maintains social structure.	"Law" will have less importance than the will of "society."

(continued)

TABLE 4-4 ■	*Lawrence Kohlberg's Theory of Development of Moral Reasoning (Continued)*		
STAGE	**"RIGHT" BEHAVIORS**	**WHY WE SHOULD DO "RIGHT"**	**WHAT IF WE DO NOT DO "RIGHT"**
LEVEL III: POSTCONVENTIONAL ("PRINCIPLED LEVEL")			
5. Social contract	"Right" or "good" is behaving according to a general consensus.	We blend together for the greatest good and the welfare of all.	May become aware that "moral" and "legal" may not be the same.
6. Universal "good"	Universal rules of justice and equality for all prevail. This is the "ideal" according to Kohlberg.	Live within the universal "good" according to own conscience.	Few people reach this, according to Kohlberg. Therefore, in his manual, the latest revisions do not measure this stage.

balance to id. Ego keeps id under control (in a mentally healthy individual) by responding in an unconscious form of "now, wait a minute" attitude. Think for a minute about that last exam you took. Pretend that it was in a subject you felt fairly confident about, so you chose to study less than you would for other exams. You went partying with friends for the weekend instead. Think about this as id behavior. As you enter the testing area, that little gnawing feeling starts to enter your consciousness. You sense "butterflies" in the pit of your stomach. You see the first question on the exam, and you go temporarily blank. That is the ego response. It's telling you there are two sides to every situation. In this scenario, the ego is telling the id, "Hmm. Maybe you aren't quite as confident as you thought you were!" To those of you who have never experienced this sensation: Congratulations! Keep it up!

The third part of the personality theory of Sigmund Freud is the superego. The superego could be called the "killjoy" of the personality. It is the conscience. It is the part of the personality that allows us to determine what is right, wrong, good, and bad. The values exhibited by the superego are not to be confused with the same terms used by Lawrence Kohlberg; according to Freud, having these values is not a matter of choice or of learning.

A person who is well-adjusted, or mentally healthy, has all three components of the personality, according to Freud. Freud would expect anyone in whom any of the components is absent or out of balance to display maladaptive behaviors. Defense mechanisms have been associated strongly with Freud's theories. Discussion of these defense mechanisms and maladaptive behaviors is found in later chapters of this book.

KAREN HORNEY (1885–1952)

Karen Horney (Fig. 4-5) was a psychoanalyst and one of very few early female theorists. Her ideas were very close to those of Freud; however, she believed that the causes of abnormal behaviors or mental illness were related to ineffective mother-child bonding.

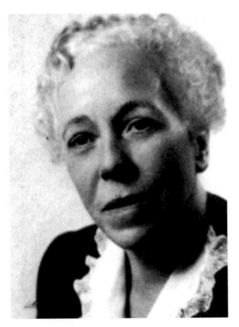

FIGURE 4-5. Karen Horney

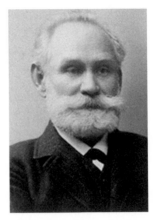

FIGURE 4-6. Ivan Pavlov

IVAN PAVLOV (1849–1936) AND B. F. SKINNER (1904–1990)

These men worked on "conditioning" or manipulating behaviors. They are called behavioral theorists because they believed that working with different behaviors and different stimuli could obtain different responses. Behavior modification is a direct result of their work.

Pavlov (Fig. 4-6) worked on involuntary responses. His well-known study was carried out with dogs, steaks, and a bell. When the dogs saw a choice piece of meat, they salivated in preparation for eating it. Pavlov incorporated the ringing of a bell when the meat was presented so that, in time, the researcher rang the bell and the dogs' association of meat with the sound of the bell stimulated the salivation response. This was a great breakthrough in the study of causes of behavior and ways in which behavior can be manipulated.

B. F. Skinner (Fig. 4-7) worked on operant conditioning, which is based on voluntary responses. Operant conditioning, very simply stated, means taking a behavior and operating on it by changing the variables or conditions surrounding the behavior. Skinner is known for the "Skinner boxes" in which he kept the animals he studied. These so-called boxes were cages big enough for the animal to move around in and contained an apparatus for the animal to operate voluntarily in response to different stimuli. There are three main parts to Skinner's the-

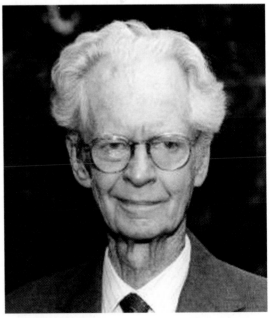

FIGURE 4-7. B. F. Skinner (Courtesy of College of Education, Northern Illinois University, DeKalb, IL.)

TABLE 4-5	*Operant Conditioning: B. F. Skinner*
SKINNER'S THEORY	**EXPLANATION**
RESPONSE	Any movement or observable behavior that is to be studied. The response is measured for frequency, duration, and intensity (e.g., chicken rings bell in cage).
STIMULUS	The event that immediately precedes or follows the operant behavior. The object is to find the stimulus that gets the chicken to ring the bell (e.g., food, noise, boredom).
REINFORCER	A variable that will cause the operant behavior to repeat predictably or increase in frequency. Sometimes this is called a "reward." The reinforcer has to be meaningful to the person whose behavior is being "operated" on (e.g., chicken pecks bell and food drops into tray; when chicken wants food, it knows that pecking the bell will produce food).

ory: response, stimulus, and reinforcer. Table 4-5 defines these parts.

Skinner's theory led to the development of what we call behavior modification. It is possible to "modify" or change any behavior by using appropriate stimuli and reinforcers to obtain the desired behavior.

Both positive and negative behaviors can be operated on. It is generally believed today that positive reinforcing is the most effective way of changing a behavior. Pointing out the positive qualities in a person or client or focusing on the abilities (positive) rather than the disabilities (negative) seems to yield the best results. For instance, let's pretend that the behavior we wish to operate on is getting a particular coworker to arrive to work on time. The supervisor has two possible paths to follow: One is positive reinforcing; the other, negative reinforcing.

Negative: "Nurse M, you are routinely late for work. This is very difficult on your patients and on the rest of the staff. One more instance of being late, and you will be fired."

OR

Positive: "Nurse M, you are still occasionally late for work. I have noticed, however, that you have been late only three times this month. If you continue to improve your timeliness, I will be able to give you a raise at your next review."

The positive reinforcement method seems to give some dignity and positive self-regard to the employee. It allows the employee to understand the consequences and to make choices about being late. It will then be up to the supervisor to follow through with whichever consequences are earned by Nurse M.

ABRAHAM MASLOW (1908–1970)

Abraham Maslow (Fig. 4-8) is one of a group of theorists described as person-centered, client-centered, or humanist. Person-centered theories involve observing and treating the whole person. Nursing is highly centered in the person-centered and behaviorist theories. One of the main ideals embraced by the nursing profession is **Maslow's Hierarchy of Needs**. This hierarchy or orderly progression of development takes in the physical components of personality development as well as the emotional components. Self-esteem is a tenet of humanistic psychology.

Maslow's Hierarchy of Needs has five levels. Maslow said that one must pass through

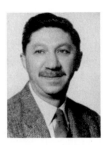

FIGURE 4-8. Abraham Maslow (Courtesy of University of Wisconsin, Madison, WI.)

these stages in order and that it is not possible for a person to move up to the next level until the previous level has been mastered. Many times this hierarchy is depicted as a large triangle or stair steps to help visualize the progression from the "basic" needs to the "higher" needs of people (Fig. 4-9). The steps are as follows:

1. Physiological needs
2. Safety and security
3. Love and belonging
4. Esteem
5. Self-actualization

Physiological Needs

These are elements people need to survive: food, water, oxygen, clothing, absence of extremes in temperature, ability for body excretions, and sexual activity. These are considered necessary for life to continue. Without food, clothing, and a shelter that is clean and of a comfortable temperature, an individual could die; without sexual activity, the species could die.

Safety and Security

It is important that people feel safe and free of fear. When individuals feel comfortable that their physical needs are being met, they begin to feel a sense of safety that they can maintain their survival. Bear in mind that having these basic needs met does not necessarily mean living in wealth or with steady employment. People who are on the street

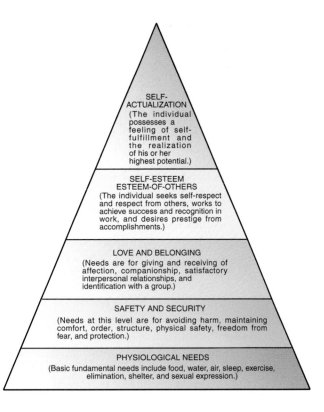

FIGURE 4-9. Maslow's Hierarchy of Needs. (From Townsend, M.C., *Essentials of Psychiatric Mental Health Nursing*, 3rd ed., F.A. Davis Company, Philadelphia, 2005, p. 4. Reprinted with permission.)

for whatever reason learn to survive and are proud of their ability to survive in conditions that most people would consider deplorable, yet for some people, street life is a choice and they meet the criteria of Maslow's hierarchy.

Love and Belonging

We have now progressed to the middle of Maslow's Hierarchy of Needs. It is a popular belief within psychology that loneliness is a major cause of depression. Quotes such as "Man does not live by bread alone" and "No man is an island" have implied this for many years; it is now being borne out more scientifically. People need to feel loved, appreciated, and part of a group. The focus of that sense of love and belonging may change over the life span. When we are babies and young children, the love needs to come from our parents or other caregivers; in adolescence and adulthood, the focus may change to a significant life partner or a peer group, or both. Regardless of the developmental stage of life, we need to feel loved.

Esteem

The "higher" needs begin with the idea that "If I am loved by someone, there must be something special and good about me." Finding that "something" and learning to accept, appreciate, and acknowledge those positive traits in ourselves is the goal of the fourth of Maslow's hierarchy: esteem or self-esteem.

Self-esteem is the ability to be confident that you are a person with good qualities and that others know and appreciate these qualities. This sounds easier to achieve than it often is. When someone compliments you on a new piece of clothing or haircut or a job well done, what is your usual response? "Oh, this old thing? Do you really think so? I think it's way too short now" or "It was nothing, really" are responses we often give. In addition to the effect it has on effective communication, responding in this manner does not show positive self-esteem. One of the most difficult things to do in our culture is

to learn to say "Thank you!" when given a compliment. "Thank you" not only acknowledges the other person's positive regard for a quality we possess, but it reinforces to our "self" that "Yes, I did do that well and I do deserve the recognition." Unfortunately, we sometimes interpret this simple response as "false pride" and consider it to be in poor taste to acknowledge ourselves in a positive manner. Women have been socialized this way for years and, although there has been some improvement over the past 20 years, there is much work yet to be done in this area.

Self-Actualization

The fifth and final rung on Maslow's hierarchy ladder is called self-actualization. This means achievement, taking risks, and working to our individual potential. The self-actualized person is a problem solver. Situations can be creatively dealt with when a person is confident enough to stretch the limits of ability. Some of you may be training in a new profession. It doesn't matter what caused you to enter nursing; the fact is you are here. You have taken a risk and stretched your boundaries. This is a form of self-actualization, even though it may not feel comfortable yet.

Gender differences have been the cause of many a discussion since the beginning of time. Men and women have always said that they just don't understand each other. Proof of that exists now. We can truthfully, confidently, and nonjudgmentally say that "Yes, there are differences in the way men and women think, communicate, and process life." Carol Gilligan, a psychologist, has studied this phenomenon (Gilligan, 1982). She has hypothesized that one of these fundamental differences appears to affect Maslow's hierarchy; women tend to value relationships as a basic need, and men tend to value achievement as a basic need. This is not an issue of right or wrong; no value statement is being made. It is important, however, when you are observing and collecting data on your patients, to understand

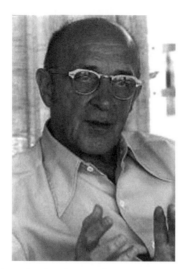

FIGURE 4-10. Carl Rogers (Courtesy of Bonnie Drumwright, PhD, Gold River, CA.)

that differences in their attitudes and responses to treatment may be related to gender issues.

CARL ROGERS (1902–1987)

Carl Rogers (Fig. 4-10) was also a person-centered or humanistic psychologist. Although he believed that all people need to be

"prized and loved," he described his theory a little differently than Maslow's. The phrase associated with Carl Rogers is "unconditional positive regard." Rogers believed that we may all have different ideas about life and the world we live in. He did not think it was appropriate to put a value on another person's perception of the world, so he said that every person deserved to be treated with respect and "unconditional positive regard" just by virtue of being a human being.

He also differed from Maslow in the area of self-actualization. Rogers believed that self-actualization was the basic motivator for people and that all people had a built-in desire to achieve their capabilities.

Nursing practice is based very strongly in Rogers' theory. His eight steps to being a helping person are listed in Table 4-6.

CARL JUNG (1875–1961)

Although he broke from some of Freud's ideas, **Carl Jung** (Fig. 4-11), a Swiss psychologist, also believed in the effects of the unconscious mind. He included in his defi-

TABLE 4-6	*Rogers' Eight Steps*
EMPATHY	"Walk in another's shoes."
RESPECT	Care for client as a *person*, not just a patient.
GENUINENESS	Helper is a sincere/authentic role model.
CONCRETENESS	Identify patient's feelings by careful listening and stereotyping.
CONFRONTATION	Discuss discrepancies in behavior.
SELF-DISCLOSURE	Share self, as is appropriate to situation.
IMMEDIACY OF RELATIONSHIPS	Helper selectively shares own feelings.
SELF-EXPLORATION	The more we explore ourselves, the greater/better the coping/adapting.

Source: Prochaska, J.O. (1984). Systems of Psychotherapy. *Pacific Grove, CA: Brooks-Cole.*

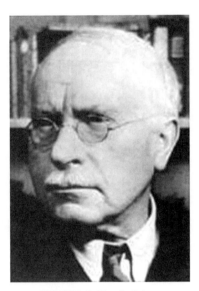

FIGURE 4-11. Carl Jung

nition of "unconscious" both repressed personal experiences and representations of universal human experiences, those experiences all of us have. He used different terminology to describe the various parts of our personality, and he believed that healthy personalities are a balance between the conscious and the unconscious. "Self" to Jung meant the deep, inner part of ourselves. He believed that males and females are different organisms but that each contains part of the other. If you recall the study of the endocrine system in your anatomy and physiology classes, you will remember that men have traces of female hormones and women have traces of male hormones. To Jung, it logically followed that this fact affects the way each of us develops our personality. Therefore, he used the term "anima" to describe the feminine tendencies in men and the term "animus" to describe the male characteristics in women.

"Mask" is a word Jung used to define the part of our personality that we present socially. It hints at the idea that our innermost self may be different from our public self.

■ STAGES OF HUMAN DEVELOPMENT

Nurses are entrusted with caring for people of all ages. Many nursing program mission statements have some reference to the concept that nursing must cover a continuum of experiences throughout the life span. It becomes the nurse's responsibility to have a working knowledge of the main physical and behavioral changes that can be expected within certain age groups. It is also important to have some idea of the complications that might occur if developmental tasks are not completed successfully. This is called the study of developmental psychology. Table 4-7 identifies the life stages, some of the expected major physical development, expected **behavioral** development, and possible outcomes of failure to meet certain developmental tasks. This chart incorporates traits from all the theorists identified in this text. It is not a substitute for knowing the concepts of the individual theorists.

Life is an accumulation of experiences. Some of those are positive, and some are not. Each of us will have to deal with gains and losses as we travel through our lives. Your patients may be in different stages of loss with their illness. Each age group has its own sets of gains and losses. Learning to deal with these ups and downs early in life can make the more significant experiences less difficult to cope with. Overuse of defense mechanisms (see Chapter 6) can be curtailed with effective stress-management techniques, which can be learned very early in life. The process of death and dying is a major loss that each of us will face at some point during our lives. What can be done to help this process?

DEATH AND DYING

Losing a loved one at any age or for any reason is a difficult experience. Separation, loss, and grief are human conditions that are unavoidable. In today's world, we have

TABLE 4-7   *Overall View of Human Development (represents traits from all theorists mentioned earlier)*

LIFE STAGE	AGE RANGE (AGES VARY SOMEWHAT ACCORDING TO THEORIST)	EXPECTED PHYSICAL DEVELOPMENT	EXPECTED BEHAVIORAL DEVELOPMENT	POTENTIAL OUTCOME OF INEFFECTIVE DEVELOPMENT
PRENATAL	Conception through 10th **lunar month** (lunar month = 28 days)	■ Cells differentiate (specialize) by the end of the first trimester ■ Intrauterine conditions of mother may affect prenatal development	■ Fetus kicks and may respond to stimuli such as familiar voices, music, and so on	■ Threats to mother's health of primary concern (e.g., smoking, drugs, malnutrition); mother's prenatal habits seem to have a strong influence on the developing baby ■ Alcohol consumption during pregnancy of special concern; can lead to a condition called fetal alcohol syndrome (FAS), which can cause physical anomalies as well as cognitive, emotional, and behavioral complications in child
NEWBORN	1st month of life	■ May have flattened nose, unevenly shaped head, bruises from the passage through the birth canal; these physical characteristics will change over the first month of life	■ Bonding (e.g., touching, talking) of parents and baby is said to be crucial to development of trust ■ Sucking reflex ■ Can see 7–10 inches ■ Likes bright colors ■ Likes to be talked to ■ Prefers female voices ■ Likes touch, cuddling, rocking, and the like ■ Will not be "spoiled" by this attention ■ Can hold head up for a few seconds ■ Follows light with eyes	■ Angry crying ■ Mistrust ■ Withdrawal ■ Stress, which slows further development

(continued)

TABLE 4-7	Overall View of Human Development (represents traits from all theorists mentioned earlier) (Continued)			
LIFE STAGE	AGE RANGE (AGES VARY SOMEWHAT ACCORDING TO THEORIST)	EXPECTED PHYSICAL DEVELOPMENT	EXPECTED BEHAVIORAL DEVELOPMENT	POTENTIAL OUTCOME OF INEFFECTIVE DEVELOPMENT
INFANT	2nd month–1½ years of life	Infants are all very much alike (physically and developmentally) until the age of 10 months	2–4 months: ■ Begins to laugh ■ Follows people's movements with eyes 5–7 months: ■ Holds head erect ■ Turns head toward voices ■ Babbles/coos ■ Drinks from a cup 8–10 months: ■ Sits up alone ■ Says "mama," "dada"; understands "no" and "bye-bye"	■ Poor parent-child relationship can lead to mistrust and poor self-concept ■ Failure-to-thrive syndrome ■ Separation anxiety
TODDLER	1½–3 years	■ Long trunk ■ Short legs ■ Brain about ¾ of full size in order to be able to support future growth and development ■ Walking	■ Toilet training ■ Learning sex roles by copying behaviors of same-sex parent ■ Self-centered ■ Doesn't share ■ Wants things now ■ Both boys and girls learning **autonomy** (independence) by using the word "no" ■ **Assimilation,** which is taking in and processing of information via the senses ■ **Accommodation,** which is the ability to adjust to new information or situations	■ Anger ■ Regression ■ Reversion to infant-age behaviors

(continued)

PRESCHOOL (EARLY CHILDHOOD)	3–6 years	■ Medical and dental examinations important ■ Nutrition can be challenging; children are starting to pick and choose their favorite foods; time to start teaching good nutrition ■ Lead poisoning still a threat: it tastes sweet and may still be found in some older plumbing or in old paint layers in housing units	■ Cognitive development is a primary activity; many questions; "Why" a frequently used word ■ Socializes ■ Play important for self-expression and anxiety relief ■ Reading is the best parent-child activity ■ Aggressive behavior (rough-housing) ■ Active imagination possibly leading to nightmares ■ Mixed feelings about going to school	■ Enuresis—the involuntary bed-wetting in preschool and school-age children who have been toilet trained; often due to poor personal relationships ■ Encopresis—involuntary bowel movements in the same population as enuresis
SCHOOL AGE	6–12 years	■ Body thinning out and growth slowing temporarily ■ Losing baby teeth and gaining permanent teeth ■ By age 6, brain almost full size; neurologic system develops from head down ■ By age 6 or 7, vision at its peak ■ Vision and hearing screening usually begun by the time the child enters school ■ Agility increases ■ Scoliosis (lateral curvature of the spine) screening possibly encouraged	■ Learning to share ■ Forming friendships with same-sex friends ■ Peer group activities (secret clubs, and so on) ■ Beginning to show acceptance of moral issues by questions and discussions ■ Reversibility: the ability to put things in an order or sequence or to group things according to common traits	■ Shyness and/or fear of school if trust and autonomy have not developed fully; may be a result of not being included in peer groups; has been defined as a "silent prison" ■ Gangs—can be the result of negative types of peer groups ■ Stuttering—repetitive or prolonged sounds or speech flow that is interrupted; seems to happen four times more often in boys; may be stress-related ■ Accidents—the leading cause of death in children; teaching safety to families and children is important ■ Child abuse/neglect noted more frequently; all health-care personnel have the duty to report abuse or suspected abuse (discussed in more detail in Chapters 5 and 21)

(continued)

TABLE 4-7	Overall View of Human Development (represents traits from all theorists mentioned earlier) (Continued)		
LIFE STAGE	**AGE RANGE (AGES VARY SOMEWHAT ACCORDING TO THEORIST)**	**EXPECTED PHYSICAL DEVELOPMENT**	**EXPECTED BEHAVIORAL DEVELOPMENT**	**POTENTIAL OUTCOME OF INEFFECTIVE DEVELOPMENT**
SCHOOL AGE *(cont'd)*	6–12 years	■ Late childhood (10–11 years old)—beginning of sexual development, especially in girls, who now are maturing about 2 years ahead of boys ■ Colds frequent, owing to social habits		
ADOLESCENT	12–18 years	■ Growth spurt (musculoskeletal system) ■ Endocrine system maturing (hormones) ■ Secondary sex characteristics developing (facial and underarm hair, males' shoulders broaden, females' hips broaden and breasts develop, and so on) ■ **Puberty**—individual is capable of reproducing ■ **Menarche**—female's first menstrual period, which happens around age 11–15 (it is important to know that nutrition and exercise affect this)	■ Learning independence ■ Learning self-sufficiency ■ Learning new social roles ■ Mood swings ■ Boredom ■ Introspection ■ Preoccupation with body image ■ Own "language" ■ Peer group very important—teens need intimacy ■ Talking on phone for hours ■ Possible experimentation with alcohol, drugs, sex ■ Communication between parent and adolescent crucial	■ Anorexia/bulimia frequent dangers for males as well as females; usually from white, middle-class families ■ Males who mature later seem to have the hardest time adjusting ■ Suicide a major concern for this age group, usually because of feeling unimportant and not being taken seriously by adults

(continued)

Stage	Age	Physical	Psychosocial
YOUNG ADULT	18–35 years	■ Body usually in optimal physical condition	■ Intimacy the main task to accomplish ■ Schooling and career planning important ■ Marriage and family decisions made
ADULT	30–60 years	■ Gradual decline in hearing and visual acuity ■ Body beginning to shorten somewhat as musculature and bone structure change ■ Lung and cardiac capacity beginning to decrease somewhat	■ Generativity, or passing down values and skills to the next generation (personally and professionally)— a major task of the adult
OLDER ADULT	60 years–death	■ Visual and hearing acuity continue to decline ■ Body becomes susceptible to an increasing number of physical and emotional illnesses	■ Acceptance of limitations on independence and physical ability ■ Acceptance of the idea of death and beginning to prepare for it ■ Acceptance of retirement ■ Increases in stress throughout the life span ■ Fear of death and dying ■ Difficulty with retirement—identity is often associated with career ■ Depression relating to aging, loss of friends, and so on

conflicting phenomena. We have a better quality of life and better health care than ever before. Because of this, the average life expectancy is in the early 70s. On the other hand, we exist in a fast-paced and competitive society, which causes high levels of stress and encourages people to make unhealthy choices in their diets and lifestyles. This results in people dying of myocardial infarctions in their 30s and 40s. Automobile accidents and recreational activities are taking the lives of children at higher numbers than ever before. Acquired immunodeficiency syndrome (AIDS) is taking the lives of many people. It is believed that 50 percent of us will have a family member or close acquaintance die of AIDS. It is easy to understand how the experts can say that death is the final stage of life.

Death is defined differently from state to state. Physical signs such as vital signs, skin color and temperature, presence or absence of activity on electroencephalogram (EEG) and electrocardiogram (ECG), and the ability to be viable, or to live without mechanical assistance, are criteria used by states to define "death." It is your responsibility to know the legal definition of death in the state you will be working in.

The nurse's responsibility in the death process also varies from state to state. For instance, in some states nurses are allowed to pronounce the death of a patient; in other states this must be done only by a physician. Other considerations for the nurse might include the existence of and state's recognition of a "living will" (wishes of the dying person that are placed on a legal document, signed by the person while competent, and witnessed), the family's wishes, and possibly the wishes of a nonfamily significant other (such as a "domestic partner" with whom the dying person has been living but to whom he or she is not legally married).

Psychologist **Dr. Elisabeth Kübler-Ross** (Fig. 4-12), who passed away in August of 2004 at age 78, was a leader in the study of the *process* of death and dying. She made her reputation by learning about the activi-

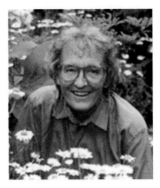

FIGURE 4-12. Elisabeth Kübler-Ross (Courtesy of Ken Ross, Scottsdale, AZ.)

ties of the mind and body at and around the time of death. Her initial studies were based on only 200 subjects, all of whom had cancer, yet her theory has survived and has spanned more than 20 years of providing care to dying patients. Her idea implies that the end result of experiencing the five stages of grief or dying is the ability to die in peace and with dignity. These stages are listed in Table 4-8.

Death, and the activities that accompany it for the dying person and those left behind, is not only physiologic; it is deeply rooted in cultural and spiritual tradition. Just as every person is unique in life, so will the rituals surrounding the activities of death be very personal and individual.

Dr. Kübler-Ross' theory also emphasizes the fact that hearing is the last sense to leave a person at death. People who are in comas or in the end stage of death may not be able to respond to verbal cues or participate in conversation, but it is widely believed that they continue to hear what is going on in their environment. For this reason, nurses must be careful in talking to the patient and the family, even immediately after the patient's death. Again, people from some cultures and religions believe that the "spirit" or "soul" remains in the room for a period of time after death. Regardless of the belief system, it is a sign of respect to the patient and the significant others to include the patient in the conversation and

TABLE 4-8	*Five Stages of Grief/Death and Dying by Dr. Elisabeth Kübler-Ross*	
STAGE	**KEY WORDS**	**EXPECTED BEHAVIORS**
DENIAL	"Not me!"	Refuses to believe that death is coming; states "That Doctor doesn't know what he/she is talking about!"
ANGER	"Why me?"	Expresses envy, resentment, and frustration with younger people and/or those who are not dying
BARGAINING	"If I could have one more chance . . ."	May become very religious or "good" in an effort to gain another chance at life or more time to live
GRIEF/ DEPRESSION	Realizes that "bargaining" is not working and death is approaching	Becomes depressed, weepy; may "give up," quit taking medications, quit eating, and so forth
ACCEPTANCE	"OK . . . but I don't have to like it!"	Enters a state of expectation; may begin to call family members near; needs to complete "unfinished business"; prepares spiritually to die

continue to speak in terms of the reality of the situation.

Children go through the same stages as adults; and as with adults, they may need special help to come to terms with losing a loved one. The help nurses give to younger patients must be age-appropriate. Infants and toddlers may not be able to understand what happened, but they do sense the change. Keep their routine as normal as possible. Provide them with physical closeness and a safe environment.

Children from 2 to 6 years of age may have the sense that death is reversible. How often do they see cartoon characters "die" and then immediately return to animated life? When the reality that Grandma or Grandpa is not coming back to life is understood, it is important that the child understand that he or she did not cause the death of the loved one.

Children ages 6 to 12 are at varying degrees of understanding. It is important to allow and encourage children to talk about their feelings. Recent incidents of violence involving this age group have provided the opportunity for grief counselors to intervene with children who have survived the ordeals.

Teens are bridging the gap from childhood to adulthood and may respond to grief and loss in many ways. Provide structure, routine, and an environment in which they may freely express their thoughts and feelings.

Controversial topics of euthanasia (sometimes called "mercy killing") and "physician-assisted suicide" are being debated in society and tested in the courts. There is a debate in the United States as to whether a person has the right to make decisions regarding his or her own life and death. People hold strong opinions on both sides of this debate. It is one of the ethical issues that will be a part of your professional career and most likely a topic that nurses will need to discuss with their patients.

Key Concepts ▫ ▪ ■

1. There are many theories about personality development in human beings. These are only theories; however, there are strong indications of validity in them all. The licensed practical nurse (LPN) and the licensed vocational nurse (LVN) must have a working knowledge of some of the more commonly accepted theories of human development throughout the life span.

2. Dr. Elisabeth Kübler-Ross has developed a theory of five stages that people go through when they are grieving or dying. These stages also apply to the significant others. Although others have presented theories on this topic, hers remains the most commonly accepted theory in nursing.

3. Each person is an individual and will go through stages of development or grief at his or her own pace. These theories are guidelines to help us understand what our patients may experience as they go through certain stages in their lives.

CASE STUDY ■ ■ ■

Mr. Y, a 24-year-old construction worker, suffered a traumatic brain injury after falling from scaffolding when his safety equipment failed. He was comatose for 8 days. During this time, family and friends kept a constant vigil. His wife was 6 months pregnant and fearful about having to raise the baby alone. Many conversations were held in his room while he was in the coma. When he awakened from the coma, he was able to tell most of what was said. He wondered why "nobody answered me when I talked to you." He especially wanted to reassure his wife that "Nothing would keep me from seeing that baby!"

1. What suggestions could a nurse have made to the family of this patient regarding patients who are comatose?

2. How can a nurse help the patient who has concerns about "memories" he or she acquired while in a coma (i.e., what is real and what is not, what things might have been said in confidence, and so forth)?

REFERENCES

Barger, R.N. (2000). *A Summary of Lawrence Kohlberg's Stages of Moral Development*, University of Notre Dame, Notre Dame, IN.

Barry, P.D. (2002). *Mental Health and Mental Illness*, 7th ed., JB Lippincott, Philadelphia.

Dennis, L.B. and Hassol, J. (1983). *Introduction to Human Development and Health Issues*. WB Saunders, Philadelphia.

Gilligan, C. (1982). *In a Different Voice: Psychological Theory and Women's Development*. Harvard University Press, Cambridge, MA.

Kübler-Ross, E. (1969). *On Death and Dying*. Macmillan, New York.

Lickona, T. (1991). *Educating for Character: How Our Schools Can Teach Respect and Responsibility*. Bantam, New York.

CRITICAL THINKING EXERCISES ■ ■ ■

1. Your patient is in a monogamous homosexual relationship and is in the final stage of life. Death is imminent, but the patient is still alert and oriented. Family and partner are in the room. The patient asks you to ask the physician to "put me to sleep." The patient's partner weeps but supports the request; the family members threaten to sue if the physician does "any such thing." What are your thoughts about euthanasia? What are your feelings about euthanasia? What will you do to help the patient? The family? The partner? What if this were your parent or child who was about to die? What would you think and feel then?

2. Jamie is a 2-year-old. Jamie's parents are becoming frustrated because Jamie is "so naughty." They say that Jamie is always saying "No!" and "Mine!" They say that Jamie is fascinated by playing with the dirty diapers in the diaper pail. They feel responsible for what they say is "disgusting" behavior and wonder what they are doing "wrong." They are quick to point out that "Jamie's older sibling never did these things. Is there something wrong with us? Is there something wrong with Jamie? Please help us!"

List the "normal" behaviors for the 2-year-old age group. From what you know of the normal development for a 2-year-old, list the helping statements for these parents.

TEST QUESTIONS ■ ■ ■

MULTIPLE CHOICE QUESTIONS

1. Your little 4-year-old patient comes into the clinic with her father. She is being checked for a recurring ear infection. As you prepare her to see the physician, she says to you, "I love my Daddy. I'm going to marry him like Mommy someday!" Which one of Freud's stages of development is she most likely demonstrating?
   A. Genital
   B. Oral
   C. Anal
   D. Phallic

2. Patient Y is 20 years old. Y is a perfectionist and very routine-oriented. Freudian theorists would say that Patient Y did not successfully complete which of the following stages of development?
   A. Genital
   B. Oral
   C. Anal
   D. Phallic

3. Patient Y (from question 2) is being treated by a behavioral psychologist. When Patient Y begins to miss meals and activities because of the need to complete routines perfectly, the staff is to intervene. Patient Y failed to come to dinner on your shift. You go to check, and you see Y carefully placing personal items in a special place in the bathroom. Your best response to Y from a behavioral and therapeutic background could be:

   A. "Y, where were you at dinner tonight?"
   B. "Y, you blew it. You didn't come to dinner and you know what that means: no pass for the weekend."
   C. "Y, I am just here to remind you it is dinnertime."
   D. "Y, it is not appropriate to miss dinner. What is the consequence of that, according to your care plan?"

4. In prenatal development, cell differentiation is normally completed by the end of the:

   A. First trimester
   B. Second trimester
   C. Third trimester
   D. First lunar month

5. The infant mortality rate is highest in mothers who are:

   A. Over 35 years old
   B. Over 30 years old
   C. Under 20 years old
   D. Under 15 years old

6. The term *anima* of Carl Jung describes:

   A. Male characteristics in women
   B. Feminine characteristics in men
   C. Male characteristics in men
   D. Feminine characteristics in women

7. According to Erikson's theory, the developmental task stage a 3- to 6-year-old needs to accomplish is:

   A. Identity
   B. Industry
   C. Intimacy
   D. Initiative

8. Infants seem to be very much alike (developmentally) until the age of:

   A. 2 months
   B. 6 months
   C. 10 months
   D. 12 months

9. A toddler's ability to take in or acknowledge changes in the environment is called:

   A. Adjustment
   B. Assimilation

C. Accommodation
D. Autonomy

MATCHING QUESTIONS
Directions
Match the theorist with the theory and the main belief or concept of that theory. Note: there is one "best" combination. There is one theory and one main belief or concept that is not correct for any of the theorists in this question.

THEORIST	THEORY	MAIN BELIEF or CONCEPT
1. Skinner	I. Moral judgment	A. Humans must be prized and loved
2. Jung	II. Hierarchy of needs	
3. Freud	III. Operant conditioning	B. All components of behavior are in the "unconscious"
4. Maslow	IV. Personality is a balance between conscious and unconscious; males and females are different organisms yet each contains part of the other	C. Inner self may be different from public self
5. Kohlberg		D. Must pass through the stages in order
	V. Person-centered	E. Stimulus, response, reinforcer
	VI. Psychoanalytic/ psychosexual	F. Interest in how people justify and support their decisions

5

Sociocultural Influences on Mental Health

Learning Objectives ■ ■ ■

1. Define culture.
2. Define religion.
3. Define ethnicity.
4. Identify parenting styles.
5. Differentiate between abuse and neglect.
6. Define stereotype.
7. Define prejudice.
8. Define homelessness.
9. Identify some possible reasons for homelessness.
10. Identify nursing care for people who are homeless.

Key Terms ■ ■ ■

- Abuse
- Culture
- Ethnicity
- Ethnocentrism
- Homeless
- Parenting
- Prejudice
- Religion
- Stereotype

Many professionals in the field of psychology believe that social and cultural environments have a great influence on the way people develop and process life. They believe that positive or negative social and cultural experiences will lead to that person's growing up to become an adult who believes and behaves in that same positive or negative manner. Part of the nurse's role is to take time to learn about traits that are common among people and those that are different. It is important to understand people's customs and beliefs to avoid unrealistic expectations of the patients. Let's take a look at some of the topics that are said to have the greatest influence on people.

■ CULTURE

Culture is a term that is often misused. Culture is a shared way of life, the combination of traditions and beliefs that makes a group of people bond together (also see Chapter 3). It is not based on color of skin or country of origin. For example, in the 1960s, a group of young people who were speaking

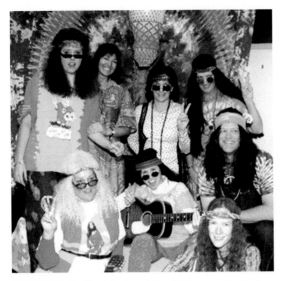

FIGURE 5-1. The hippies of the 1960s represented their own unique culture. (Courtesy of Montana Heritage Project, Townsend, MT.)

out against the politics and morals of their parents began living in groups (Fig. 5-1). The area they chose to start this movement was the Haight-Ashbury district in San Francisco. They called themselves "hippies," and they shared a way of life that consisted of experimenting with drugs; living together without benefit of marriage (or "free love," as it was termed); dressing in ripped, dirty clothing; not bathing enough or cutting their hair; and doing just about everything else that was directly opposite to the values of the "older generation." This group believed in loving everyone, regardless of race, creed, and color—as long as the individual embraced the beliefs of the group. The group's symbols were the daisy and the "peace sign," and "flower power" and "power to the people" represented some of the ideals they followed. Much to the chagrin of the over-30 age group, these young people fit the definition of "culture." It was called a "subculture" or "counterculture" at the time. Today, we might equate the "goth" statement many youth are making to the statements of their parents or grandparents in the 1960s.

A psychoanalyst named Karen Horney proposed the theory that some cultural tra-

ditions and beliefs cause disturbances in personal relationships and that this can lead to some forms of emotional disturbances. Today, we can look at other groups who have a shared belief system and a shared way of life. How many of these cultures can you think of?

Religious belief is often included in discussions of culture; however, it is important to note that the religion is *not* usually the culture. In people who practice Judaism or Islam, the relationship between the religious beliefs and the cultural beliefs is so entwined that it is hard to separate those traits. However, the hippie group contained people raised in many different religions.

Religion is the belief in a higher power of some sort. This belief system can be very strong—so strong that people have fought wars over religion—and it is often the subject of **stereotype.** A stereotype is a fixed notion or conviction about a group of people or a situation. Rituals or worship services are usually included in organized religions.

Native American groups worship different gods or spirits. Certain numbers are sacred, and special qualities are attributed to the four directions of north, south, east, and west. Of course, it is improper to categorize all Native Americans into one large group; there are many nations and many tribes, each with its own set of beliefs. Spirituality and religion are extremely important to some patients and unimportant or nonexistent to others. As nurses, we must be comfortable talking to patients about spiritual needs without pushing our own values on these patients. A person's success at recuperating from an illness or a surgical procedure may be deeply tied to his or her spirituality. Nurses who are not comfortable in these situations should offer to call the chaplain in the facility or a spiritual leader of the patient's choice.

Some religions involve items considered sacred to the patient and his or her belief system. Items may be in book form (Bible, Koran) or may be an item of jewelry (brooch, pin), or it may be the person's dress (headwear, loose fitting clothing) or other type of personal effect. It is generally believed that patients should be allowed to keep these items when at all possible. In situations where a patient may be in poor mental health and possession of these items are of actual or potential danger to the patient or others in the area, it may be necessary to remove the items. If that becomes necessary, enlisting the assistance of a representative from the particular religion may be helpful.

■ ETHNICITY

Ethnicity defines one's more personal traits. Language, country of origin, and skin color are parts of one's ethnicity. There can be different ethnic groups within a culture. For example, when you see a blonde, blue-eyed woman walking in front of you, you see characteristics of her ethnic background. What can you say about her culture by looking at her appearance? Probably nothing definitely; that would require speaking to her and obtaining some information. People are generally very proud of their culture and ethnicity. Many communities have festivals that celebrate their different cultures and ethnic groups. These festivals do much to educate the community about the various people living together. Sometimes we can learn a lot about a group of people by the kind of food they eat, and these celebrations are usually overflowing with foods of the particular group. Education helps eliminate **prejudice**, which is judging a person or situation before all the facts are known. Prejudice is a destructive behavior; it is hurtful and it shuts the door on the enrichment of the society. Laws in the United States are intended to minimize displays of prejudice relating to race, creed, gender, age, and so on. Unfortunately, it is impossible to legislate the beliefs of individual people. Nurses are in a perfect position to teach and model interpersonal relationships and,

it is hoped, to make great strides in eliminating prejudgment of others.

Health care may not be completely free of guilt in the area of race. A study was conducted at Emory University School of Medicine in Atlanta, Georgia (*Annals of Emergency Medicine*, 2000). They studied 217 patients who came in to be treated for long bone fractures. The study continued for 40 months. Of these patients, 127 were black and 90 were white. Nurses know that patients with this type of fracture usually require some type of medication for pain. The study showed that, even though the injuries and pain levels were similar, 43 percent of the black patients received no pain medication, compared to 26 percent of white patients. We are not certain from this study of the exact rationale for the outcome; did some patients refuse medication? Did some not ask? Was it a cultural choice? Did medical staff make assumptions about drug misuse in some people? Be wary of statistics. Be careful as well about silent stereotypes.

The hurt of prejudice has led to an emergence of **ethnocentrism**, which is people believing that their particular ethnic or religious group has rights and benefits over and above those of others. Gangs, supremacist groups, and terrorist groups may have had their roots in hate and prejudice.

Sadly, society is reminded of the plight of the Jewish people, who have lived through the horror of the concentration camps. The United States shows the scars of the inhumane treatment of the African and African-American people, who have been fighting for their civil rights for over 200 years. It remains a topic of debate today; the validity of affirmative action is being questioned and, in fact, being called by some a form of discrimination against other people. Religion, culture, and ethnicity, as well as prejudice caused by any of those characteristics, are deeply personal and deeply felt by members of the respective groups. It is important to keep the lines of communication open. People learn by sharing with each other, so it is much better to ask a person about something you do not know than to make an assumption about it. Making such an assumption is stereotyping, which ends a helping relationship between nurse and patient.

Many mental health professionals believe that people raised in an atmosphere of prejudice and stereotype tend to become angry, hateful, and aggressive adults. There is no proof that *all* people who are subjected to prejudice and stereotype develop into adults with such negative attitudes. This is one of the dangers in reading statistics on these topics: Statistics can be very misleading and can, in fact, support the negative stereotypes.

■ NONTRADITIONAL LIFESTYLES

The definition of "family" is changing (Fig. 5-2). Gay marriage and civil unions have opened very active debates. It is becoming more common in schools and clinics for children to have "two mommies" or "two daddies." People having gay, lesbian, bi-

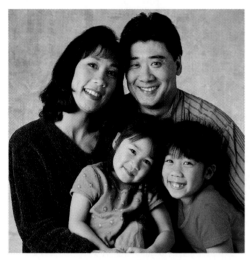

A

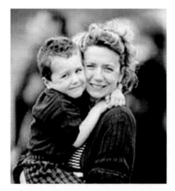

B

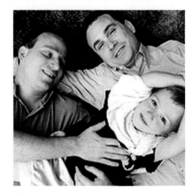

C

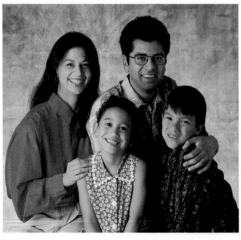

D

FIGURE 5-2. The definition of "family" is changing. A, Traditional family, with a mother, father, and their biological children. B, Single-parent family. (Courtesy of The Dr. Spock Company, drspock.com, Methuen, MA.) C, Gay family. (Courtesy of *USA Today,* McLean, VA.) D, "Blended" family, in which each spouse has his or her own children, whom they bring into a new family.

sexual, and transvestite (GLBT) lifestyles are "out" and are living life as normally as the more traditional father/mother/children families of decades earlier. All age groups are affected. Confusion, moodiness, depression, and changes in personality are some behaviors that may affect a person who is struggling with this part of who they are and with how acknowledging they may be "different" will affect relationships with family, friends, and colleagues.

People have been leading these lifestyles all along but were far less comfortable professing that in years past. Aging happens to all, regardless of lifestyle preference. By the year 2030, according to the National Gay and Lesbian Task Force, there will be approximately four million gay elders who will be requiring social services and who will be living in long-term care facilities. How will that change the way nurses provide care? Overtly, probably very little; good nursing care will remain good nursing care. However, learning to alter communication styles in order to ask for and accept people's preferences for roommate, type of clothing to wear, or activities to attend may need to be altered. Activities may cross gender barriers in a different way than they do today. Who shares bathrooms may become a different priority. Clearly, in the not too distant future, nurses practicing in clinics and long-term care or assisted living facilities can expect some changes in the clientele as well as the way in which those people will require our assistance.

Additionally, more individuals are choosing to start and raise families as single parents. Parents are choosing to adopt children from other countries, other ethnicities, and other races. One family may now include parents and siblings with assorted skin tones and languages. The global family is rapidly and constantly evolving.

■ HOMELESSNESS

Homelessness is not a mental illness (Fig. 5-3). It receives brief mention in this text

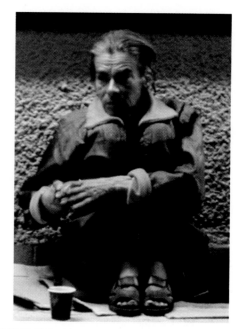

FIGURE 5-3. Homelessness is not a mental illness, but many homeless people face threats to their mental health. (Courtesy of Telecom Pioneers, Nova 5 Chapter #5, Brooklyn, NY.)

because many of the people in the United States who are **homeless** also have some threat to their mental health.

Some people are working full time but are homeless. They are victims of the economy, housing, or other situations not related in any way to having a mental illness. A small number of people choose to live on the streets. They are making a statement about the priorities of a nation that they think is not serving its people as it said it would. A large number of people who use community-based mental health services are the poor, especially the homeless poor (Barry, 2002).

Some people are homeless as an indirect result of the health-care delivery system. Mentally ill people constitute approximately 50 percent of the homeless in the United States. Many of these are people with schizophrenia. Because of the diagnostic criteria, the availability of benefits for the mentally ill, and the nature of the illnesses, people with certain illnesses have a difficult time trying to live independently with their illness. They end up out of work, out of money, and out of a home.

In the 1950s, deinstitutionalization led to the discharging of people who were technically able to be "in the community" but who were not always able to cope with the stresses of caring for themselves, caring for their families, and maintaining employment. For some mentally ill people, this kind of pressure and competition is the factor that keeps them ill. The Urban Institute Study of 2000 estimates there are approximately 3.5 million people annually who are homeless. Approximately one-third of those are children. (See Box 5-1.)

In 1987, the Health Resources and Services Administration–Health Care for the Homeless (HRSA-HCH) was formed to provide information and help create plans to help the homeless. The problem was that funding of federal programs depends on statistics, and it is extremely difficult to get accurate numbers because they change markedly approximately every 2 months (*Society Magazine,* 1994).

Most experts, however, agree that upwards of 50 percent of adult homeless people have a mental illness. Schizophrenia is a major problem among the homeless population. Put in simple terms, approximately one-third of the homeless population in the United States is mentally ill. Patients may be brought to a facility through the emergency department or by a law enforcement agency. Sometimes medication is given to stabilize the person, and he or she is returned to the community; other times the patient is admitted to a medical unit.

Shelters of varying types do exist in many cities. They are funded and staffed in differ-

---

BOX 5-1	*Homeless in America. Who Are They?*

Group	Approximate Percentage
Families	30%–50%
Children under the age of 18	25%–40%
People between the ages of 31 to 50	50%–60%
People ages 55 to 60	Difficult to determine. 2%–20%
Single females	14%–16%
Single males	40%–45%
Veterans of wars	25%–40%
African-American	55%–65%
Caucasian	35%–45%
Hispanic	12%–16%
Native American	2%–8%
Asian	1%–5%

Note: these numbers are approximations and will vary according to the study and the area of the country. Average time that families are spending in shelters has increased from approximately 4–5 months in the mid-1990s to approximately 1 year in the early 2000s.

Data from United States Department of Health and Human Services-Substance Abuse and Mental Health Services Administration (SAMHSA) http://www.mentalhealth.org/cmhs/Homelessness/facts.asp; Macomb Intermediate School District, Clinton Township, MI http://www.misd.net/Homeless/statistics.htm; National Coalition for Homeless Veterans http://www.nchv.org/page.cfm?id=81; National Coalition for the Homeless —Who Is Homeless? http://nationalhomeless.org/who.html

ent ways. For example, some are church funded and some rely on grants and underwriting by large businesses. Some are completely run by volunteers and some have some paid staff. Depending on the resources available, shelters for homeless people provide anything from meals and overnight shelter to health care, dental care, and assistance with job placement.

Often, however, behavioral conditions exist. Homeless people may be required to stay drug and alcohol free and to show proof that they are compliant with medications or some other criteria to help them return to an improved lifestyle.

What techniques do nurses need to help patients who may be homeless and physically or mentally compromised?

1. Treat the whole person, not the homelessness.
2. Treat the person as any other person on the unit.
3. Maintain all patient rights.

■ ECONOMIC CONSIDERATIONS

Rich versus poor: which is better? The debate will go on for all time. It would be logical to expect the response to that question to be "It really doesn't matter." Experts would have us think twice about that. For example, a study by Eron and Peterson in 1982 found that the lower the socioeconomic status, the higher the incidence of abnormal behavior in United States society. That statement, however, is not accurate in all cases. The study showed that the statement applies more strongly to patients with schizophrenia than it does to those with mood disorders. The implication is that there are always other variables besides socioeconomic status. For example, people who live in poverty or underprivileged circumstances will very likely have greater stressors than will those of higher socioeco-

nomic status. So, is it the lack of money or increased stress that leads to the disorder? Such questions make it very difficult, if not impossible, to make absolute statements about the correlation between disease and any variable. Behaviorists will be quick to remind you that people always have a choice. If the foregoing statements about poverty and illness were completely true, then it would follow that *all* people in that same circumstance would be mentally ill.

We know this is simply not the case. What variable allows some people to be ill and others not to be ill? Is it choice? Is it genetic? Is it learned behavior? This is part of the intrigue of the study of the mind.

■ ABUSE

Abuse is misuse of a person, substance, or situation. Sometimes people say that they cannot be abusing, as they consider themselves to know what they are doing. This is not true. Anyone who misuses or overuses a person, a substance, or a situation (such as gambling or power) is displaying abusive behavior.

Some individual forms of abuse disorders are discussed in Chapter 21. Abuse in general is a growing phenomenon in our society. People debate about whether a higher incidence of abuse actually exists now or whether people are just talking about it more openly. There is new speculation that multiple personality disorder may be caused at least in part by physical or sexual abuse. Violence is a learned behavior. It is well documented that, in the majority of physical abuse situations, the abuser was abused at some point. In the case of abuses such as alcoholism, the findings are not quite as conclusive. Some studies indicate that this type of abuse may be genetic, learned, or possibly due to a chemical imbalance in the body. A phenomenon called the "addictive personality" is defined as grouping abuse disorders together. It is important for nurses to understand that there may be more than one cause for a particular mental health problem. Good communication and data-collecting skills will help you find some potential causes for each patient's mental health problem.

■ POOR PARENTING

What is a "good" parent? Is it the parent who lets the child do anything the child wants? Is it the parent who buys all the newest fads for the child? Is it the parent who teaches strict values and ethics? Maybe it is the parent who is with the child at all times. **Parenting** is the method or methods of raising children, used by parents or other primary caregivers. Parenting is a learned behavior; babies do not come with instruction books. So, how do parents *learn to be* parents? Typically, one tends to parent based on the way he or she was parented. That means all the cultural and religious values that have been planted in one parent's belief systems are brought out in the open and blended with those values from the other parent's upbringing. Then, it is up to the parents to take one day at a time and learn from their mistakes. Sometimes parenting is learned from friends and neighbors. Sometimes schools, health-care facilities, and communities offer classes for parents.

American society is experiencing more single-parent families and same-sex parent families. Reactions to altered parenting styles are varied. Again, there is no "perfect" situation or guarantee of being "good" parents. Parenting is stressful. No matter what your patients are concerned about during their hospitalization, it is almost certain that their children will be a paramount focus of attention. Nurses can best help parents not only through the stress of being hospitalized and apart from their children but also with the stresses of parenting in general by helping the parent choose healthy lifestyles. Healthy nutrition, moderate exercise, and "adult time" apart from the children can be effective stress relievers.

Diana Baumrind (1971) has developed a classification of types of parents. They are described as follows:

1. *Authoritarian Parent:* This parent sets up very strict rules. The child has little or no voice in family decisions. Sometimes our society jokes about this style of parenting as evidenced by clothing imprinted with the saying, "Because I'm the Mommy/Daddy, that's why!" This authoritarianism can lead to a rebellious, hostile child who may enter adulthood angry, violent, unwilling to obey laws, and unable to make consistent decisions.

2. *Authoritative Parent:* This style of parenting has firm, consistent rules and limits, while allowing for discussion and occasional flexibility of those rules, according to special circumstances. Children are allowed some freedom, within set limits, and some voice in decisions. Researchers think that this is the preferred style of parenting. It offers a balance between rules and responsibilities, which allows the child to learn to make appropriate choices and accept the outcomes of those choices.

3. *Permissive Parent:* This may be the type of parent we wanted as we went through adolescence. This style of parenting provides little structure and few guidelines. The child is not sure of the boundaries. If one does not learn boundaries, it becomes difficult to learn how to control oneself and how to behave in certain situations. Permissive parents can be in danger of being accused of neglect.

Key Concepts ■ ■ ■

1. Culture, ethnicity, sexual orientation, and religion are basic deeply rooted human experiences. They are not "good" or "bad"; they are different for each individual or group of individuals who claim membership in that culture, ethnic group, or religion.
2. People have many more similarities than they have differences. It is important for nurses to concentrate on the similarities among people and to be comfortable asking questions about the background of their patients and coworkers. Role modeling cooperative relationships can be very helpful in teaching others about cultural sensitivity.

CASE STUDY: M ■ ■ ■

M is a 21-year-old woman from Turkey. She was flown to a medical center in the United States because of orthopedic complications that could not be treated properly in her country. M traveled with her mother. Neither of the women spoke English, and their understanding of English was minimal.

M's surgery was successful and routine, according to the surgical report; however, the nurse's charting reflected a patient who was not easily aroused for postoperative checks. The nursing staff validated understanding with M's mother and were satisfied that, when she nodded her head "yes," she actually understood what the nurses were saying to her. When M was asked questions by the nurses, her mother answered for her. Her mother answered in her own language, and the nurses could not understand her responses. M was not eating, and her IV was a source of concern to her mother. M slept most of the time; her mother would not allow the nurses to get M out of bed for walks or other positioning.

After a week of trying, nursing and social service staff members were able to find a translator for M. The staff learned that it was the norm for M's mother to care for her "sick" daughter. The mother considered the male nurses that had been assigned to M unacceptable because M was unmarried and remained a virgin; therefore, it was considered improper for a man to touch her for any reason. Communication was opened up among M, her mother, and the nursing staff. Hospital routines and legal issues were explained to M and her mother, and compromises were made by all parties. M's mother was allowed to "help" the nurses with M's care. A new plug with a grounding prong allowed for a hot plate to be brought into the room so that traditional food could be prepared for M. Within 2 weeks, M had improved in her postsurgical course to the point that she was discharged from the hospital.

What nursing techniques would you use to facilitate cooperation and understanding with this patient and mother? How might you alter activities such as exercise, nutrition, and other basic needs in order to satisfy both the cultural concerns and requirements for health maintenance for this patient?

Using the suggested nursing diagnoses listed here (or others you can think of), complete a nursing process for M.

Suggested Nursing Diagnoses

1. *Adjustment*
2. *Management of therapeutic regimen*
3. *Verbal communication*

CASE STUDY: TONY ■ ■ ■

Tony is a 22-year-old male. He has been admitted to the young adult unit in the long-term care facility in which you are the evening shift nurse. Tony is six feet two inches tall, weighs two hundred pounds and is in excellent physical condition, except that he has become quadriplegic from a recent diving incident. He and his friends had been celebrating his upcoming graduation from college. They had been drinking moderately. The group had met at a local swimming area. Two groups of young men challenged each other to a diving competition, but the water was not as deep as they had anticipated. Tony was the first diver. He sustained severe high cervical injury and will be paralyzed for the remainder of his life. Many people, male and female, visit Tony. He is very popular. He seems to have a special relationship with a particular young female. You wait to help with his evening cares until you see the young woman leave, you knock, walk in, and find Tony and another young male together in Tony's hospital bed kissing. What will you do? What is your initial "gut" response as you read this scenario? What questions might you need to ask Tony in order to help you provide nursing care to fit his needs?

Using the suggested nursing diagnoses listed here (or others you can think of), complete a nursing process for Tony.

Suggested Nursing Diagnoses

1. *Sexuality patterns*
2. *Body image*
3. *Coping*

CASE STUDY: HAROLD ■ ■ ■

Harold is a 76-year-old nursing home resident. He has type I diabetes and gives himself his own insulin. He has the diagnosis of paranoid schizophrenia but has been asymptomatic for 1 year. Harold is also a severe alcoholic, and he periodically leaves the nursing home against medical advice and is gone for 2 to 3 days. He has friends "on the street" because, before being institutionalized, that is where he lived. Harold goes to the local shelter for meals and knows he can go to the hospital to get his insulin. He has no family in the vicinity who can participate in his care.

He no longer meets the criteria for skilled-care nursing. A decision must be made about his future, as he will no longer be eligible to remain in this nursing home. Harold wishes to be his own advocate and is found to be legally capable of making his own decisions. The outcome for this patient was that he chose to "take my chances" and return to the streets. He had not been seen again by any of the nursing home staff. No further information is available about this patient.

Considering Maslow's Hierarchy of Needs, how would you classify Harold? What are the arguments both for and against his decision to leave the nursing home? Do you consider Harold to be mentally healthy and competent? Why or why not?

Using the suggested nursing diagnoses listed here (or others you can think of), complete a nursing process for Harold.

Suggested Nursing Diagnoses

1. *Health maintenance*
2. *Nutrition*
3. *Self-care*

CASE STUDY: KATRINA ■ ■ ■

Katrina is a 22-year-old single mother of two children, ages 2 and 3. Katrina has a high school education and had been working as a telemarketer until 6 weeks ago, when she was laid off due to consolidation of services at her place of employment. Katrina has a history of marijuana and alcohol abuse. She was evicted from her apartment because she had not been paying the rent.

You are the LPN/LVN staffing the local homeless shelter today when Katrina and her children arrive. She and the children appear dirty, and she states they have not eaten for 2 days. She has discoloration on her cheeks and her upper arms. You note a sweet odor about her, and you think you detect dilation of her pupils. She asks for help.

This shelter is able to provide many services, including medical, dental care, clothing, and personal supplies, etc. The shelter has a strict policy of not assisting anyone who is actively using drugs or alcohol or who is suspected to be under the influence of drugs or alcohol. The shelter governance thinks it is an issue of safety not only for that individual, but also for others in the shelter.

What are your nursing priorities for Katrina and her children? What communication skills will be necessary? How will you help her and her children and maintain the shelter's policy relating to use of drugs and alcohol?

Using the suggested nursing diagnoses listed here (or others you can think of), complete a nursing process for Katrina.

Suggested Nursing Diagnoses

1. *Risk for suicide*
2. *Parenting*
3. *Coping*

REFERENCES

Barry, P.D. (2002). *Mental Health and Mental Illness,* 7th ed. JB Lippincott, Philadelphia.

Baumohl, J. and Huebner, R. (1991). *Alcohol and Other Drug Problems Among the Homeless: Research, Practice, and Future* http://www.knowledgeplex.org/kp/text_document_summary/scholarly_article/relfiles/hpd_0203_baumohl.pdf.

Social science and the citizen: Counting homeless (1994, November/December). *Society Magazine.*

Baumrind, D. (1971). Current patterns of parental authority. *Developmental Psychology* (monograph 1), *4,* 1–103.

Cummins, H.J. (June 22, 2003). Coming out, moving on. *Star Tribune,* Minneapolis, MN.

Eron, L.D. and Peterson, R.A (1982). Abnormal behavior: Social approaches. In M.R. Rosenzweig & L.W. Porter (Eds.) Annu. Rev. of Psychol *33,* 231-65.

Galanti, G. (1991). *Caring for Patients from Different Cultures—Case Studies from American Hospitals.* University of Pennsylvania Press, Philadelphia.

Kaplan, B.J. (November 2002). Gay elders face uncomfortable realities in LTC. *Caring for the Ages,* American Medical Directors Association (November 2002), Vol. 3, No. 11.

Martin, M.L. (2000). Ethnicity and Analgesic Practice: An Editorial. *Annals of Emergency Medicine, 35,* 77–81.

Purtilo, R. and Haddad, A. (2002). *Health Professional and Patient Interaction,* 6th ed. W.B. Saunders Company, Philadelphia.

Todd, K.H., Deaton, C., D'Adamo, A.P., and Goe, L. (2000). Ethnicity and Analgesic Practice. *Annals of Emergency Medicine, 35,* 11–16.

WEBSITES

http://www.bphc.hrsa.gov/homeless
http://www.amda.com/caring/november2002/gayelders.htm

CRITICAL THINKING EXERCISES ■ ■ ■

1. Your patient is from a different country and speaks only minimal English. Your translator has seen the patient and has gone over the hospital routines, rules, and patient's rights. The patient's mother insists on staying in the room 24 hours a day and refuses to let you perform assessments and cares on the patient. The patient is in pain, but the mother will not allow pain medication to be given. The patient will not accept the food from the hospital. You smell food cooking and enter the room to find the mother cooking on a hot plate, which is a fire code violation. What can you do in this situation?

2. You are home one evening and you hear the 18-month-old child of your upstairs neighbors. The child has been crying for 3 hours. You have heard no footsteps in the apartment. The answering machine picks up each time you attempt to call. You become concerned and call the building supervisor to open the apartment. When you get in, you find unsanitary conditions, and the parents are not in the apartment. You look outside and see the parents several apartments down, partying with friends. What are your responsibilities? How will you respond to the parents? Whom will you notify? The parents tell you to mind your own business. What will you say to them? What will you do if it happens again?

3. Read the case study of M on page 87. List as many situations as you can think of from this example that may be culturally related. What could you do to help this patient and her mother that the nurses did not do? What legal issues would you anticipate for the patient as well as for yourself as a nurse in this situation?

4. Review your facility's policies on caring for the homeless. You are the administrator of your facility and also a nurse. You are responsible to your board of directors as well as for the welfare of your patients. What suggestions can you make to improve the treatment they receive? How will you adjust your budget (which is already stretched to the limit) to accommodate your building, your patients, your staff, and the special needs of a growing population of chronically ill homeless?

5. You are the only source of income for your family. You are laid off because of a merger of two agencies. How long can you survive with no income? How will you pay for insurance? Jobs are not plentiful; the outlook for comparable employment in the near future is bleak. How close are you to living on the street? What will be the plan of action for you and your family?

ACTIVITIES

1. Interview a person who is from a religion or a culture different from your own. You may use the interview format from Chapter 7. Present the results orally or in writing. This will reinforce the information presented in Chapter 7, as well as provide firsthand information pertinent to this chapter.

2. Have a culture celebration day. Dress in clothing traditional for your religion or culture. Make the day an *event*—have traditional ethnic foods, music, games, and the like.

3. Choose someone you know who is a parent. This can be a family member, friend, neighbor, or anyone you feel comfortable with. Using the parenting definitions of Diana Baumrind, complete the following chart and decide what basic parenting style you think this parent uses.

AUTHORITARIAN	AUTHORITATIVE	PERMISSIVE

What type of parenting style do you think this parent uses most consistently? Pretend that your subject is stating a desire to change his or her parenting style. Choose one of the alternative styles and develop a nursing process to assist the subject to begin to make the desired change. Several nursing diagnoses are suggested, but you may choose others from your NANDA list.

SUGGESTED NURSING DIAGNOSES

1. *Parenting, altered*
2. *Knowledge deficit (parenting)*
3. *Parental role conflict*

4. *Decisional conflict (independent living versus nursing home living)*
5. *Health maintenance, altered*
6. *Injury, risk for*

ASSESSMENT/ DATA COLLECTION	NURSING DIAGNOSIS	PLAN/ GOAL	INTERVENTIONS/ NURSING ACTIONS	EVALUATION CRITERIA

4. Participate in the evening-out sleepouts that many major communities participate in as a fund-raiser for shelters and food shelves.

TEST QUESTIONS ■ ■ ■

MULTIPLE CHOICE QUESTIONS

1. The concepts of space, time, and waiting are:
   A. Religious
   B. Cultural
   C. Economic
   D. Ethnic

2. The condition of judging a person or situation before all the facts are known is called:
   A. Hatred
   B. Abuse
   C. Prejudice
   D. Stereotype

3. Homelessness is being blamed, in part, on:
   A. Deinstitutionalization
   B. Access to community services
   C. Mental illness
   D. All of the above

4. Nurses who care for patients who are homeless understand that in the United States:
   A. Homelessness is classified as a mental illness.
   B. Approximately one-third of the homeless are mentally ill.
   C. All the homeless have some form of mental illness.
   D. People must be mentally ill to choose to be homeless.

5. A patient is admitted with the diagnosis of paranoid behavior. The patient claims to be of a religion requiring wearing of very heavy necklaces. You research the religion and determine this to be true, but the patient has been seen violently flinging the necklace at his or her roommate. Your best nursing action is:
   A. Call an assistance code.
   B. Remove all religious items.
   C. Do nothing: it is his or her religious right.
   D. Enlist the assistance of a religious representative to negotiate removal of the item(s) in question.

6. A set of parents accompany their ill 8-year-old child to the clinic. The child was diagnosed last month with type I diabetes and is insulin dependent. The parents admit they are not administering the insulin, as their religious belief does not allow for foreign substances in any form for any reason. A check of the chart clearly indicated diabetes teaching had been done with this family unit at last month's visit. Your initial nursing action is:
   A. Report these parents for child endangerment, as nurses are mandatory reporters.
   B. Inform the parents this child could die without the required insulin.
   C. Leave the room and call for a doctor or RN to the room stat.
   D. Collect information pertaining to what the religion would allow and facilitate discussion with the doctor.

7. When collecting data during an intake interview, the nurse understands:

SELECT ALL ANSWERS THAT APPLY

A. Most homeless people are unemployed.

B. Culture is a shared belief system.

C. Prejudice exists within the health-care delivery system.

D. It is likely that nursing home residents may profess a homosexual lifestyle.

E. There is no correlation between mental illness and the condition of homelessness.

Coping and Defense Mechanisms

Learning Objectives ■ ■ ■

1. Define coping.
2. Differentiate between effective and ineffective coping.
3. Define defense (coping) mechanisms.
4. Identify main defense mechanisms.

Key Terms ■ ■ ■

- Coping
- Defense mechanisms
- Effective
- Ineffective

■ COPING

"Deal with it." "Get a grip." "Don't make a mountain out of a molehill." These are pieces of advice that most people may have heard or given at some point. But what do they mean? What is **coping?** Coping is the way one adapts to a stressor psychologically, physically, and behaviorally. It is the ability one develops to deal consciously with problems and stress. Webster defines to "cope" as to fight or contend with (something) successfully. Individuals have different methods of coping or dealing with their stressors. What makes some people very successful at handling stress and others not successful at all? What allows some people to have a drink or run to reduce their stress and causes others to become addicted to the same behavior?

Cultures, religions, and individual belief systems seem to be the lead factors in this mystery. Personal choices also play a supporting role. It is not the value of a behavior that we assess as nurses; it is the desired outcome that is important. The short-term and long-term goals of a change in behavior emphasize demonstration of specific effective coping skills. What is an effective coping skill, and how will you observe and measure it?

Effective coping skills are those that are specifically identified to offer healthy choices to the patient. Hospitalization is a stressful experience for patients and families, with so many unknown and unfamiliar things, so many noises and interruptions.

The patient may not understand the illness or the implications of the treatment plan. Mealtimes may be different from the routine at home. It is very common to see patients use coping mechanisms to help deal with hospitalization. It is helpful if patients and families can be active participants in the treatment plan (Fig. 6-1). The patient should be included in the decision making as to which new behaviors are acceptable and which ones are not. Practicing these new behaviors in a safe place, such as a hospital or organized group setting, is the secret to success. This will probably require a lifestyle change for the patient, and it will be hard work. As the saying goes, "Old habits die hard," but old habits can die and healthy new ones can replace them. This process of effective coping is sometimes called "adaptation." Allowing the patient to "practice" the new coping techniques will promote confidence and decrease the stress that can accompany change. The patient will adapt to the stress by using the new tools.

Often, the dividing line between effective and ineffective coping is in the degree of the

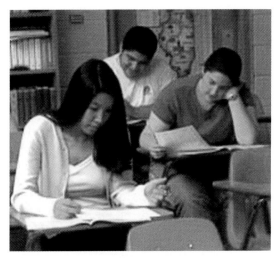

FIGURE 6-2. A little anxiety can be a positive thing. (Courtesy of Three Rivers Community College, Norwich, CT.)

technique used. For instance, a little worry or anxiety can be a positive thing. Most of the time when there is a little tension, we are more alert and ready to respond (Fig. 6-2). The "fight or flight" mechanism can actually help us adapt to a new situation. Too much

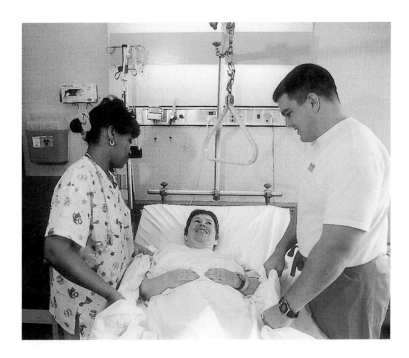

FIGURE 6-1. Involving patients and families in the treatment plan can go a long way toward reducing the stress of hospitalization. (From Williams, LS, and Hopper, PD: *Understanding Medical Surgical Nursing*, 2nd ed. Philadelphia, FA Davis Company, 2003, p. 27. Reprinted with permission.)

worry begins to cloud the consciousness and interferes with our ability to make appropriate choices and recall the new adaptive tools we have learned.

One of the most helpful actions a nurse can take is to listen to the patient's thoughts and feelings about the stressor and then provide information that will reinforce the patient's positive feelings. Providing honest, positive feedback about the patient's progress in a given lifestyle change will let the patient know that others are noticing the hard work that he or she has done.

Ineffective coping is another story. When the conscious techniques we try are not successful, we often allow ourselves unconsciously to fall into habits that give us the illusion of coping. These habits are called **defense mechanisms** (or coping or mental mechanisms).

■ DEFENSE MECHANISMS

Defense mechanisms are mental pressure valves. They give the illusion that they are helping alleviate the stress level, when, in reality, they mask the stress and can actually end up increasing it. Defense mechanisms come out of the ego mechanism of Freud's theory of personality. Although they appear to be very purposeful, they exist, for the most part, on the unconscious level.

The purpose of defense mechanisms is to reduce or eliminate anxiety. Surprisingly, when used in very small doses, they can be helpful. It is when they are overused that they become ineffective and can lead to a breakdown of the personality. Again, people are not born with these behaviors; they are learned as responses to stress. Many times, they are developed by the time we are 10 years old.

Because the main purpose of defense mechanisms is to decrease anxiety, people tend to have their own repertoire of them and to use them (unconsciously) over and over. Periods of high stress are not the times to try something new, so the psyche allows people to use the old "standbys" to get over yet another hump in life. Some of the commonly used defense mechanisms are shown in Table 6-1.

Key Concepts ■ ■ ■

1. Stress and people's responses to it are very individualized. We are not all stressed by the same things, nor do we deal with our stress in the same ways.
2. Defense mechanisms are believed to be part of the ego of Freud's description of personality. They are based in the unconscious, for the most part, but they can appear to be very deliberate.
3. Use of defense mechanisms for a short period can be helpful. The mechanisms act like a pressure valve and allow the psyche to put the stress into perspective. If the patient then deals with the problem, the outcome can be an effective coping technique; if not successful, the patient's anxiety level may increase.

TABLE 6-1 ▪ Defense Mechanisms

MECHANISM	DESCRIPTION	EXAMPLES	OVERUSE CAN LEAD TO …
DENIAL	Usually the first defense learned and used. Unconscious refusal to see reality. Is *not* consciously lying.	The alcoholic states, "I can quit any time I want to."	Repression, dissociative disorders.
REPRESSION (STUFFING)	An unconscious "burying" or "forgetting" mechanism. Excludes or withholds from our consciousness events or situations that are unbearable. A step deeper than "denial."	"Forgetting" a loved one's birthday after a fight.	
DISSOCIATION	Painful events or situations are separated or dissociated from the conscious mind. Patients will often say, "I had an out-of-body experience" or "It happened to someone else, but it was as though it happened to me."	1. Patient who had been sexually abused as a child describes the situation as if it happened to a friend or sibling. 2. Police visit parent to inform parent of death of child in car accident. Parent tells police, "That's impossible. My child is upstairs asleep. You must have the wrong house."	One of the dissociative disorders, such as multiple personality disorder.
RATIONALIZATION	Use of a logical-sounding excuse to cover up true thoughts and feelings. The most frequently used defense mechanism.	1. "I did not make a medication error; I followed the physician's order." 2. "I failed the test because the teacher wrote bad questions."	Self-deception.

(continued)

Mechanism	Definition	Examples	Disadvantages
COMPENSATION	Making up for something we perceive as an inadequacy by developing some other desirable trait.	1. The small boy who wants to be a basketball center instead becomes an honor roll student. 2. The physically unattractive person who wants to model instead becomes a famous designer.	Failure to resolve internal conflicts.
REACTION FORMATION (OVER-COMPENSATION)	Similar to compensation, except the person usually develops the *exact opposite* trait.	1. The small boy who wants to be a basketball center becomes a political voice to decrease the emphasis of sports in the elementary grades. 2. The physically unattractive person who wants to be a model speaks out for eliminating beauty pageants.	
REGRESSION	Emotionally returning to an earlier time in life when there was far less stress. Commonly seen in patients while hospitalized. *Note:* Everyone does not go back to the same developmental age. This is highly individualized.	1. Children who are toilet trained beginning to wet themselves. 2. Adults who may start crying and have a "temper tantrum."	May interfere with perception of reality. May interfere with progression and development of personality.
SUBLIMATION	Unacceptable traits or characteristics are diverted into acceptable traits or characteristics.	1. Burglar teaches home safety classes. 2. Person who is potentially physically abusive becomes professional sports figure. 3. People who choose to not have children run a day-care center.	The "socially accepted" behavior might actually reinforce the negative tendencies, and the person may still show signs of the undesirable behavior or trait.

(continued)

TABLE 6-1 ░ Defense Mechanisms (Continued)

MECHANISM	DESCRIPTION	EXAMPLES	OVERUSE CAN LEAD TO ...
PROJECTION (SCAPEGOATING)	Blaming others. A mental or verbal "finger-pointing" at another for the problem. *Memory tool:* Think of a projector at the movie theater. It "points" the images of the film onto the screen, just as a person using this defense mechanism "points" blame on another person or situation.	1. "I didn't get the promotion because you don't like me." 2. "I'm overweight because you make me nervous."	Finds faults in everything and everyone. Fails to learn to take personal responsibility. May develop into delusional tendencies.
DISPLACEMENT (TRANSFERENCE)	The "kick-the-dog syndrome." Transferring anger and hostility to another person or object that is perceived to be less powerful.	Parent loses job without notice; goes home and verbally abuses spouse, who unjustly punishes child, who slaps the dog.	Loss of friends and relationships. Confusion in communication.
RESTITUTION (UNDOING)	Makes amends for a behavior one thinks is unacceptable. Makes an attempt at reducing guilt.	1. Giving a treat to a child who is being punished for a wrong-doing. 2. The person who sees someone lose a wallet with a large amount of cash does not return the wallet but puts extra in the collection plate at the next church service.	May send double message. Relieves the "doer" of the responsibility of honesty in the situation.
ISOLATION	Emotion that is separated from the original feeling.	"I wasn't really angry; just a little upset."	Avoids dealing with true feeling; can increase stress.
CONVERSION REACTION	Anxiety is channeled into physical symptoms. *Note:* Often, the symptoms disappear soon after the threat is over.	Nausea develops the night before a major exam, causing the person to miss the exam. Nausea may disappear soon after the scheduled test is finished.	Anxiety not dealt with can lead to actual physical disorders such as gastric ulcers and possibly some cancers.
AVOIDANCE	Unconsciously staying away from events or situations that might open feelings of aggression or anxiety.	"I can't go to the class reunion tonight. I'm just so tired, I have to sleep."	

WEBSITES

Understanding Defense Mechanisms, Lynn M. Levo, Vol. VII, No. 4 September/October 2003: http://www.sli.org/page_110_defense_mechanisms.htm

Personality (no other title or author credited): http://www.psychweb.pdx.edu/ Course%20Notes/Personality-webnotes.doc http://childstudy.net/cdw-old.html http://childstudy.net/FREUD.html

CRITICAL THINKING EXERCISE ■ ■ ■

Nurse D, LVN, has been routinely calling in "sick" on his weekends to work. This has created a hardship for the patients and the staff. On Monday, Nurse D reports for the assigned work shift but is called to the nurse manager's office. The nurse manager informs Nurse D of the pattern that has developed in his attendance and gives him a chance to explain the situation. Nurse D says, "Well, I am a single parent and I need to take care of my children. You should assign single people without families to work the weekends. If you cared a little more about your employees, we wouldn't have to call in so often."

Nurse D is quiet for a second and then says with a shaky voice, "You make me so nervous that I've started needing a couple of drinks at night so I can sleep. I could quit any time if you'd just let me have my weekends off."

What defense mechanisms do you hear Nurse D using? How many of them have you used? If you were the nurse manager, what would you say to Nurse D? Using three of the suggested nursing diagnoses listed here (or others you can think of), complete a nursing process for Nurse D.

SUGGESTED NURSING DIAGNOSES

1. Coping
2. Denial
3. Role performance
4. Thought processes
5. Caregiver role strain
6. Adjustment
7. Self-care

NANDA CHOICE	SUPPORTING INFORMATION FOR NANDA CHOICE

ACTIVITIES

1. List three situations that were very uncomfortable for you. What defense mechanisms did you use? How will you respond to each of these situations in a more effective manner? List three situations in which you observed someone else using defense mechanisms. How can you help him or her to cope in a more effective manner?

2. Perform the first activity on someone else. It can be a family member, friend, classmate, or anyone you choose. Identify who it was easier to do this assignment on—yourself or the "other" person—and discuss the rationale for these feelings.

3. Continue to work with the person you chose in activity number 2. Have the person choose one defense mechanism that he or she would like to eliminate. Create a nursing process for that defense mechanism behavior change. Suggested nursing diagnoses are supplied here, but you may choose others from the NANDA list.

SUGGESTED NURSING DIAGNOSES

1. *Coping, individual, ineffective*
2. *Thought processes, altered*
3. *Self-esteem, disturbance*

ASSESSMENT/ DATA COLLECTION	NURSING DIAGNOSIS	PLAN/ GOAL	INTERVENTIONS/ NURSING ACTIONS	EVALUATION CRITERIA

TEST QUESTIONS ■ ■ ■

MULTIPLE CHOICE QUESTIONS

1. A person who always sounds like he or she is making excuses is displaying:
   A. Denial
   B. Fantasy
   C. Rationalization
   D. Transference

2. The alcoholic who says, "I don't have a problem. I can quit any time I want to; I just don't want to" is displaying:

   A. Denial
   B. Fantasy
   C. Dissociation
   D. Transference

3. Your young male patient who tells you that he may not be big enough for the basketball team, but "that's no problem because I'm a 4.0 student and on the principal's list," is displaying:

   A. Denial
   B. Transference
   C. Dissociation
   D. Compensation

4. Mr. V. becomes angry that Mrs. V. spent the whole day shopping with her friends. Upon her return home, he hits her and tells her "It's your own fault. Stay home once in a while!" Mr. V is displaying:

   A. Repression
   B. Regression
   C. Dissociation
   D. Projection

5. You overhear someone jokingly repeating the social cliché "Stop Smoking, Lose Weight, Exercise, Die Anyway" as they order a big burger and super-sized fries. That cliché is an example of:

   A. Rationalization
   B. Repression
   C. Regression
   D. Rebellion

6. Yesterday, Tara became drunk and inappropriate at a family function. Tara's 16-year-old daughter was embarrassed and in tears. Today, Tara bought two expensive concert tickets for her daughter and a friend. This is an example of:

   A. Denial
   B. Undoing
   C. Symbolization
   D. Conversion

MATCHING QUESTIONS

Directions

Match the statement or example in Column A with the defense mechanism in Column B. On your answer sheet, write the letter of the response from Column B next to the corresponding number of Column A. Use each response only once; there is an extra response you will not use.

COLUMN A	COLUMN B
1. Compensation	**A.** Painful ideas/feelings/events separated from awareness.
2. Repression	**B.** Believable, false story.
3. Regression	**C.** Also called *escapism*.
4. Denial	**D.** Retreat to earlier, less stressful time.
5. Conversion	**E.** "I can quit drinking anytime I want to."
6. Projection/ scapegoating	**F.** "I'm overweight because you make me so nervous I have to eat."
7. Dissociation	**G.** "I might be too short for basketball, but I'm in music."
8. Fantasy	**H.** Anxiety that is channeled into physical symptoms.
	I. "Stuffing" of painful thoughts/feelings.

7

Nursing Process in Mental Health

Learning Objectives ▪ ▪ ▪

1. Define the role of the LPN/LVN in the five steps of the nursing process.
2. Identify the components of a mental health status assessment.
3. State the need for the nursing process in mental health issues.
4. State the concepts of patient interviewing.
5. Prepare a patient interview.
6. Collaborate in creating a nursing process for a given, hypothetical patient.
7. State the concepts of patient teaching.
8. Prepare and implement a teaching exercise.

Key Terms ▪ ▪ ▪

- Affect
- APNA
- Awareness
- Data collection
- Evaluation
- Implementation
- Judgment
- Memory
- Mood
- NANDA
- Nursing diagnosis
- Nursing process
- Orientation
- Patient interview
- Patient teaching
- PES
- Plan of care
- Thinking/Cognition
- NIC
- NOC

The **nursing process** is a tool used throughout all areas and levels of nursing. It is a formula for nurses to learn to think about patients and how to organize and implement their care in a systematic, universal way. It is part of the culture of nurses.

There are different models or theories of nursing diagnosis. Scope of practice, how-

ever, determines that the registered nurse (RN) and the licensed practical nurse/licensed vocational nurse (LPN/LVN) play different parts in the nursing process. In the early 1950s, Hildegard Peplau hypothesized that nurses are a tool best utilized in relationship to the patient and the environment and in collaboration with other nurses and health-care professionals. She stressed the phases of a working relationship that included a termination phase where nurses prepare both themselves and their patients for termination of the relationship. Her model is still widely used in nursing process and nursing practice today.

In the early 1970s, the American Nurses Association (ANA) developed Standards of Practice for RN- and LPN/LVN-prepared nurses. The association differentiated between the RN's role and the LPN's role in the nursing process. Individual state Nurse Practice Act and Boards of Nursing may also offer their own interpretation of the ANA guidelines relating to the role and scope of practice for the LPN/LVN-prepared nurse in the nursing process.

■ STEP 1: ASSESSING THE PATIENT'S MENTAL HEALTH

The role of the LPN/LVN in this first step of the nursing process is to *assist* with assessment. **Data collection** (or assessment) is made during every contact a nurse has with a patient. It is essential to the well-being of the patient and in assisting the medical team in making the best choices concerning that person. Nurses collect data about the patient and his or her condition. In most cases, this is accomplished with the help of a form that is used by the facility. Nurses also use nonverbal communication skills to assess the patient's attitude, tone of voice, facial expression, and so on. The problem with many of these generic forms is that they are written in closed-ended format. They are very impersonal and may not reflect the specific information needed about that patient.

It is during the data collection/assessment part of the nursing process that the mental status exam is performed. The mental status exam is a series of questions and activities that check eight areas: the patient's level of awareness and reality orientation, appearance and behavior, speech and com-munication, **mood** and **affect, memory, thinking/cognition,** perception, and **judgment.** These examinations are of varying lengths and formats, but they all assess the patient's mental capabilities.

Table 7-1 lists areas to be assessed during a mental status examination. It also suggests the type of assessment made and ideas for questions or commands used by members of the health-care team to make the assessments, as well as some parameters for responses of a person with normal and abnormal mental functioning.

There are many ways to improve the quality of our data collection. Two ideas for improving data collection in the form of interviews are listed here. Remember, this is not an exhaustive list of reasons to interview patients.

INTERVIEWING TECHNIQUES

For purposes of this text, the word *interview* pertains to any nurse-patient interaction that requires a nurse to obtain specific information from a patient. The **patient interview** is usually the primary method of data gathering used in health care. It is important to collect data about the whole person. Data related to thoughts and feelings are as important to any nurse-patient interview as the physical data collected.

INTAKE/ADMISSION INTERVIEW

Most facilities have developed standard interview forms that suit their particular needs. The forms are written in a very matter-of-fact way and are usually in a closed-ended format. Patients who are frightened, angry, or just too ill at the moment may easily refuse to answer those closed-ended questions. The patient may have heard the questions before and feel frustrated by what he or she perceives to be inefficiency or poor communication among the staff. This can set both the nurse and the patient up for a difficult time. It is up to the nurse to rephrase the questions in an open-ended format that

TABLE 7-1 ■ *Mental Health Status Examination*

AREA OF ASSESSMENT	TYPE OF ASSESSMENT	SUGGESTED METHODS OF ASSESSMENT AND NORMAL PARAMETERS	ALTERATIONS TO NORMAL PARAMETERS
APPEARANCE AND BEHAVIOR	Objective and subjective observations about dress, hygiene, posture, and so on; and about the patient's actions and reactions to health-care personnel.	Clean, hair combed; clothing intact and appropriate to weather or situation. Teeth in good repair. Posture erect. Cooperates with health-care personnel.	Displays either unusual apathy or concern about appearance. Displays uncooperative, hostile, or suspicious-type behaviors toward health-care personnel.
LEVEL OF AWARENESS AND ORIENTATION	Subjective and objective assessment of the patient's degree of alertness (wakefulness) and the degree of patient's knowledge of self.	*Awareness* is measured on a continuum that ranges from unconsciousness to mania. "Normal alertness" is the desired behavior. There is usually a standard guideline for helping with this assessment, but subjective observations can be documented as well, if the patient cannot stay awake for even short intervals or is overly active and has difficulty staying in one place for any period of time. *Orientation* measures the person's ability to know who he or she is, where he or she is, and the day and time, usually within 1 or 2 days of the actual day and time. Measurement techniques are accomplished by asking the patient, "What is your name?" "Where are you right now?" and "Tell me what the day and date are." Asking "Who is the president of the United States?" is used here as well. Nurses frequently document this as "oriented × 3," but it is best to also write down the objective data on which this routine answer is based.	Outcome is not within normal limits if the patient is difficult to arouse and keep awake or finds it difficult to feel calm. Abnormal results of orientation are the patient's inability to correctly answer questions pertaining to the patient or to commonly known social information.

(continued)

TABLE 7-1	Mental Health Status Examination *(Continued)*		
AREA OF ASSESSMENT	TYPE OF ASSESSMENT	SUGGESTED METHODS OF ASSESSMENT AND NORMAL PARAMETERS	ALTERATIONS TO NORMAL PARAMETERS
THINKING/CONTENT OF THOUGHT	Subjective assessment of what the patient is thinking and the process the patient uses in thinking.	Formal testing may be undertaken by the psychologist or psychiatrist to determine the patient's general thought content and pattern. Nurses may contribute to the assessment of thought by documenting statements the patient makes regarding daily cares and routines.	Behaviors including flight of ideas, loose associations, phobias, delusions, and obsessions may become apparent. These alterations in "normal" thought processes are defined and discussed in future chapters that relate to specific illnesses.
MEMORY	Subjective assessment of the mind's ability to recall previously known recent and remote (long-term) information.	*Recent memory:* Recall of events that are immediately past or up to within 2 weeks before the assessment. One measurement technique is to verbally list five items. After 1 minute, patient can recall 4–5 of those items. Continue with assessment and at 5 minutes, patient should be able to recall 3–4 of the items. *Remote memory:* Recall of events of the past beyond 2 weeks prior to assessment. Patients are often asked questions pertaining to where they were born, where they went to grade school, and so on.	Inability to accurately perform recent or remote recall exercises within parameters; may indicate symptom of delirium or dementia.
SPEECH AND ABILITY TO COMMUNICATE	Objective and subjective assessment of aspects of patient's use of verbal and nonverbal communication.	Patient can coherently produce words appropriate to age, education, and so on. Rate of speech reflects other psychomotor activity (e.g., faster if patient is agitated). Volume is not too soft or too loud. Stuttering, repetition of words, and words that the patient "makes up" (neologisms) are also assessed.	Limited speech production; rate of speech is inconsistent with other psychomotor activity. Volume is not appropriate to situation (speaks in very loud volume even when asked to speak more quietly).

(continued)

SPEECH AND ABILITY TO COMMUNICATE *(cont'd)*		Stuttering, word repetition, or neologisms may indicate physical or psychological illness.
MOOD AND AFFECT	Subjective and objective assessment of the patient's stated feelings and emotions. Affect measures the outward expression of those feelings.	*Mood* is the stated emotional condition of the patient and should fluctuate to reflect situations as they occur. Facial expression, body language (affect) should match (be congruent with) stated mood. *Affect* should change to fluctuate with the changes in mood.	Mood and affect do not match (e.g., facial expression does not change when stating opposite feelings).
JUDGMENT	Subjective assessment of a patient's ability to make appropriate decisions about his or her situation or to understand concepts.	Give patient a "proverb" to interpret, such as "You can't teach an old dog new tricks." Patient should be able to give some sort of acceptable interpretation such as "old habits are hard to break" or "it is hard to learn something new." *Or* give the patient a situation to solve. For example, ask the patient what he or she would do if a small child were lost in a store. An appropriate response might be "to call the manager" or "to try to calm the child."	Patient cannot interpret the sayings in an acceptable manner. Patient cannot complete problem-solving questions appropriately. The patient might answer very literally. "Dogs can't learn anything when they get old" or "I would go through the child's pockets to see if there were any phone numbers in them."
PERCEPTION	Assesses the way a person experiences reality. Assessment is based on the patient's statements about his or her environment and the behaviors associated with those statements. Nurses and health-team members must document this often-subjective information in objective terms.	All five senses are monitored for interaction with the patient's reality. Patient's *insight* into his or her condition is also assessed.	Presence of hallucinations and illusions. These are discussed further in Chapter 13 (Schizophrenia). Individuals who are not within normal boundaries of judgment or insight will not be able to state understanding of the origin of the illness and the behaviors associated with it.

will seem more individualized to the patient.

EXAMPLE

Standard forms probably say, "Married? _____ YES _____ NO."

Nurse interviewer can ask, "What is your marital status?"

OR

Standard form: "Do you smoke or use alcohol? _____ YES _____ NO."

Nurse interviewer: "I am required to provide you with information about the hospital's policies on the use of tobacco and alcohol." This statement might then be followed by the standard closed-ended question, "Do you use any tobacco or alcohol?"

Questions can be changed from the closed-ended type to open-ended in most cases. Practice and patience on the part of the nurse interviewer will make this a more profitable experience for both the nurse and the patient.

HELPING INTERVIEW

The helping interview is used to determine or isolate a particular concern of the patient and to help the patient learn to help herself or himself (Fig. 7-1). Patients may trust nurses because nurses have built a rapport and are usually more easily accessible than physicians. It is always important to remember, though, to not help to the point of actually interfering with the patient's ability to help herself or himself.

Consider, nurses, that your patient may not be progressing according to a "normal" postoperative course. You notice the patient weeping and sense that a need is not being met. You can use this opportunity and observation to begin obtaining information from the patient that may help explain the delayed postoperative progress.

Guidelines for Nurse-Patient Interviewing

1. *Be honest:* Tell the patient the purpose of the interview.
2. *Be assertive:* If the interview is mandatory (intake, preoperative, and so on), the patient must understand that it is required. Contract for a mutually acceptable time to conduct the interview so that the patient will be prepared.
3. *Be sensitive:* Sometimes the questions are very difficult or embarrassing for the patient to answer. Assure the

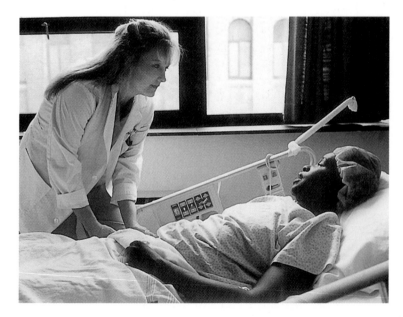

FIGURE 7-1. The helping interview allows the nurse to determine a patient's special needs and concerns. (From Williams, LS, and Hopper, PD: Understanding Medical-Surgical Nursing, 2nd ed. Philadelphia, FA Davis Company, 2003, p. 23. Reprinted with permission.)

patient that, as the nurse, you understand his or her feelings and that the information shared by the patient is part of his or her medical record. Only the patient, the patient's designee, and people who are involved in his or her care-giving will have access to this information.

4. *Use empathy:* Let the patient know that you are interested in what is being said and that, as the nurse, you are there to be helpful. Acknowledge the feelings of the patient but do not judge them.

5. *Use open-ended questions:* Personalize the questions as much as possible. Use this time to discuss and clarify as much information as you can to avoid having to repeat parts of the interview later.

■ STEP 2: DEFINING PATIENT PROBLEMS

Processing the collected data is a function of the registered nurse, according to the ANA. Guidelines for these nursing diagnoses have been published by the North American Nursing Diagnosis Association (**NANDA**). The American Psychiatric Nurses Association (**APNA**) has published a set of nursing diagnoses specific to psychiatric disorders.

In most cases, it is currently the responsibility of the registered nurse to assimilate the data that have been collected and choose one or more potential nursing diagnoses for the patient. The LPN/LVN needs to understand the function of the **nursing diagnosis,** however. In collaborative nursing practice, LPN/LVN-prepared nurses can make suggestions and offer rationales to the RN that may be incorporated into the patient's **plan of care** (Fig. 7-2).

An emerging format for writing a diagnostic statement for a patient's plan of care is the P.E.S. Model. The components for this model are: "P" the problem or need, "E" the etiology or cause, and "S" the signs, symptoms or risk factors. The nurse blends these components into a "neutral" statement that avoids value-laden or judgmental language.

■ STEP 3: PLANNING CARE

The LPN/LVN's role is again as a partner in care planning. The ANA believes that the RN has the primary responsibility for this step

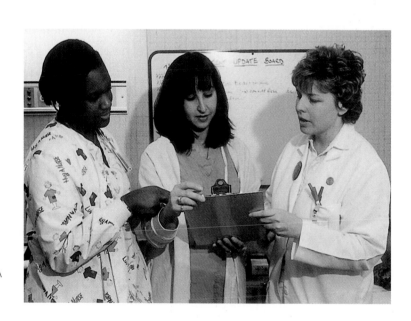

FIGURE 7-2. LPNs collaborating with an RN on a nursing care plan. (From Williams, LS, and Hopper, PD: Understanding Medical-Surgical Nursing, 2nd ed. Philadelphia, FA Davis Company, 2003, p. 5. Reprinted with permission.)

of the nursing process. Planning care involves setting short-term and long-term goals from the patient's perspective, not from the nurse's perspective. It is for this reason that the patient and significant others must be involved in the plan of care. Recovery will happen much more quickly if the patient plays an active role in decision making and does not have the impression that treatment is being done *to* or *for* him or her but rather collaboratively *with* the person.

Prioritizing the goals is the second part of planning care. This is one area in which the patient and the nurse might not see things the same way. Nurses and patients look at the same problem from two different perspectives, and the patient's priority may be quite different from the nurse's priority. Whenever possible, the patient's priority should be considered. When there is a threat to life or health that is a direct response to the patient's priority, however, the nurse must intervene and explain the reason that the patient's wishes will have to wait a while.

The aim of selecting goals that will improve mental health status is to keep the mind-body connection intact. It is estimated that about 95 percent of physical healing is related to a positive mental attitude (PMA). It will be of great help to the patient if the nurse is able to detect alterations in that mental attitude and set goals with the patient to maintain the best outlook and strongest possible effective coping skills.

■ STEP 4: IMPLEMENTATIONS/ INTERVENTIONS

The LPN's role is to assist with identifying and carrying out the specific steps that will help the patient reach the goals. Nurses are able to provide input about new interventions that may be helpful, and the LPN/LVN is often the person who begins to help adapt certain procedures to assist the patient. A nurse may use this opportunity to conduct some new patient teaching or to reinforce prior teaching. Relaying information about **implementation** (putting the care plan into action) and patient progress to the RN will provide the information to allow the team to offer the best possible care for your patient. Nurses also need to understand the rationale (reason) for the implementations that are selected and be prepared to explain them to patients and families.

Many implementations or interventions that are helpful to the patient involve **patient teaching.** Frequently, facilities have special teams or departments to carry out certain teaching, but teaching is becoming a bigger part of a nurse's responsibility. This is true at all levels of nursing preparation. The doctor is still responsible for the initial information giving, but the nurse does the "fine tuning" required to send patients home safely. Nurses teach about medications, central IV lines, adaptive equipment, and anything else the patient requires, not only for the period of hospitalization, but also for the time when he or she leaves the facility. Individual states and facilities set the guidelines regarding teaching responsibilities for doctors and nurses.

Everyone needs a little help to get started with teaching, regardless of what sort of teaching will be done. Like the forms used for the patient interviews, each facility may use standardized classes or teaching sheets. This practice helps ensure that continuity exists in teaching and that the critical information has been given to the patient. There are some legal ramifications to teaching as well. Even with standardized teaching tools, nurses still need to be aware of some principles of teaching and learning. As nurses, you have an advantage in teaching because, with the exception of nursing diagnosis, the same format you learned for nursing process can be used for setting up a teaching plan.

Teaching in any form is most effective when it is started as soon as possible after admission. Nurses teach patients in different ways. Teaching falls under the categories of either formal teaching or informal teaching.

Formal teaching is any situation in which a class is scheduled or a specific objective must be met. The instructor is often a staff nurse who has worked in the specific area being taught. Formal teaching involves a nurse instructor and one or more patients (Fig. 7-3). Usually a preset curriculum is used in all of these classes. The time to teach in the formal setting will most likely be limited by the facility according to staffing needs, because the nurse instructor probably also has a patient assignment. Examples of formal teaching include diabetic teaching and back-care classes.

Informal teaching, or adjunctive teaching, happens anytime, anywhere, whenever the patient needs information. The patient may see you in the hall, or you may notice that he or she is working with the colostomy bag or reading the exercise pamphlet. These are excellent times to reinforce what the patient has learned or to make gentle suggestions for improving his or her technique.

Nurse-teachers need a basic understanding of the principles of teaching and learning. Some of these principles are listed here.

States differ in the role the LPN plays in outcome statements or performing "evaluation" of interventions. In much the same way NANDA developed problem or nursing diagnostic standards, work is being done to standardize outcome statements. Nursing Interventions Classifications (NIC) is a comprehensive standardized language. It provides a number of direct and indirect intervention labels with definitions and possible nursing actions. The interventions address general practice and specialty areas (Doenges and Moorhouse, 2003).

Nursing Outcome Classifications (NOC) is also a standardized language, which provides outcome statements; a set of indicators describing specific patient, caregiver, family, or community states related to the outcome; and a five-point measurement scale to facilitate tracking patients across care settings. It can help demonstrate client progress even when outcomes are not fully met. These also are applicable in all care settings and specialties (Doenges and Moorhouse, 2003).

Not everyone is yet using that model. This text still works in terms of the NANDA format.

PRINCIPLES OF LEARNING

1. Each person learns differently. Some people process information visually, others by hearing, and still others by hands-on (tactile) learning.
2. Each person learns at his or her own pace. The larger the class, the more levels of ability the nurse will have to

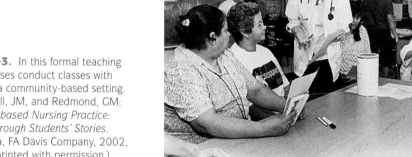

FIGURE 7-3. In this formal teaching session, nurses conduct classes with patients in a community-based setting. (From Sorrell, JM, and Redmond, GM: *Community-based Nursing Practice: Learning Through Students' Stories.* Philadelphia, FA Davis Company, 2002, p. 234. Reprinted with permission.)

work with. Some patients catch on more quickly than others.

3. People learn best when the information is *meaningful* to them. Think of your own education: The things you are interested in are the things you work harder at. Subjects that you don't like seem to be hard or boring, yet they are required for you to graduate. Your patients may not see the importance of the class that they may be required to attend as a criterion for discharge.

4. Learning is most effective when the information is presented in small segments. This may be dictated by the facility, but when the nurse can be flexible, it is best to present only as much as the patient can absorb.

5. *Success breeds success:* Positive reinforcement, in whatever way you can give it, will help your patient succeed at learning the required task. The stronger the positive reinforcement, the greater the learning. Once patients have been successful, they will want to continue to learn.

PRINCIPLES OF TEACHING

1. *Know the patients:* What are their abilities? What is their prior level of knowledge? What are the cultural or language differences in the class you will teach?

2. *Know the material:* It is not as important to give a perfect lecture or demonstration as it is to be able to interpret the questions your patients may have. Sometimes you will need to adapt the curriculum to meet someone's need in the class. A nurse-teacher who is not comfortable with the material will be less helpful to the patient than one who can individualize the curriculum to the needs of the class.

3. *Have a teaching plan:* A good teaching plan will improve a nurse's confidence and delivery of the material. A teaching plan is constructed in much the same way as the nursing process. A very simple format such as APIE for the nursing process may be easily transformed into a teaching format. An example of the APIE format follows.

■ **A** = **Assessment.** What is the need for the teaching? Who are the patients? How much time is available? Assessing the need to teach can be as simple as one or two statements. For example, "Good afternoon, everyone. My name is Sandy. This is the class on colostomy care, and it is open to anyone with a colostomy and their significant others."

■ **P** = **Plan.** In true nursing process, this is often called the goal. Nurse-teachers need to ask themselves a few questions, such as: What do you plan to accomplish in the session? How do you think you will do it? Again, this can be accomplished in one or two statements. For example, "This is the first in a series of three classes, and the task for today is to learn about the different types of appliances and equipment you have available to you."

■ **I** = **Implementation.** This is the step-by-step method nurse-teachers use to accomplish the plan. It is similar to the implementation portion of the nursing process. You will have as many or as few steps as you need. In prepared curricula, the steps are written out, but it may or may not be necessary to perform each step. This will depend on the patient group. Chances are good that a class or skill will never be taught exactly the same way twice. There will, however, be critical items that nurses need to cover with all patients to meet legal and safety issues.

■ **E** = **Evaluation.** In a teaching plan, nurses evaluate the patient's learning as well as the teaching performance. Some questions that nurse-teachers need to reflect on for this part of the teaching plan are: How do you know the patient has grasped the concepts and skills from the class? What do you look for? Do you need to ask for a return demonstration? Does it need to be perfect? How did you do? Did you achieve the plan? Did you have enough time? Too much time? What will you do differently next time? How did your students evaluate the session? Evaluation criteria may change from time to time as well.

4. *Be flexible:* To the extent that the facility's program allows, be familiar enough with the material to be able to build in extra practice time for the tactile learners, extra videos for the visual learners, or time to review verbally for the auditory learners. Be able to teach in several different styles.

5. *Be able to evaluate the learning:* In health teaching in the facility, evaluation can be in the form of a question-answer session, a short quiz, or a return demonstration.

6. *Plan to allow a few minutes after the class for questions:* Even though the nurse may ask for and welcome questions during the session, there are always people who are not comfortable asking questions in a group. These people will want your time in private, so allow some time to clarify their concern at the time or to set up a time to help that person later in the day.

Once the plan has been developed, the nurse needs to think about how to implement the teaching. This requires an idea of some commonly used methods of teaching.

Teachers tend to teach according to the method of learning they prefer. For instance, if nursing students prefer lecture classes, they probably feel most comfortable teaching in a lecture format. If a specific nursing instructor was particularly helpful to you as a student, you may prefer to role-model that teacher's methods when teaching patients. No teaching method is better or worse than any other method. What makes the difference is the learning style of the patients and the rapport that nurses build with them. Because classes in facilities generally have more than one "pupil," the nurse-teacher will need to be able to use different methods of presenting. Because people's personalities are all different, each group will have a different dynamic and each class will be different.

The typical methods used in health teaching are lecture and demonstration.

1. *Lecture:* This is a method designed for information giving. It is very unilateral; the nurse talks, and the patients listen. It is interactive only when there is some form of question-answer period or brainstorming. Lecturing is an excellent method of introducing a topic to patients and giving them some theory. It is a way to explain the significance so the material becomes meaningful.

   In preset programs, the lectures are usually prepared either in text or outline form, so the nurse-teacher has to invest minimal time researching, writing, or setting up for the lectures. Lecture classes may include videos, slides, or charts. Learning from the lecture method is traditionally evaluated through quizzes or question-and-answer sessions. Because not all patient participants are comfortable answering in a group, it may be difficult to assess how much learning each individual achieves.

2. *Demonstation:* Demonstration is an excellent technique to follow in an introductory lecture. For visual and tactile learners, it is a preferred method of learning.

   In prepared programs, the demonstration outline will be prepared. The nurse-teacher is responsible for having the equipment ready for each patient. In diabetic teaching, for example, the nurse needs to have the syringes, sterile saline for injection, gloves, injection pad, and any other equipment that agency uses.

Demonstrations are effective because, after the initial demonstration, the nurse-teacher can go around to each individual and give one-on-one help or redemonstration. This allows the nurse to make more objective assessments of the patient's learning and therefore predict the safety of the patient to perform the technique after discharge. It also allows the nurse to individualize the technique or provide options to the patient.

Evaluation for the method of teaching is usually the redemonstration. The nurse watches each patient perform the technique at a level that is safe for the patient to perform when at home and not under the guidance of the health-care professional.

In American society, it is customary to assess eye contact and to equate eye contact with interest and attentiveness. It is important for the nurse-teacher to remember that this is a cultural behavior. Not all cultures believe that eye contact is a positive thing; indeed, many cultures consider direct meeting of eyes a sign of blatant disrespect for people who are older or in a position of respect or authority. Nurses and teachers are respected in those cultural groups, and it would be a mistake on the part of the nurse to assume that the lack of direct eye contact is a sign of disinterest or disrespect for the material.

3. *Be honest:* Nobody said a nurse must have all the answers. If you as a nurse-teacher do not know something, admit it. Go look it up and either bring the information to the individual who asked or bring it to the next session of the class.

4. *Have fun!* Teaching can be a very rewarding part of nursing. There is no better way to reinforce your own nursing knowledge than to teach it to someone else. It is one way of being generative, and it is one way in which nurses can keep the nursing culture alive.

■ STEP 5: EVALUATING INTERVENTIONS

In this final step of the nursing process, the LPN/LVN plays an assisting role. The LPN/ LVN's observations and documentation about the effect of the interventions on the patient and progress in attaining the goal are of great importance. Accuracy in verbal and written reporting of the patient's progress will help determine whether the interventions are helpful or whether they need to be re-evaluated and changed.

Key Concepts ▪ ▪ ▪

1. Nursing process is an example of collaborative nursing practice. RNs are primarily responsible for the steps of the nursing process; LPN/LVN-prepared nurses assist in data collection, planning, implementing, and evaluating the nursing process.
2. Nurses are conducting more interviewing and teaching on a daily basis. Entry-level nurses need a basic knowledge of both skills. Your state and facility set the guidelines of teaching within the scope of your practice.

3. Nursing process is a helpful tool for preparing a teaching plan.
4. The ANA has set guidelines that dictate the roles of the RN and the LPN/LVN in collaborating in the nursing process.
5. New models for collaborative nursing and nursing outcome statements are being developed.

REFERENCE

Doenges, M.E., and Moorhouse, M.F. (2003). *Application of Nursing Process and Nursing* *Diagnosis: An Interactive Text for Diagnostic Reasoning*, 4th ed. F.A. Davis Company, Philadelphia.

CRITICAL THINKING EXERCISES

1. Your state Nurse Practice Act allows you, the LPN/LVN, to oversee care and function as a charge nurse, as long as a registered nurse is on call. Your medical patient has gone out on a 3-hour pass with relatives and returns to your agency refusing to perform the interventions as stated in the care plan. Your patient is argumentative but answers questions appropriately. Your data collection includes fruity odor on breath, mood swings, and hunger. You need to make corrections or additions to the care plan but are unable to make contact with the RN on call. What would you consider to be appropriate nursing diagnoses? What interventions can you perform and still remain within your state's scope of nursing practice?

2. Assist in preparing a nursing process. With the information given further on, complete the steps of the nursing process as requested. Your instructor may have more examples for you. There can be more than one solution.

3. Pick a student partner to interview. Select any topic and develop a 5-minute interview. Write it twice: once with only closed-ended questions and aggressive statements and once with only open-ended questions and assertive statements. Compare the two versions. How was it different as the interviewer and how was it different for the interviewee?

4. Select a topic to teach the class. This can be any topic you are comfortable with. You have 10 minutes (classroom instructor may choose own time limit) to teach your topic. Develop a teaching plan. Teach your topic. Evaluate your teaching. What would you do differently the next time?

ACTIVITIES

A. INTERVIEW SKILL SHEET

This interview skill is designed to be a hands-on exercise to help learn to develop and execute an effective interview that can be used in future nursing-related interviews. You will be graded in three areas: use of the APIE process format, style and quality of questions/communication techniques, and time factor.

Suggested Grading

1. APIE Format

_____ Assessment statement (1 point possible)

_____ Plan statement (1 point possible)

_____ Implementation (5 points possible)

_____ Evaluation statement (1 point possible)

2. Style and Quality of Questions

_____ Relevant to assessment and goal of interview (4 points possible)

_____ Open-ended questions (4 points possible)

_____ Nonverbal communication reflects verbal communication (4 points possible)

3. Time Factor

_____ (5 minutes allowed, at 1 point per minute = 5 points possible)

B. TEACHING SKILL

OPTION A *Single Teaching*

1. Pick a topic—nursing-related is preferred but can be anything student is comfortable with.

2. Plan for 10 minutes; time is crucial for nurses!

3. Complete teaching plan.

4. Hand in the completed teaching plan as you finish your teaching.

5. If you need something from your instructor, please request it in writing at a time of the instructor's choosing.

Or OPTION B *Team Teaching (Collaborative Exercise)*

1. Sign up in pairs.

2. Pick a topic—nursing-related is preferred but can be anything that team is comfortable with.

3. Plan for 15 minutes; time is crucial for nurses!

4. Complete teaching plan. Work is to be mutually agreed upon as being equally distributed. This is a collaborative project.

5. Contract for the amount of points you are working for if your instructor has assigned points.

6. Hand in the completed teaching plan as you finish your teaching.

7. If you need something from your instructor, please request it in writing at a time of your instructor's choosing.

TEACHING PLAN FORM

Name: _____

Names (if team teaching): _____

_____

Topic: _____

Time Started: _____ Time Stopped: _____ Time Used: _____

Assessment:

Plan:

Implementation:

Evaluation:

Suggested Grading (possible 10 points total)

Assessment:	0–2
Plan:	0–2
Implementation:	0–2
Evaluation:	0–2
Time:	0–2

(10 minutes for single teaching; 15 minutes for team teaching)
Team teaching only: We are contracting for ____ points.
We have agreed that the foregoing expectations were completed and that the work was equally distributed.

Points Earned: _____

C. NURSING PROCESS PAPER

Student Name: _____

Directions: You will be assigned a case study. You will have *minimal* information about the client in the case study. Treat the case study as if the client were in your clinic and you were compiling information to collaborate with the RN in charge. From the information presented in your case study, write your nursing process paper. Use a separate sheet of paper. There will be enough information to fill in all the blanks that follow. There is more than one right solution to the case study.

 I. Present the social history (2 points)

 II. Present the medical history (past and/or present) (2 points)

III. Describe the behaviors you see (4 points)

IV. Define previous behaviors in nursing diagnosis terms (must be complete nursing diagnosis) (2 points)

V. Write a care plan proposal for the two previous nursing diagnoses (10 points)

Complete this chart, as shown earlier.

1. PROBLEM	GOAL	NURSING INTERVENTIONS
		1.
		2.
		3.
		4.
		5.

2. PROBLEM	GOAL	NURSING INTERVENTIONS
		1.
		2.
		3.
		4.
		5.

VI. Describe your *feelings* about caring for a patient showing this behavior. How will you need to adapt or change your communication skills in order to be therapeutic for this patient? (5 points)

    Two or more spelling and/or documentation errors = −1 point (TOTAL 25 points)

CASE STUDY 1: MRS. PENN

Mrs. Penn, age 44, is admitted to the hospital for diagnostic studies. Her physician suspects peptic ulcer as the cause of her symptoms. At the time of her admission, Mrs. Penn appears pale, underweight, and in generally poor health. Diagnostic tests ordered by her physician include a complete blood count, gastric analysis, and an upper gastrointestinal (GI) series.

The evening before the gastric analysis is scheduled, you tell Mrs. Penn that, in preparation for the x-ray examination, she will not be allowed to eat or drink anything after midnight. She becomes very apprehensive and tells you she has never heard of a GI series. She asks what they will do to her in the x-ray department and why she has to have the test.

Mrs. Penn tells you that she has recently been divorced from an alcoholic husband and she wonders if the emotional upsets she has suffered have any bearing on her present physical condition.

Mrs. Penn's physician initially decided to treat the ulcer medically. He ordered a bland diet and Maalox every other hour. Because of continued tension in Mrs. Penn's daily life and her obvious inability to stay within the limits of her diet even in the hospital, the doctor has now decided to perform a subtotal gastrectomy, vagotomy, and jejunostomy. Before her surgery, a nasogastric tube will be inserted and gastric decompression will be accomplished by attaching the tube to suction.

CASE STUDY 2: JAKE

Jake, a computer programmer, is 36 years old, married, and the father of twin sons, who are 3 years old. Jake has been moody for the past few months, and his wife states that he has become withdrawn and does not volunteer to spend time with his sons. "I don't understand it. He used to love to take the boys out with him when he went target shooting and fishing. Now he just watches television." Jake is not volunteering any information to you at this time, except to tell you that he thinks "The world would be better off if I weren't here. My wife has a good job. She and the boys would be just fine." As you continue to assess Jake's condition, you find out that he was laid off from work 1 month ago in a downsizing move by his company. He did not tell his wife because he thought he could find another job. He finds that he is either overqualified or underqualified for the jobs he has applied for. "I am just worthless," he says. "I wish I were dead."

CASE STUDY 3: MR. FEAR

Mr. Fear is a 72-year-old man with chronic obstructive lung disease/chronic obstructive pulmonary disease (COLD/COPD). He has been hospitalized for an exacerbation of the illness. In addition, he has asthma and has been a heavy smoker since "the war."

Mrs. Fear has been at his bedside during this hospitalization. She is his primary caregiver. Neither of them wants Mr. Fear to be "put in a home." Mrs. Fear expects to take her husband home. She seems attentive and asks many questions. She seems reluctant to touch the tissues, which are laden with nasal secretions. She becomes visibly upset when she helps her husband with his bronchial secretions. She tells you that she has heard "people can get AIDS from this," and she points to the sputum in the tissue she holds.

After 10 days of treatment, the doctor has ordered Mr. Fear's discharge to his home. As they are checking out, Mrs. Fear says, "I don't want to take him home yet. I don't think he should leave here."

CASE STUDY 4: MARK

Mark is a 15-year-old student who has recently quit attending his high school classes. Mark has always been a straight-A student who participated in many social and athletic activities at his school.

Today, Mark's friend Tony brings Mark to the clinic that is part of your community's hospital. Tony tells you that Mark "got in with a bad group. He's been doin' the stuff real bad. He's been doin' the needles and the smokin'. He's been with me for two days, man, and he's real sick. Help him, man . . . ."

You and the physician undertake an assessment of Mark and find that he has yellowing of his sclera. He has a fruity odor on his breath and is vomiting copiously. Mark's level of consciousness is guarded; he is in and out of coherence and is not a reliable source of information about himself at this time.

The physician notifies Mark's parents and explains that Mark may have several conditions, including but not limited to serum hepatitis.

Meanwhile, you continue to admit Mark to the hospital for further testing and medical care. He is placed in enteric isolation as a precaution. An IV is started and you begin to explain the hospital routines to Mark. After you tell him that he must remain in his room for now and that his visitors will be limited during the time of the isolation precautions, he becomes angry. He conveys to you that this is "an invasion of his privacy" and that "you nurses are all part of the conspiracy."

D. MENTAL STATUS EXAM

Clinical Activity

1. If you are at a point in your curriculum that places you in clinical care, complete a simple mental status exam. You can perform this on any patient. You may use a generic form used by the clinical site, or you may ask the questions in your own words. You must address all eight areas of the exam in some way:

   ■ Level of awareness/orientation
   ■ Appearance and behavior
   ■ Speech/communication
   ■ Affect
   ■ Thinking
   ■ Perception
   ■ Memory
   ■ Judgment

2. If you can, and if your clinical affiliates will allow, arrange to follow with a nurse from the mental health unit. Write a summary of the experience. Include observations of the nurse-patient relationship, such as communication, rapport, patient responses, and so on.

TEST QUESTIONS ■ ■ ■

MULTIPLE CHOICE QUESTIONS

1. The nursing process is a method for:
   A. Systematic organization and implementation of patient care
   B. Documenting patient needs
   C. Differentiating RN role from LPN/LVN role
   D. Data collection

2. You are assisting in collecting data on a new patient to your unit. The physician suspects alcohol abuse. You want to learn the patient's history and frequency of alcohol use. Your best choice for collecting these data might be:
   A. "Do you use alcohol?"
   B. "How often do you get drunk?"
   C. "How many times a week would you say you drink alcohol?"
   D. "Why do you use alcohol? It's bad for you."

3. When conducting patient teaching, the best method to evaluate the success of the patient is:
   A. Lecture
   B. Redemonstration
   C. Implementation
   D. Assessment

4. The mental status exam takes place in what part of the nursing process?
   A. Assessment
   B. Plan
   C. Implementation
   D. Evaluation

MATCHING QUESTIONS
Directions
Choose all the statements in Column B that apply to the component of nursing process in Column A. Each answer will only be used once.

COLUMN A	COLUMN B
1. Nursing Process	A. Formula to help nurses organize and implement care in a systematic, universal way
2. Nanda	
3. PES	
4. NIC	B. Putting the plan of care into action
5. NOC	C. Five-point measurement scale to facilitate tracking patients across care settings
6. Data Collection	
7. Nursing Diagnosis	
8. Planning Care	D. Address general practice and specialty areas
9. Interventions or Implementation	E. Intake interview
	F. Specific actions

G. Involves setting short- and long-term goals
H. Method of writing a diagnostic statement that involves a problem, cause and symptom, or risk factor
I. Standardized language providing outcome statements and indicators describing specific conditions related to outcome
J. Teaching
K. Mental Status Exam
L. May demonstrate client progress even if outcomes are not fully met
M. Tool used in all areas and levels of nursing
N. General classifications of potential patient problems, published by the North American Nursing Diagnosis Association
O. Comprehensive standardized language
P. Provides direct and indirect intervention labels with definitions and possible nursing actions
Q. Applicable in all care settings and specialties.
R. North American Nursing Diagnosis Association
S. Patient and significant others should be involved
T. Theory is recovery will happen quicker if the patient plays an active role

CHAPTER

8

Treating Mental Health Alterations

Kathy Neeb, RN, BA and Brenda Agee, RN, MSN

Learning Objectives ■ ■ ■

1. Describe a therapeutic milieu.
2. Identify classifications, uses, actions, side effects, and nursing, as well as considerations for selected classifications of psychoactive medications.
3. Describe psychoanalysis.
4. Describe behavior modification.
5. Describe rational-emotive therapy.
6. Describe humanistic/person-centered therapy.
7. Identify the nurse's role in counseling.
8. Describe three types of counseling.
9. Describe concepts of group therapy.
10. Describe electroconvulsive therapy and the nurse's role in it.
11. Define crisis.
12. Identify the five phases of crisis and the nurse's role in them.
13. Define and discuss terrorism as it relates to mental health in today's world.

Key Terms ■ ■ ■

- Antidepressants
- Antimanic agents
- Antiparkinson agents
- Antipsychotics
- Behavior modification
- Cognitive
- Counseling
- Crisis
- ECT
- Hypnosis
- Milieu
- Monoamine oxidase inhibitors
- Person-centered
- Psychoanalysis
- Psychopharmacology
- Rational-emotive
- Stimulants

People who have alterations to their mental health have special needs related to treating those alterations. When emotional health is threatened, many other daily activities can be altered as well. **Cognitive** ability (the ability to think rationally and to process those thoughts) can be decreased. Emotional responses can be decreased or even absent in some conditions. These alterations can be extremely frightening to a patient who may already feel unable to control his or her life; this can lead to a deepening of the mental disorder or even the development of another disorder.

Accurate and timely observations and data collection by the nurse may be the instrument that keeps the patient from traveling a swift downward spiral. Hospitalized patients can develop a sense of helplessness and hopelessness about themselves and their conditions.

Nurses can be the tools that help the patient regain control. You may be observing your patient's treatments and therapies, or you may be an active part of them. Either way, as a nurse, you will be making observations about the patient's reactions and participating in the plan of care. This chapter discusses some of the more frequently used methods for treating alterations in mental health.

■ MILIEU

One of the areas that nurses have some control over is the therapeutic environment itself. In mental health terminology, this therapeutic environment is called the **milieu,** or therapeutic milieu. It is believed that the environment has an effect on behavior. Think about it for a minute: Have you ever gone to an event such as a concert or a ball game that you may not have felt excited about? How long after you arrived at the event did you begin screaming or singing along and generally getting into the spirit of things?

The milieu is the setting that will provide safety and help during the patient's stay. The milieu, or milieu therapy, is intended to combine the social environment and the therapeutic environment. In that way, every contact between nurse and patient gives the opportunity for a therapeutic interaction. The milieu must be comfortable and safe. Patients need to feel accepted as they learn new behaviors. It is best to have the milieu as appropriate to the situation as possible. Obviously, nurses cannot move walls and change decorating themes in the hospital, but we can allow the patient to choose the room for therapy or move to an area where the patient is more comfortable. If the patient is on a psychiatric unit rather than a medical or surgical unit, he or she is usually allowed to walk from area to area on the unit. A nurse can keep the area calm and quiet and arrange for roommate changes if needed. There are many things a nurse can and must do to maintain a milieu that is conducive to a patient's progress. As the patient progresses, the milieu will be changed to allow the patient to take on more responsibility.

■ PSYCHOPHARMACOLOGY

Since the introduction of the phenothiazines in the 1950s, the number of medications available for treating patients who have mental health disorders, comprising the field of **psychopharmacology,** has increased greatly. The reasons for using medications are twofold: First, the medications control symptoms, thus helping the patient to feel more comfortable emotionally. Second, the medications are usually used in connection with some other type of therapy. The patient is generally more receptive and able to focus on therapy if medications are also used. Several classifications of psychoactive drugs are discussed below; however, there are far too many drugs to discuss individually in this text. In most cases, only the most commonly seen information is presented about a medication. Nurses find it necessary to consult a pharmacology or drug reference book for more specific information before administering these medications or instructing patients on their use.

ANTIPSYCHOTICS (NEUROLEPTICS/MAJOR TRANQUILIZERS)

Action: Typical antipsychotic agents act on the central nervous system (CNS). Their main action is to block the dopamine receptors. Dopamine is a neurochemical that our bodies contain naturally. However, if it is overproduced or utilized incorrectly, it can cause someone to exhibit psychotic behavior. Atypical antipsychotic agents block both serotonin (a neurochemical) and dopamine.

Uses: Treatment of schizophrenia and other acute or chronic psychotic behavior that is violent or potentially violent. Typical antipsychotic agents treat the positive symptoms of schizophrenia such as hallucinations, delusions, and suspiciousness. Atypical antipsychotic agents also reduce the negative symptoms of schizophrenia such as flat affect, social withdrawal, and difficulty with abstract thinking.

Side Effects: **Antipsychotics** have many unpleasant side effects. Sometimes people are reluctant to take these medications because they are afraid that the side effects will be worse than the illness. Some of these side effects are certain blood dyscrasias, photosensitivity (especially with Thorazine), darkening of the skin from increased pigmentation, neuroleptic malignant syndrome (NMS), and a group of side effects called extrapyramidal side effects (EPSEs). There is less risk of EPSEs with the atypical agents, but early observation and reporting of any possible EPSEs is crucial to minimizing these effects on the patient. The EPSEs include:

1. *Drug-induced Parkinsonism (pseudoparkinsonism).* Symptoms appear 1 to 8 weeks after the patient begins the medication. The major symptom is akinesia, manifested as shuffling gait, drooling, fatigue, mask-like facial expression, tremors, and muscle rigidity.

2. *Akathisia.* Symptoms appear 2 to 10 weeks after the patient starts taking the medication. Symptoms are agitation and motor restlessness, and they seem to appear more frequently in women. There is no absolute reason for this, but it is suggested that it may be due to hormonal interaction with the medication.

3. *Dystonia.* Symptoms appear 1 to 8 weeks after the patient starts taking the medication. Symptoms manifest as bizarre distortions or involuntary movements of any muscle group. Tongue, eyes, face, neck, or any larger muscle mass can become tightened into an unnatural position or have irregular spastic movements.

4. *Tardive dyskinesia (TD).* Symptoms appear within 1 to 8 weeks after the patient starts taking the medication. The frequently seen manifestations are rhythmic, involuntary movements that look like chewing, sucking, or licking motions. Frowning and blinking constantly are also common. TD is irreversible.

   Neuroleptic malignant syndrome (NMS) is an uncommon but potentially fatal reaction to treatment with neuroleptic medications. Symptoms include muscle rigidity, hyperpyrexia, fluctuations in blood pressure, and altered level of consciousness. Early recognition and immediate medical care is important.

Contraindications: Antipsychotics should be used carefully in patients who are hypersensitive to medications or who have brain damage or blood dyscrasias.

Nursing Considerations: Careful teaching by doctors and nurses can help the patient to understand that these are very strong medications. The possibility of seizures increases in patients who require antipsychotic medications. Observe for any sign of EPSEs or NMS and carefully monitor blood work for abnormal results. Careful instruction to the patient and family regarding wearing a wide-brimmed hat, covering all exposed skin, and using a sunscreen when in the sun will help lessen chances of the patient's suffering sunburn, especially if the patient is using Thorazine. Body temperature is harder to maintain; therefore, temperature extremes should be avoided. Patients should be taught to avoid alcohol. Other medications, including over-the-counter (OTC) products, should not be taken without doctor approval. It is important to instruct the patient not to alter the dose without first discussing it with the doctor.

This classification of medication should be discontinued slowly. If medication is ordered once daily, teaching patients to take the medication 1 to 2 hours before going to bed works well and promotes sleep. Antacids decrease the absorption of antipsychotics, so these types of medications should be taken 1 to 2 hours *after* oral administration of antipsychotics.

Commonly Used Antipsychotic Agents: Typical: Thorazine (chlorpromazine), Haldol (haloperidol), Stelazine (trifluoperazine), Mellaril (trioridazine), Loxitane (loxapine), and Prolixin (fluphenazine); Atypical: Risperdal (risperidone), Clozaril (clozapine), Seroquel (quetiapine), Zyprexa (olanzapine), Geodon (ziprasidone), and Abilify (aripiprazole)

ANTIPARKINSON AGENTS (ANTICHOLINERGICS)

Action: Inhibit the action of acetylcholine. Acetylcholine increases as dopamine decreases at its receptor sites (the cholinergic effect). When the amount of acetylcholine available to interact with dopamine is decreased, there is a better balance between the two neurochemicals, and the symptoms of parkinsonism decrease.

Uses: Help decrease the effects of drug-induced and non-drug-induced symptoms of parkinsonism.

Side Effects: Blurred vision, dry mouth, dizziness, drowsiness, confusion, tachycardia, urinary retention, constipation, and changes in blood pressure.

Contraindications: Patients with known hypersensitivity should not use these medications. People with glaucoma, myasthenia gravis, peptic ulcers, prostatic hypertrophy, or urine retention should not take these medications. These agents should be avoided in children under the age of 12 years and used with caution with the elderly.

Nursing Considerations: Monitor blood pressure carefully (at least every 4 hours when beginning treatment). Encourage using hard, sugarless candy to combat the effects of dry mouth.

Commonly Used Antiparkinson Agents: Akineton (biperiden), Cogentin (benztropine), Artane (trihexyphenidyl), Mirapex (pramipexole), Benadryl (diphenhydramine)

ANTIANXIETY AGENTS (ANXIOLYTICS/MINOR TRANQUILIZERS)

Action: Depress activities of the cerebral cortex.

Uses: Decrease the effects of stress, anxiety, and mild depression. They can be used preoperatively to help promote sedation.

Side Effects: Can cause physical and psychological dependence. Other side effects include drowsiness, lethargy, fainting, postural hypotension, nausea, and vomiting. If discontinued abruptly, severe side effects, including nausea, hypotension, and fatal grand mal seizures can occur anywhere from 12 hours to 2 weeks after the drug is stopped.

Contraindications: Patients with known hypersensitivity should not use these medications. People with a history of chemical dependency are not good candidates for this classification of drug because of the potential for addiction.

Nursing Considerations: Nurses must monitor blood pressure before and after giving this medication. When possible, these types of drugs should be given at bedtime to help promote sleep, minimize side effects, and allow a more normal daytime routine. Administer intramuscular (IM) dosages deeply and slowly into large muscle masses. The Z-track method of IM administration is preferred. It is important to teach the patient and family that it is not safe for the patient to drive or use alcohol while using this classification of medication. The patient should rise slowly from sitting or lying positions to prevent a sudden drop in blood pressure.

Commonly Used Antianxiety Agents: Xanax (alprazolam), BuSpar (buspirone), Librium (chlordiazepoxide), Serax (oxazepam), Klonopin (clonazepam), Valium (diazepam), Ativan (lorazepam), and Atarax or Vistaril (hydroxyzine)

ANTIDEPRESSANTS (MOOD ELEVATORS)

Antidepressants have several subdivisions. Different drug references subdivide the antidepressants differently. There are similarities and differences among the subgroups.

Selective Serotonin Reuptake Inhibitors (SSRIs) (Bicyclic Antidepressants)

Action: Increase the availability of serotonin, which is decreased in the brains of depressed individuals.

Uses: Treatment of depression, anxiety, obsessive disorders, impulse control disorders.

Side Effects: Dependence, suicidal tendencies, sedation, dry mouth, agitation, postural hypotension, headache, arthralgia, dizziness, insomnia, confusion, and tremors.

Contraindications: Patients with known hypersensitivity should not use these medications. People using MAOIs or within 14 days of being taken off MAOIs should not use these medications. People using certain herbal preparations including but not limited to St. John's wort, ginseng, brewer's yeast, vitamin B6, and ginkgo biloba should not use SSRIs without consulting their physician.

Note: In October of 2004, it became mandatory for producers of SSRIs to place a boxed-in warning on the medication container cautioning about the danger of increased chance for suicidal tendencies, especially in children and adolescents, while taking this medication.

Nursing Considerations: Do not abruptly discontinue the medication. Caution should be used with driving or activities that require alertness. Alcohol and CNS depressants should be avoided. Hard, sugarless candy can be used for dry mouth. The patient should change positions slowly to avoid a sudden drop in blood pressure. Monitor the patient for suicide ideation.

Commonly Used SSRI Agents: Celexa (citalopram), Prozac (fluoxetine), Zoloft (sertraline), Luvox (fluvoxamine), Paxil (paroxetine), Lexapro (escitalopram)

Tricyclic Antidepressants

Action: These drugs increase the level of serotonin and norepinephrine, thereby increasing the ability of the nerve cells to pass information to each other. Patients with depressive disorders generally have decreased amounts of these two neurochemicals.

Uses: Treatment of symptoms of depression, including (but not limited to) sleep disturbances, sexual function disturbances, changes in appetite, and cognitive changes.

Side Effects: Sedation, lethargy, dry mouth, constipation, tachycardia, postural hypotension, urine retention, blurred vision, weight gain, and changes in blood glucose.

Contraindications: Patients with known hypersensitivity should not use these medications. Women who are pregnant or breastfeeding and individuals with kidney disease, liver disease, or a recent myocardial infarction should not take these medications. Anyone who has asthma, seizure disorders, schizophrenia, benign prostatic hypertrophy, or alcoholism should use tricyclic antidepressants with extreme caution.

Nursing Considerations: Patients should not stop using these medications abruptly. Medications (including over-the-counter medications such as cold preparations) that contain antihistamines, alcohol, sodium bicarbonate, benzodiazepines, and narcotic analgesics can increase the effects of tricyclic antidepressants. Nicotine, barbiturates, and the hypnotic chloral hydrate decrease the effect of the tricyclic antidepressant.

Commonly Used Tricyclic Antidepressant Agents Elavil (amitriptyline), Tofranil (imipramine), Pamelor or Aventyl (nortriptyline), Asendin (amoxapine), Norpramin (desipramine), Anafranil (clomipramine), Sinequan (doxepin)

Tetracyclic Antidepressants (Heterocyclic Antidepressants)

The actions, uses, contraindications, side effects, and nursing considerations for the tetracyclic antidepressants are similar for those of the SSRIs and tricyclic antidepressants.

Commonly Used Tetracyclic Agents: Ludiomil (maprotiline), Wellbutrin or Zyban (bupropion), Remeron (mirtazapine), Desyrel (trazodone)

Serotonin Norepinephrine Reuptake Inhibitors (SNRIs)

Action: Increases the availability of serotonin and norepinephrine, which are decreased in the brains of depressed individuals.

The uses, contraindications, side effects, and nursing considerations for the SNRI antidepressants are similar for those of the SSRIs.

Commonly Used SNRI Agents: Serzone (nafazodone), Effexor (venlafaxine)

Monoamine Oxidase Inhibitors (MAOIs)

Action: Prevents the metabolism of neurotransmitters by an enzyme, monoamine oxidase. Too much monoamine oxidase can lead to destructive, psychotic behaviors.

Uses: Generally used for patients with varied types of depression who have not been helped by other antidepressants.

Side Effects: Postural hypotension, photosensitivity (sunburn potential), headache, dizziness, memory impairment, tremors, fatigue, insomnia, weight gain, and sexual dysfunction.

Contraindications: Patients with known hypersensitivity should not use these medications. MAOI medications should be given carefully to patients who have asthma, congestive heart failure, cerebrovascular disease, glaucoma, blood pressure conditions, schizophrenia, alcoholism, liver or kidney disorders, or severe headaches, as well as those who are over 60 years old or pregnant. There are many drug-drug interactions that may occur if MAOI agents are combined with other medications. Other prescriptions and over-the-counter products should be taken only after consulting a doctor or a pharmacist.

Nursing Considerations: Teach patient to avoid foods containing the amino acid tyramine, a precursor of norepinephrine, while taking these medications. MAOIs block the metabolism of tyramine, resulting in increased norepinephrine. A hypertensive crisis may occur. Foods containing significant amounts of tyramine include

- Aged cheese (cheddar, Swiss, provolone, blue cheese, parmesan)
- Avocados (guacamole)
- Yogurt, sour cream
- Chicken and beef livers, pickled herring, corned beef
- Bean pods
- Bananas, raisins, figs
- Smoked and processed meat (salami, pepperoni, and bologna)
- Yeast supplements
- Chocolate
- Meat tenderizers (MSG), soy sauce
- Beer, red wines, caffeine

Commonly Used MAOI Agents: Nardil (phenelzine), Parnate (tranylcypromine), Marplan (isocarboxazid)

NURSING CONSIDERATIONS FOR ALL ANTIDEPRESSANTS

Reinforce the teaching that these medications take 2 to 3 weeks to become effective. Encourage patients to continue taking the medication during this time, although they may not feel any change in their mood right away. All antidepressant medications should be tapered gradually rather than abruptly discontinuing to prevent withdrawal symptoms. It is imperative that all patients receiving antidepressant medications be monitored for suicide potential throughout treatment.

Alternative Treatments for Depression

People are seeking alternatives to the prescription antidepressant drugs available through traditional American medicine. Some reasons they seek alternatives include cultural preferences, cost of medications, insurance issues, and unpleasant side effects they may experience with the medications they have used.

One such alternative is a chemical called SAMe ("sammy"). SAMe is a combination of an amino acid (methionine) and ATP. It is used as an antidepressant and sold in the United States as a dietary supplement. Other alternative forms of therapy are explored in Appendix F.

The nurse's role is the same with these alternative choices as it is with prescription medications. Nurses must encourage their patients to discuss the use of supplements with their physicians and to provide as much information as possible to allow the patient to make safe, informed choices.

ANTIMANIC AGENTS (MOOD STABILIZING AGENTS)

Lithium carbonate was the drug of choice for treatment and management of bipolar mania for many years. In recent years, several other medications have become treatment options. Other medications being used as mood stabilizers are classified as anticonvulsants or calcium channel blockers.

Lithium Carbonate

Action: The exact action of lithium is not completely known at this time. It is not metabolized by the body. One hypothesis about the action of lithium is that there seems to be a connection between lithium and constancy of sodium concentration, which might help regulate and moderate information along the nerve cells, thus preventing mood swings. Another possibility is that lithium increases the reuptake of norepinephrine and serotonin, thereby decreasing hyperactivity.

Uses: For the manic phase of bipolar depression and sometimes for other depressive or schizoaffective disorders.

Side Effects: Side effects can be numerous. Some of the more common ones are thirst and dry mouth, nausea and vomiting, abdominal pain, and fatigue.

Contraindications: Consistent with those of the other categories listed earlier.

Nursing Considerations: Encourage patient to keep all appointments for blood work and evaluation of drug effectiveness. Therapeutic serum levels are 0.6 to

1.5 mEq/L. Symptoms of lithium toxicity begin to appear at blood levels greater than 1.5 mEq/L. Signs of toxicity include severe diarrhea, persistent nausea and vomiting, muscle weakness, tremors, blurred vision, slurred speech, and seizures. Lithium crosses the placenta and milk barriers, so each woman of childbearing years may need to be counseled regarding the effects of this drug on her pregnancy. Dehydration and fevers can cause increased danger of toxicity. Adequate fluid and sodium intake are essential. Patients should not decrease their dietary intake of salt (unless instructed to do so by the physician) and should be taught to inform the physician immediately if they are ill. Hard, sugarless candy can be helpful to decrease dry mouth and thirst.

Commonly Used Antimanic Agents: Eskalith, Lithonate, Lithane, Lithobid (all are lithium carbonate)

Anticonvulsants

Action: The action is not clear.

Uses: To stabilize the manic episodes in bipolar disorders.

Side Effects: Nausea, vomiting, indigestion, drowsiness, dizziness, prolonged bleeding, headache, confusion.

Contraindications: Patients with known hypersensitivity should not use these medications. People with bone marrow suppression should not take these medications. Caution should be used with renal, cardiac, or liver disease. Caution should also be used with the elderly and children.

Nursing Considerations: Do not stop the medication abruptly. The medication should be tapered when therapy is discontinued. Teach patient to avoid alcohol. Nonprescription medications should not be used without doctor approval. Do not drive or operate dangerous equipment until the effects of the medication are known.

Commonly Used Anticonvulsants: Tegretol (carbamazepine), Depakene (valproic acid), Depakote (divalproex)

Calcium Channel Blockers

The action, uses, side effects, contraindications, and nursing considerations are similar to anticonvulsants. Postural hypotension and bradycardia are additional side effects. The patient should rise slowly from sitting or lying positions to prevent a sudden drop in blood pressure.

Commonly used calcium channel blockers: Calan or Isoptin (verapamil)

STIMULANTS

Stimulants are readily available over the counter as well by prescription. They are found over the counter in diet preparations, pills to prevent sleep, in cigarettes, and in beverages such as coffee and soda. They are used medically to combat narcolepsy and attention deficit disorder in children.

Amphetamines are one type of stimulant. Amphetamines can be abused, and they have many "street names," including "uppers," "speed," and "bennies." The ease with which they are available should not diminish the power and potential danger of the drug.

Action: Direct stimulation of the central nervous system (CNS).

Uses: Promote alertness, diminish appetite, and combat narcolepsy (sleep disorder related to abnormal rapid eye movement sleep). Used in the treatment of attention deficit hyperactive disorder (ADHD).

Side Effects: Increased or irregular heart rates, hypertension, hyperactivity, dry mouth, hand tremor, rapid speech, diaphoresis, confusion, depression, seizures, suicidal ideation, and insomnia.

Contraindications: Patients with known hypersensitivity should not use these medications. Pregnant or lactating women should not use this classification of drugs. Because these are chemicals that increase stimulation of the CNS and respiratory systems, they should not be given to people who are alcoholic, manic, or who display suicidal or homicidal ideations. People who have heart disease or glaucoma also should not use these drugs because of the potential dilating effect of the medications. Elderly people and patients who have diabetes, hypertension, or other cardiovascular conditions should use these drugs cautiously and with careful monitoring.

Nursing Considerations: Tolerance and physical and psychological dependence can occur with CNS stimulants, especially with long-term use. Do not discontinue medication abruptly. Monitor for suicide potential. Diabetic patients who take amphetamines should be informed that the amphetamines may cause changes in their insulin requirements. These medications can also cause changes in judgment; therefore, people should be counseled to use extreme caution when driving or operating equipment and should avoid these activities if possible. Encourage frequent rinsing of mouth with water or use of hard, sugarless candy to relieve dry mouth.

Commonly Used Stimulant Agents: Dexedrine (dextroamphetamine), Desoxyn (methamphetamine), Ritalin (methylphenidate), Cylert (pemoline)

Table 8-1 summarizes the medications previously mentioned.

■ PSYCHOTHERAPIES

Psychotherapy is the term used to describe the form of treatment chosen by the psychologist or psychiatrist to treat an individual. The goals of psychotherapy are to

1. Decrease the patient's emotional discomfort.

2. Increase the patient's social functioning.

3. Increase the ability of the patient to behave or perform in a manner appropriate to the situation.

These goals are achieved in a variety of ways including therapeutic relationships, open and honest venting of feelings and thoughts, allowing the patient to practice new coping skills, helping the patient to gain insight into the problem, and consistency in the team approach to the patient's care and treatment. Positive reinforcement of progress is encouraged.

Several types of therapy are typically used. Nurses may or may not be actively involved in the therapy, but, to provide continuity in the care of the patient, they must understand the basic ideas of the types of therapy.

PSYCHOANALYSIS

Psychoanalysis is the form of therapy that originated from the theory of Sigmund Freud. In psychoanalysis, the focus is on the cause of the problem, which is buried somewhere in the unconscious. The therapist tries to take the patient into the past in an effort to determine where the problem began. Chances are, according to Freud, that it had something to do with poor parent-child relationships and ineffective psychosexual development.

It is typical for the psychoanalyst to be positioned at the head of the patient and slightly behind, so that the patient cannot see the therapist. This decreases any kind of nonverbal communication between the two people. The patient is typically on the "couch," relaxed, and ready to focus on the therapist's instructions.

Some of the techniques used in psychoanalysis are as follows.

Free Association

In free association, the patient is allowed to say whatever comes to mind in response to a word that is given by the therapist. For example, the therapist might say "mother"

TABLE 8-1 ■ *Medications Used for Alterations in Mental Health*

CLASSIFICATIONS	COMMON TRADE NAMES	USES	SIDE EFFECTS	NURSING CONSIDERATIONS	PATIENT TEACHING
ANTIPSYCHOTICS	Thorazine, Haldol, Mellaril, Prolixin, Risperdal, Clozaril, Zyprexa, Seroquel	Treatment of schizophrenia and violent or potentially violent psychotic behavior	Blood dyscrasias, photosensitivity, darkening of skin, neuroleptic malignant syndrome (NMS), and extrapyramidal side effects (EPSEs): parkinsonism, akathisia, dystonia, tardive dyskinesia.	Observe for any sign of EPSEs or NMS. Monitor blood work for any abnormality. Discontinue slowly. Antacids will decrease absorption of antipsychotics.	Wear a wide-brimmed hat, cover all exposed skin, and use a sunscreen when in the sun. Avoid alcohol. Use other medications only with doctor approval. Avoid temperature extremes. Do not alter dose before discussing it with the doctor. Take antacids 1–2 hours after oral doses of antipsychotics.
ANTIPARKINSON AGENTS	Cogentin, Artane, Akineton	Decrease the effects of drug-induced and non-drug-induced symptoms of parkinsonism	Blurred vision, dry mouth, dizziness, drowsiness, confusion, tachycardia, urinary retention, constipation, and changes in blood pressure.	Should be avoided in children under 12 years of age. Use with caution with the elderly. Blood pressure should be monitored carefully.	Use hard, sugarless candy to combat the effects of dry mouth. Increase dietary roughage to maintain bowel functioning. May cause drowsiness, so should not drive or operate equipment until the response to medication is established.
ANTIANXIETY DRUGS	Xanax, BuSpar, Valium, Ativan, Librium, Klonopin	Decrease the effects of stress or mild depression without causing sedation	*Can cause physical and psychological dependence,* drowsiness, lethargy, fainting,	Administer intramuscular (IM) dosages deeply, slowly, and into large muscle masses. Z-track	Teach the patient and family that it is not safe to drive or use alcohol while using this classification of medication.

(continued)

ANTIANXIETY DRUGS *(cont'd)*			postural hypotension, nausea, and vomiting.	method of IM administration is preferred. Discontinue slowly.	Instruct to change positions slowly.
ANTIDEPRESSANTS	Elavil, Tofranil, Pamelor, Prozac, Zoloft, Celexa, Paxil, Asendin, Ludiomil, Parnate, Nardil, Marplan	Treatment of depression and some anxiety disorders	Dependence, drowsiness, dry mouth, agitation, postural hypotension, vertigo, constipation, urine retention, weight gain, blurred vision, photosensitivity, and suicidal tendencies.	Encourage patients to continue taking the medication during this time, although they may not feel any change in their mood for up to 3 weeks after beginning the medication. Discontinue slowly. Observe for suicidal ideation.	Instruct to protect from sunburn. Teach to change positions slowly. Teach diet restrictions with MAOIs. Use other medications only with doctor approval.
ANTIMANIC AGENTS	Lithium, Tegretol, Depakote, Calan	To stabilize the manic phase in bipolar disorder	Thirst, dry mouth, fatigue, nausea, abdominal pain, tremors, headache, drowsiness, and confusion.	Observe for signs of toxicity: severe diarrhea, muscle weakness, persistent nausea and vomiting, and seizures. Dehydration and fever can cause toxicity.	Instruct patient to have periodic lab tests to monitor for lithium blood levels. Teach patient to have adequate fluid and sodium intake. Teach patient the signs of toxicity and to notify the doctor if any indication of toxicity. Hard, sugarless candy can be helpful for dry mouth and thirst. Instruct patient that pregnancy and breast-feeding are not recommended while taking these medications.

(continued)

TABLE 8-1 Medications Used for Alterations in Mental Health (Continued)

CLASSIFICATIONS	COMMON TRADE NAMES	USES	SIDE EFFECTS	NURSING CONSIDERATIONS	PATIENT TEACHING
STIMULANTS	Dexedrine, Ritalin, Cylert	Promotes alertness, diminishes appetite, and combats narcolepsy. Treatment of attention deficit hyperactivity disorder (ADHD).	Rapid or irregular heart rates; hypertension, hyperactivity, hand tremor, rapid speech, confusion, depression, seizures, and suicidal thoughts.	Tolerance, physical and psychological dependence, especially with long-term use. Amphetamines can cause changes in insulin requirements in diabetic patients. Monitor for suicide potential. Do not discontinue medication abruptly.	Diabetic patients should monitor insulin carefully and inform the physician of any changes. Patients should use extreme caution when driving or operating equipment. Patients should not stop medication without consulting physician. Patients should use hard, sugarless candy to relieve dry mouth.

or "blue," and the patient would give a response, also typically one word, to each of the words the therapist says.

The therapist then looks for a theme or pattern to the patient's responses. So, if the patient responds "evil" to the word "mother" or "dead" to the word "blue," the therapist might pick up one potential theme, but if the patient responds "kind" and "true" to the words "mother" and "blue," the therapist might hear a completely different theme. The theme may give the therapist an idea of the cause of the patient's emotional disturbance.

Dream Analysis

Because Freudians believe that behavior is rooted in the unconscious and that dreams are a manifestation of the troubles people repress, what better way to get an idea of the problem than to monitor and interpret dreams? The patient is asked to keep a "dream log." The person is asked to train himself or herself to awaken immediately after a dream and to write the dream down right away in a notebook kept next to the bed. Easier said than done! On the other hand, how many times have you had a particularly troubling or wonderful dream, yet when you awaken, you can remember only bits and pieces of it? Psychoanalysts believe that dreams truly are the mirror to the unconscious and that it is possible to train the self to awaken long enough to record the dream. The dreams are then interpreted in much the same way as free association. Significant people or situations in the dreams are explored with the patient, and possible meanings are offered by the therapist.

Hypnosis

Many people are afraid of **hypnosis.** For many years, it was reputed to be quackery and presented in stage shows in which people did things such as cluck like chickens, which served as entertainment. Granted, this sort of thing can happen. Fraternity and sorority members love to invite stage performers to hypnotize pledges during rush.

Certainly, people like the entertainer David Copperfield have made comfortable livings with hypnosis.

Hypnotherapy, as the professional therapists prefer to call it, is used for certain people in certain instances. It is not a magic solution to problems. It takes practice on the part of the patient. It can, however, be a very effective tool for unlocking the unconscious or for searching further into a technique called "past life regression."

Hypnosis is very deep relaxation. If you have listened to a relaxation tape and felt the effects of it or if you have been driving your car and notice that 20 minutes have passed that you can't account for (which is *not* a good idea, by the way), you have been hypnotized.

In hypnotherapy, the relaxation is *guided* by the therapist, who has been trained in techniques of trance formation and who then asks certain questions of the patient or uses guided imagery to help picture the situation in an effort to find the cause of the problem (Fig. 8-1). At the end of the session, the therapist will leave some helpful hints for the patient. These are called posthypnotic suggestions and typically include positive, affirming statements for the patient to think about as well as instructions to help the person accomplish self-hypnosis.

Of course, just as there are unethical people in all walks of life, a small number of therapists may abuse this relationship. It is very uncommon. People do not generally lose control when under hypnosis; they will, in most cases, still realize what is comfortable and acceptable to them personally, and they will not allow themselves to go deeper into hypnosis or to perform behaviors that they find objectionable.

Hypnosis and hypnotherapy are discussed in more depth in Chapter 9.

Catharsis

Catharsis is "the act of purging or purification" or "elimination of a complex (problem) by bringing it to consciousness and affording it expression" (Merriam Webster

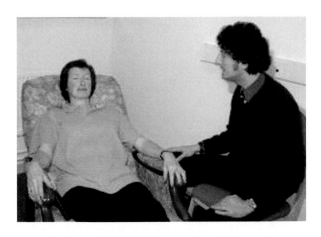

FIGURE 8-1. In hypnotherapy, a patient in a state of very deep relaxation is guided by the therapist. (Courtesy of South East Cancer Health Centre, Purley, United Kingdom.)

Online 2005). In psychoanalysis, the therapist helps the person see the root of the problem and then, by talking or some other means, allows the patient to learn to evacuate this problem from the psyche. This can take place in conjunction with other forms of psychoanalysis.

These therapies are undertaken on a one-on-one basis between patient and therapist. The nurse can be helpful in the treatment process by allowing the patient to talk about the experiences in therapy and by carefully documenting the responses of the patient.

Behavior Modification

The treatment method known as **behavior modification** is based on the theories of the behavioral theorists (Skinner, Pavlov, and others). It is a common treatment modality used in long term care facilities and facilities that treat patients with alterations in mental health.

The purpose of behavior modification is to eliminate or greatly decrease the frequency of identified negative behaviors. One of the basic beliefs of behavior modification is that, whenever a behavior is removed, it must be replaced by another behavior. Therefore, replacing the negative behaviors with ones that are more desirable is a major function of this type of psychotherapy.

As Skinner and Pavlov showed, behaviors can be learned and unlearned. The process of finding the appropriate stimuli and rein-

forcers determines the effectiveness of the change in behavior. According to some behaviorists, it takes approximately 20 repetitions of a behavior to make it a part of our lifestyle. Anyone who has tried to lose weight or stop smoking might have a rebuttal to that theory!

Behavior can be changed, according to behavior modification theory, by either positive or negative reinforcement. Positive reinforcement is the act of rewarding the patient with something pleasant when the desired behavior has been performed. For instance, if Mrs. P has the habit of using foul language in an attempt to have a need met, it might be assumed that the desired behavior change would be to come to a staff member and ask quietly for what she needs. Mrs. P loves to be outside but is not allowed out except at supervised times. A suitable positive reinforcer might be to allow 15 additional minutes outdoors when she remembers to ask for her needs quietly. Generally, when the behavior is exhibited by Mrs. P, the staff would either ignore it (because correcting it would in itself be a form of reinforcing the behavior) or quietly tell her that is not acceptable behavior and then acknowledge her only when the desired change has been demonstrated.

Negative reinforcement is interpreted by some as punishment. Great care must be taken when performing behavior modification with certain populations of people. It can look like an infraction of the Patient Bill of Rights and could be reported by someone who does not understand the situation.

Negative reinforcement is the act of responding to the undesired behavior by taking away a privilege or adding an unwanted responsibility. Critics of the legal system in this country sometimes cite the system of imprisonment and capital punishment as forms of negative reinforcement. Parents who "ground" a child after the child behaves unacceptably are using negative reinforcement; requiring that child to perform extra household tasks for a stated period of time is reinforcing the fact that the negative behavior has consequences. The child may not repeat the negative behavior after either of these parental choices.

Whatever option is chosen, it is important to have the behaviors and consequences clearly stated. In a facility, this will be incorporated into the plan of care. At home, it can be stated in family meetings, agreed upon verbally by the family members, or made known by some other method of clear communication. It is required that the patient have the ability to understand the ramifications of the behavior to be changed and the purpose for the type of consequence that is chosen. If the person is not capable of understanding the situation or is not able to remember due to some other problem, behavior modification could be considered a questionable alternative to other kinds of treatment.

COGNITIVE THERAPIES

Rational-Emotive Therapy (RET)

Dr. Albert Ellis, a "reformed" psychoanalyst, and other cognitive therapists have developed theories proposing that people teach themselves to be ill because of the way they think about their situations. *Cognitive* means "of, relating to, or being conscious of mental activity (as thinking, remembering, learning or using language)" (Merriam Webster Online 2005). Cognitive therapy emphasizes ways of rethinking situations.

The therapist confronts the patient with certain behaviors and then works out ways of thinking about them differently.

Rational-emotive therapy (RET) is probably the best-known cognitive therapy. Dr. Ellis's theory is based on an A-B-C format:

■ A is the *activating* event, or the subject of the faulty thinking.
■ B is the *belief* system a person has adopted about the activating event.
■ C is the *consequence* to continuing the belief system.

Dr. Ellis has made up terminology that he uses with his therapy, such as "musturbation" (the act of insisting that something *must* go a certain way), "awfulizing" (the belief that something is not just inconvenient or unpleasant, but the extreme of "awful"), and "catastrophizing" (at which point, one has lost control of the situation). In RET, there are no "musts" or "shoulds." Feeling sad about an unpleasant experience (such as the death of a loved one) is acceptable and normal, but becoming depressed about the death is "awfulizing" and therefore considered by him to be unhealthy.

RET and other forms of cognitive therapies are gaining in popularity because they are usually significantly more short term than psychoanalysis and therefore less costly to the patient. It is common for RET to be performed in groups. The patients are given homework to complete in the period between sessions. The outcome is that we will no longer "disturb ourselves by the way we think" (Ellis, 1988).

Person-Centered/Humanistic Therapy

The theorists Abraham Maslow and Carl Rogers are most frequently credited with the concept of **person-centered,** or humanistic, therapy. In this form of treatment, all caregivers are to focus on the whole person and to work in the "present." It is not important in humanistic treatment to understand the cause of the problem or what happened in the person's past; what is important is the here and now.

Unconditional Positive Regard

This is the phrase used by therapists who follow Rogerian theory. Unconditional positive regard means full, nonjudgmental acceptance of the patient as a person. It also means that the patient must work at accepting himself or herself. Being self-aware and having feelings that are congruent (equal) to that self-concept are some of the goals of humanistic therapy.

Rogers believed that people who care for other people must have three qualities. These qualities are empathy (the ability to identify with the patient's feelings without actually experiencing them with the patient), unconditional positive regard, and genuineness (honesty). Although nurses may not be active participants in the actual therapy sessions with our patients, it is important for us to maintain these three qualities in *all* our therapeutic relationships. When a patient feels betrayed, it usually results in deterioration of the nurse-patient relationship and loss of credibility for the nurse in that situation.

COUNSELING

Counseling is licensed and regulated differently not only state by state, but sometimes municipality by municipality. Some states require that a person be prepared at a PhD level to practice therapy independently; in some areas, only certain types of therapy are licensed. Nurses prepared at an LPN/LVN level or at an RN level can, in some localities, practice forms of treatment. It is up to you to make the appropriate phone calls to determine your rights, responsibilities, and regulations in your locality, if counseling is a path you wish to pursue. Nurses may be asked or required to accompany their patients to counseling sessions at times. You may be asked to facilitate (lead) a group discussion sometime. If you have the opportunity, take it. It is very interesting to see the dynamics of the group and the way the facilitator guides patients through issues. *Remember:* These are confidential sessions, even if they are group oriented. Patients are

there to work; others are there by invitation for special reasons.

Pastoral or Cultural Counseling

Some people prefer to obtain assistance or counseling from their church or spiritual leaders. Sessions are often free, or on a "free-will" or "ability to pay" status. The person who provides therapy in this time or circumstance may or may not be trained in traditional mental health theories and modalities.

In some Christian faiths, nurses may have an opportunity to serve in ways they could not in a traditional setting. For example, "parish nurses" are licensed nurses who work through their church and perform tasks ranging from simply visiting a homebound church member to actually performing care and counseling or referrals for that individual (Fig. 8-2). Depending on the particular church organization, nurses who serve as parish nurses may serve in a volunteer capacity or in a paid position. Training sessions are offered in some locales for nurses who wish to provide this service,

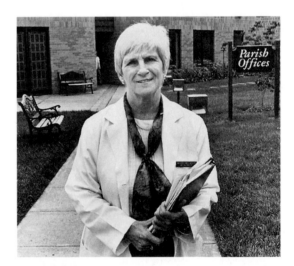

FIGURE 8-2. A parish nurse works through a church to provide counseling services. (From Sorrell, J.M. and Redmond, G.M. *Community-Based Nursing Practice: Learning Through Students' Stories.* Philadelphia, FA Davis Company, 2002, p. 417. Reprinted with permission.)

although many churches do not yet require formal training for all their nurses.

Patients who profess Judaism, especially if those individuals observe kosher practices, may have concerns about dietary selections, may refuse to have certain procedures done between sundown Friday and sundown Saturday, and may insist on being admitted to a Jewish hospital if one is available.

Patients of Islamic faith follow rituals that may conflict with schedules and routines within the hospital. Prayer times are proscribed by their faith and are strictly followed; therefore medication times, treatment times, or attendance at therapy may meet with some conflict on the part of that patient. Islamic belief follows holy times that are different from the traditional holidays or holy days celebrated in the social calendar in the United States or those traditionally celebrated within Christianity or Judaism. Nurses need to be aware of the potential conflicts between hospital routines and the religious obligations of their patients. Nurses of Islamic faith may find their own challenges working within this belief system. Women of Islamic faith wear head scarves that completely cover the hair. In the often sterile world of health care, some practitioners are concerned for the safety of the nurse and the people under her care: What if the scarf becomes tangled in the electric bed? What if the patient and nurse tangle in the scarf during a transfer? What infection control concerns might arise if a nurse wears her scarf on the job? To date, no dangerous situations have been documented. However, nurses who wear head scarves should be alerted to the possibility of a supervisor's asking questions and expressing concern for the safety of the nurse and her patients.

Some Native American patients may have healing traditions that conflict with traditional Western medicine. Remember, especially, that it is not appropriate to label all Native Americans as one group; many tribes have their own unique beliefs and traditions. Shamans, healers, and medicine men are examples of people who may be present in the room with the Native American patient.

Box 8-1 examines a number of concepts that may affect certain cultural groups' willingness to seek and comply with mental health treatment.

Group Therapy

Group therapy is a very broad topic. Groups are formed for many reasons; they can be ongoing or short term, depending on the needs of the patients or the type of disorder (Fig. 8-3). For example, Alcoholics Anonymous (AA) and similar 12-step groups are well established, ongoing groups. They are held not only in the treatment facility but also in several places in the community. Meeting times are established and published so that people know when and how to access them. As a rule, AA meetings are "closed" meetings; that is, only alcoholics are welcome. Sometimes, maybe once a month or once quarterly, a meeting is advertised as "open," so that other interested persons (and students) are welcome. Many people who have experienced alcoholism or other chemical dependencies have benefited from this 12-step approach to healing, and it is said that this type of peer group help is the most beneficial for this type of illness.

Family counseling sessions are often set up with individual therapists with a specialty in the problem area for that family. It is expected that the whole family attend, but there may be times when only certain members are asked to attend or when the individuals will "break out" with another therapist and then return to the family group later.

Marriage counseling is set up either with an individual counselor or in a group with other couples. Many times, peer counselors are used. These are people who have experienced similar obstacles in their marriage and found creative, effective ways to manage their conflicts. Sometimes, people choose to seek help from a spiritual leader.

It is important for us to remember that the therapists and counselors are tools. They do not heal the patient; the patient

| BOX 8-1 | *Concepts that May Affect Certain Cultural Groups' Seeking or Complying with Mental Health Treatment.* |

CONCEPTS

CAUCASIAN
- Stigma remains attached to mental illness but is weakening somewhat.
- Generally have more access to health insurance and availability to mental health professionals.
- Tend to be more receptive to taking medications than other groups may be.

AFRICAN AMERICAN
- More likely than whites to receive initial treatment for mental health in emergency rooms (it is thought this may be because this population delays treatment).
- Approximately 20–30 percent of African Americans do not have health insurance.
- More likely to receive treatment from primary health care provider rather than a mental health specialist.
- If any treatment is rendered, may be substandard.
- Statistics may be skewed to show over-representation of African Americans having mental illness.

HISPANIC
- Mental illness among Hispanics is about equal to Caucasians.
- Currently the highest group not having health insurance (approximately 35%).
- Language barriers. Approximately 4% of Hispanic patients say they do not have strong English skills.
- Young Hispanics tend to have higher rates of depression, anxiety disorders, and suicide.
- Hispanics born in the United States tend to be diagnosed with a mental illness more frequently than those born in Mexico.

AMERICAN INDIANS
- Suicide rate approximately 50% higher than the general U.S. population.
- Mental health treatment options very limited.
- Lack of research into mental health issues for Native Americans. Also difficult to design and provide effective mental health care.
- Cultural stigmas.

ASIAN AMERICANS
- Cultural stigmas; depending on the group, the stigma is expressed differently.
- Language barriers.
- Tend to seek mental health services at lower rates than Caucasians.
- Goal is to restore balance in life; often accomplished through exercise or diet rather than a mental health system.

Community education can modify attitudes. Emphasize that talking about problems can help, that early diagnosis is crucial, and that by law, providers must keep problems confidential.

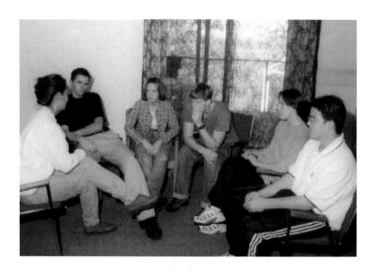

FIGURE 8-3. Group therapy can be a very helpful treatment method for many patients. (Courtesy of Willow Crest Hospital, Inc., Miami, OK.)

heals himself or herself. Patients must take the suggestions given by the therapist, try them, and see what works for them (Fig. 8-4). Nurses can help patients by reinforcing the good work they do in learning to keep themselves healthy. We can also help by reminding patients gently that they do their own healing. Sometimes, when the road to healing gets rocky, patients may use the therapist as a scapegoat. Rather than agree or disagree with the patient, the nurse needs to remember the therapeutic communication skills, empathize with the hard work that is being done by the patient, and encourage the patient to discuss the frustration with the therapist.

Electroconvulsive Therapy

Electroconvulsive therapy **(ECT),** or electroshock therapy, as it is sometimes still called, is another form of treatment that is frightening to some patients. They envision the old movies in which the patient flopped relentlessly on the table. Relax, nurses; those days are gone.

First of all, we know more about the procedure itself. Patients are generally given a sedative before the treatment. Nurses carefully monitor blood pressure and pulse before and after treatment. The amount of electric energy used is individualized to the patient. A treatment usually lasts only a few minutes, and if you are slow to look, you might miss seeing a patient's so-called convulsion. Often, only a toe or a finger may twitch slightly; there are no more uncon-

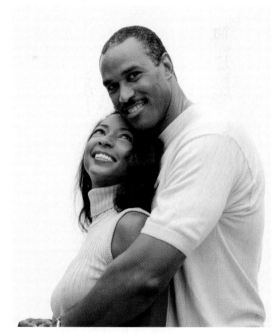

FIGURE 8-4. This obviously happy couple is a reminder that people can find creative, effective ways to manage conflicts within their relationships. A therapist may help them with suggestions, but they must try those suggestions themselves and find what works for them.

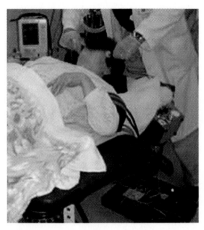

FIGURE 8-5. Electroconvulsive therapy is no longer the frightening procedure many people imagine, but it is still usually used only when other therapies have not been successful. (Courtesy of Osaka City University Medical School, Osaka, Japan.)

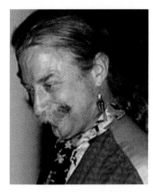

FIGURE 8-6. Dr. Hunter "Patch" Adams has made pioneering efforts in the field of humor therapy. (Courtesy of Steve Wilson and Company, Columbus, Ohio.)

trolled seizures on the treatment table (Fig. 8-5).

ECT has a few side effects that can be fairly unpleasant. The patient may feel confused and forgetful immediately after the treatment. This can be from a combination of the ECT itself and the pretreatment medication. If there has been a stronger seizure, the patient may have some muscle soreness. Patients are secured with restraints during the treatment, however, so movement is minimal. Because of the possibility of confusion and forgetfulness, it is common to restrict activity for 24 hours after a treatment, and it is recommended that the nurse stay with the patient until the patient is oriented and able to care for himself or herself. ECT is not used indiscriminately as it once was. Today, it is used when other therapies have not been helpful, and it is usually reserved for severe or long-term depression and certain types of schizophrenia.

The nurse's responsibilities include careful monitoring of vital signs and accurate documentation relating to the patient's subjective and objective response to the treatment. The patient should have nothing by mouth (NPO) for at least 4 hours before a treatment. Reminding the patient to empty his or her bladder and to remove dentures, contact lenses, hairpins, and so on is also important. Ensuring that the patient is kept safe after therapy is also a major concern.

Humor Therapy

Many studies have been done over the years showing the effects of smiles, hugs, and laughter on mental health as well as physical conditions such as cancer.

The movie *Patch Adams,* based on a real-life doctor-clown, portrayed the potential of humor therapy. Viewers saw breakthroughs take place in patients previously thought untreatable (Fig. 8-6).

Humor therapy uses many media, from clowns to movies to just 10 good "belly laughs" daily. Whatever the medium, laughter alters outlooks and neurochemical production. Patients can show remarkable progress. In fact, this kind of intervention has brought responses such as singing, hand clapping, and laughter from dementia patients who do not usually respond to other programming.

The danger in humor therapy is that what some people find funny, others find offensive. Humor therapy must be sensitive to such varied reactions. Also, some people are fearful of clowns.

Smiles are always appropriate. A brave nurse wearing a red rubber nose into the room of an appropriate patient could ease that person's pain—either mental or physical—even if only for a short while.

Crisis Intervention

Crisis can happen at any time to anyone. It can involve your child, your next-door neighbor, or your patient. What do you do when you get the call? What skills must you remember?

Crisis is defined in several ways. In the health fields, a crisis is a sudden, unexpected event in a person's life that drastically changes his or her routine. Crisis has been defined as a state in which the body is out of homeostasis. It is thought of as a situation in which a person may "lose control of feelings and thoughts, thus experiencing an extreme state of emotional turmoil" (Shives and Isaacs, 2002).

A person in crisis is at risk for physical and emotional harm inflicted by self or by others. Examples of people who may be experiencing a crisis are those who have lost a job suddenly or were divorced recently, are in an abusive relationship, have had a loved one die, are chemically dependent or otherwise mentally challenged, or are contemplating or attempting suicide. An important concept to remember is that each person has a different set of stressors and a different way of dealing with stress. What is crisis for one person may be simply a minor nuisance for another person.

Many employers recognize the potential for crisis and offer some type of employee support service. The service is confidential, and usually at least the initial call is free to the employee. The services all vary in what they are able to provide and may act as a referral service for the employee. Nurses should ask the patient if his or her employer provides this benefit.

PHASES OF CRISIS

Although crisis is a highly individual situation, most experts agree that people experiencing a crisis pass through the five phases described in Table 8-2.

TABLE 8-2	*The Five Phases of Crises*
PHASE	**BEHAVIORS**
PRECRISIS	Person feels "fine." Will often deny stress level, and, in fact, state a feeling of well-being.
IMPACT	Person feels anxiety and confusion. May have trouble organizing personal life. High stress level. Person will acknowledge feeling stress but may minimize its severity.
CRISIS	Person denies problem is out of control. Withdraws or rationalizes behaviors and stress. Uses defense mechanism of projection frequently. This may last varied amounts of time.
ADAPTIVE	Crisis is perceived in a positive way. Anxiety decreases. Person attempts to regain self-esteem and is able to start socializing again. Person is able to do some positive problem solving.
POSTCRISIS	Surprisingly, both positive and negative functioning may be seen. Person may have developed a more positive, effective way of coping with stress *or* may show ineffective adaptation, such as being critical, hostile, depressed, or may use food or chemicals such as alcohol to deal with what has happened.

GOALS OF CRISIS INTERVENTION

Nurses at an entry level have the unique opportunity of often being present for the first three phases of the crisis and not for the outcome. In many agencies, we are not involved with longer-term treatment, but we may very easily be the one who walks into the room during a suicide attempt or who may take the call at the nursing station of a distraught parent who is about to hurt his or her child.

The goals of crisis intervention change according to the degree of treatment you will be involved in. Crisis intervention for the health-care provider is obviously provided at a different level than it would be from a law enforcement or emergency dispatch viewpoint. Since this text is meant to be an overview to prepare nurses at an entry level of practice, we will look at the goals of crisis intervention from a health-care perspective.

1. *Ensure safety:* Assess the situation. If you or the patient is in physical danger, signal for help. *Do not* leave the patient unless danger to yourself is imminent. It may sound harsh, but you will be no good to anyone if you are hurt, or worse. Take care of your own safety; then take care of the patient's safety.

2. *Diffuse the situation:* Do this verbally, when at all possible. A person in crisis is most likely not in control of his or her thoughts, feelings, or actions. Physical attempts at restraining or calming are best left until all verbal attempts have been made, and only when there is enough help to do it safely for the patient and the staff.

3. *Determine the problem:* Attempt to find out from the patient's viewpoint the cause of the crisis. It is very important that you *not push* the patient to give you reasons and that you *remain calm* during the intervention. The last thing the person in crisis needs is a nurse in panic. There is time for us to talk about our feelings when the patient is safe.

4. *Decrease the anxiety level:* Your adrenaline level will probably be at an all-time high, but it won't be even close to that of the person in crisis. Make every attempt to reassure the patient that he or she is in a safe place. Let the person know you are concerned and want to help. Gently but firmly tell him or her that you will do whatever you can to make the situation more comfortable but that you do need his or her help and cooperation. *Caution:* Be very careful with physical contact at this point. Touch as a nonverbal communication skill may be interpreted inaccurately as aggression or sexual innuendo by a person whose thoughts and feelings are in turmoil.

5. *Return patient to precrisis (or better) level of functioning:* You may be able to calm the person to the point that he or she is able to understand what just happened; you may not. It might take a longer-term session of treatment to help the person gain that kind of insight. No matter what level of intervention the patient requires, the ultimate goal is for him or her to learn the skills necessary to cope with stress in a more positive way than was used before the crisis. Much of that learning will come from the role modeling from the nurses. How we handle ourselves in high-stress times and how we demonstrate positive coping skills will represent the 70 percent of nonverbal communication that speaks louder than our words.

■ TERRORISM

September 11, 2001, changed life in the United States. Citizens of the United States became aware of a way of life experienced routinely by some of our global neighbors. Suicide bombers, anthrax, sarin gas, and tainted water and food sources—American citizens suddenly have a new kind of connection to those in other countries who have been falling victim to terror for generations. Reality was attached to that which many of us only knew from movies or the evening news. That way of life, that behavior, is called terrorism. Terror, according to Webster Online (2004) is "1: a state of intense fear; 2a: one that inspires fear b: a frightening aspect c: a cause of anxiety d: an appalling person or thing; 3: violence (as bombing) committed by groups in order to intimidate a population or government into granting their demands."

These words will appear frequently as you progress through this text. They define terrorism, but they are also symptoms of many mental illnesses. Perhaps the most frightening part of this definition is that humans do not always know the source of the terror and thus are unable to defend themselves. They may feel a loss of personal control over their life and safety. It is difficult for adults to accept and deal with what has become an ever-present possibility in what we Americans had always assumed was a safe place to live; how, then, do we help our children to process the potential dangers in our world at the same time they are moving through the normal stages of growth and development? How can we convey the message that while bad things happen, people are basically good and not to fear them? How do we as adults, parents, teachers, and health-care professionals prepare to help with others who experience crisis, post-traumatic stress, depression, and other potential effects of terror? Suggestions will be offered in various chapters throughout this text; however, to borrow an idea from the sports world, the best defense is a good offense. We need to be ready for the possibility of patients experiencing some effect of terrorism and we must be willing to discuss the situation with that patient. As with so many other areas of nursing, it means nurses must take stock of their own thoughts and feelings about the topic.

■ LEGAL CONSIDERATIONS

We are living in a litigious society. It is easy to be tempted to stay uninvolved when people call out for help. In some states, nurses, physicians, and anyone else in the health fields are required by law to help. Some localities require health-care professionals to post identifying insignia on their vehicles. Most states do not require this yet, but many are considering it. This puts nurses in a sensitive position. We want to help. Nursing curriculum at the entry level provides very little in the way of hands-on crisis intervention technique. What if something goes wrong? It is suggested in literature related to crisis intervention that nurses risk a higher liability if we fail to try to help. In other words, it is safer legally for you to do something to help than to do nothing.

Exactly what you, as a nurse, are able to do depends greatly on your locale, your level of preparation, your state's nurse practice act, and your comfort level. Staying within the legal parameter of your nursing licensure is of major importance; do only what you know and what is legal. The truth is that anyone can sue anyone for anything. The good news is that most states will find in favor of the medical professional who has, in good faith and in accordance with his or her licensure, made an effort to help a person in a crisis situation. The Good Samaritan law is there for our protection as well. The Good Samaritan law *does not* generally cover us within the confines of our employment, however; only when acting to assist in a crisis or emergency situation are we protected. *Remember:* Crisis intervention has something in common with the rule of thumb about cardiopulmonary resuscitation (CPR): Once you start and make that commitment to help, you cannot quit until you are physically no longer able to continue. Starting to provide help and then changing your mind can be interpreted as neglect or abandonment, and in such an instance, the nurse could be found at fault.

What happens to the person experiencing the crisis? Because of the nature of crisis, we understand that the person probably does not have a valid insight into the situation. The individual is very likely to be concerned about personal safety. On top of that, the fear and inability to perceive the situation as it really is will interfere with communication. In most instances, the medical staff will encourage the person to accept some form of treatment. The patient then has two choices: voluntary or involuntary commitment.

Voluntary treatment happens when the patient gives informed consent to be hospitalized or accept some formal treatment program. *Informed* consent means that the person has been made aware of his or her behaviors, the implications of the behaviors, and expectations from the treatment. Informed consent can be verbal, nonverbal, or written. *Implied* consent allows people who are unconscious to be treated in such a way as to preserve life. If the patient is an adult of legal age who is considered to be competent in the eyes of the law (or an adolescent who has acquired legal emancipation), this patient can also sign himself or herself out at any time.

Involuntary commitment varies somewhat from state to state. Many states have the capability to place a "hold" on the patient, usually for 48 to 72 hours. During this time, the person is confined to the treatment setting. Usually a social worker is assigned to visit the patient and act as an advocate for that person. The goal of the hold period is for the patient to see the need for help with his or her crisis and then consent to voluntary treatment. If, at the end of the hold period, the person does not consent to treatment, he or she is free to leave the facility, as long as no other manifestation of crisis has surfaced during the hold.

In either instance, patients maintain all civil rights while in the treatment setting. The Patient Bill of Rights is covered with the patient, and most often the patient keeps a copy of the rights.

The Community Mental Health Centers Act made provisions for community-based treatment. Communities develop centers and provide treatment according to the needs of the area; not all centers provide all types of treatment or 24-hour service. However, the community is supposed to provide some method of emergency psychiatric treatment to help people in crisis as well as those who are chronically mentally ill. These centers can be in the form of free-standing crisis centers or walk-in clinics, and many are connected with the community hospital.

The concepts of mental illness and its treatment are changing as we learn more about what mental illness is. Crisis is a form of mental illness that, if treated in an appropriate and timely way, is usually temporary. Crisis intervention theories are changing to try to keep up with the current concepts of illness. Nevertheless, people will always be experiencing crisis. When it happens, it is important that the person who is there to help understands that this is a very frightening time for the person in turmoil. We nurses must understand that we are in a special position to be able to have some knowledge of crisis and communication skills and be able to help, yet we must always be aware of the legal ramifications of intervention. These patients deserve the best and safest care we can provide.

Table 8-3 summarizes treatment modalities that may be used alone or in conjunction with medications. The common uses, desired outcomes, nursing actions, and patient teaching are also included for the areas to which they apply.

TABLE 8-3 Summary of Commonly Used Treatment Modalities

TREATMENT MODALITY	USES	DESIRED OUTCOMES	NURSING ACTIONS	PATIENT TEACHING
PSYCHOTHERAPY	For treatment of various alterations to mental health.	1. Patient states improvement in emotional discomfort. 2. Patient returns to comfortable social functioning. 3. Patient behaves in a manner appropriate to the situation.	Positive reinforcement of patient's progress. Honest communication.	Practice new coping behaviors. Help patient develop insight into his or her illness.
BEHAVIOR MODIFICATION	To remove or greatly diminish behaviors that are inappropriate or unhealthy.	Former undesirable behaviors have been replaced by new, healthy behaviors.	Positive reinforcement of new behaviors. Clearly stated expectations and appropriate behaviors. Consistently upholding the patient's care plan.	Communication skills are important. Ensure patient's understanding of the reasons for the changes in behavior.
COGNITIVE THERAPY RATIONAL-EMOTIVE THERAPY (RET)	For any mental health alteration that is consciously controlled.	Patient will be able to remain "undisturbed" as a result of rethinking activating events, belief system, and consequences.	Patients will probably not be inpatients.	Perform "homework." Avoid the words "must" and "should."
PERSON-CENTERED/HUMANISTIC	All aspects of patient care	Patient will feel accepted as a human, which will allow patient to be self-aware and self-accepting.	Maintain the three basic qualities of Rogerian theory 1. Empathy 2. Unconditional positive regard 3. Genuineness	Remain centered in the present. Practice accepting self unconditionally.

(continued)

149

TABLE 8-3 *Summary of Commonly Used Treatment Modalities (Continued)*

TREATMENT MODALITY	USES	DESIRED OUTCOMES	NURSING ACTIONS	PATIENT TEACHING
COUNSELING	All forms of mental health alterations.	Patient will gain insight to situation and receive tools to make changes in his or her life.	May be facilitator. Nurse-counselor licensing requirements vary by state. Confidentiality is mandatory.	Patient must work at gaining confidence to try options.
PASTORAL COUNSELING OR CULTURAL COUNSELING	All forms of mental health alterations.	Patient gains tools from a religious/cultural background to be able to make changes in his or her life.	May act as "parish nurse" (or similar title) or representative of a specific religion or cultural group in home visits or health facility visits. May be a paid or volunteer position.	Patient works with teaching from religious or cultural affiliation to regain mental health.
GROUP THERAPY	Many uses, including those for short-term or long-term treatments. AA and RET are examples.	Patient gains knowledge that there are others with similar problems. Patient learns from peers and helps others.	Facilitation. Patient advocacy.	Patient heals self; facilitators and counselors are tools for the patient.
ELECTROCONVULSIVE THERAPY (ECT)	Depression or schizophrenia that does not respond to other treatments.	Patient will state and exhibit appropriate mood and affect or a measurable improvement in mood and affect.	Monitor vital signs before and after treatment. Maintain safety after treatment. Premedicate if ordered.	May be disoriented after treatment. May lose short-term memory. Side effects last about 24 hours.

(continued)

HUMOR THERAPY	All forms of mental health alterations and physical conditions.	Patients respond and react to the humor. Patients interact. Patients may show improvement in physical condition.	Assist in determining appropriate patients. Assist in the humor "application."	Patient identifies how humor improves situation. Patient helps in seeking out opportunities to apply humor in his or her life.
CRISIS INTERVENTION	For states of extreme emotional or physical turmoil in which patients feel out of control of self or situation.	Patient returns to precrisis (or higher) level of functioning.	Assess for the level of crisis patient is experiencing. Assess suicide potential. Use verbal and nonverbal communication skills to diffuse situations.	Determine stressors. Work with new coping techniques. Access support system before stress reaches crisis.

Key Concepts ■ ■ ■

1. The place in which treatment is given must be conducive to therapy. *Milieu* is the word used to describe the environment of the treatment area.
2. Psychopharmacology is very important to the effective treatment of the patient. There are many classifications of psychoactive medications and many individual medications within each classification. It is our responsibility as nurses to consult a drug reference regarding all the psychotropic medications we give our patients. It also is part of our role to reinforce teaching about the medications to the patient.
3. Psychotherapy, sometimes in conjunction with medications, is often used to treat patients. There are several methods of psychotherapy, including psychoanalysis, behavior modification, rational-emotive therapy, and humanistic, or person-centered, therapy.
4. Counseling is carried out in different ways, depending on the patient's needs and type of illness. Counseling may be licensed and the nurse's role in counseling regulated differently from state to state and municipality to municipality. Counseling is given individually or in group settings, according to the situation.
5. ECT is used for specific situations. Premedication is usually ordered. It is the role of the nurse to monitor vital signs, maintain safety, and document posttreatment observations.
6. Crisis intervention is very individualized. Crisis has five phases, and each person experiences them differently.
7. Employee support systems are becoming more accessible through employers. They are confidential and free or reasonably priced.
8. Pastoral or cultural counseling may be the treatment of choice for an individual. Nurses must do all they can to help that patient receive care that is personally meaningful.

REFERENCES

CNN.com/Health. Report: Minorities lack proper mental health care. Dr. David Satcher, US Surgeon General. August 27, 2001.

Ellis, A. (1988). *A Guide to Rational Living*. From the video series *Thinking Allowed*. Oakland, CA: InnerWork.

Meadows, M. (1997, September). Closing the Gap: Mental Health and Minorities. *Cultural Considerations in Treating Asians*. A Newsletter of the Office of Minority Health.

Webster Online http://www.merriam-webster.com (2005).

Shives, L.R. and Isaacs, A. (2002). *Basic Concepts of Psychiatric-Mental Health Nursing*, 5th ed. Philadelphia: JB Lippincott.

WEBSITES

http://www.omhrc.gov/ctg/mhm-01.htm
http://www.mhafc.org/minorities.htm

CRITICAL THINKING EXERCISES ■ ■ ■

1. Look in your city's telephone book for agencies that handle crisis intervention. Contact one or more either by phone or in person. Inform them that this is a school project and you wish to ask them a few questions such as, Whom do they service? What are their hours of operation? How are they funded? What does the emergency care cost the patient? Who is their staff? Write a short report of your findings. If possible, appoint someone to compile all the information so that each student nurse has a "starter set" to be able to help others.

2. With a student partner, role-play one or more of the following potential crises (or think up your own). Think about your communication techniques. Do they change when dealing with crisis? If so, how? What about your non-verbal communication techniques?

   - Parent whose child has been abducted at the mall
   - Man who calls the clinic, stating he has just killed his wife
   - Woman who is frantically seeking shelter from an abusive relationship
   - Adolescent friend of your son or daughter who is slashing his or her wrists as you are talking, while you are alone at home
   - Alcoholic, the main wage earner for the family, who has just been fired from job

3. Maya is a new employee on your medical floor. Maya is Muslim. She has been given permission to wear her head scarf. Maya "disappears" at odd times in addition to her assigned breaks. Today is exceptionally busy. Staffing is short, and there are new patients on the floor. The patient in the private room down the hall is deteriorating; she has the potential for stroke and is waiting to be transferred to the Emergency Department. Where is Maya? You find her on her knees deep in prayer. You try to tell her that things are very critical right now. She is needed; can't she pray later? Maya tells you she needs to pray now and that she will only be a few more minutes. What priorities must be addressed? Whose priorities are they? What potential problems could arise from this situation? What are some potential resolutions?

4. You are on vacation with your family. There are three adults and two children in your vehicle. You have chosen a road trip to a major theme park. You are within 15 minutes from the gate when you see smoke on the horizon. The radio in your vehicle alerts you that your theme park has just experienced an explosion. Details are sketchy, but there are numerous injuries. The park has been closed. As you approach what was the entrance to the park, you witness many individuals running, injured, crying. People are on fire and rolling. There is a very unpleasant odor. Police, firefighters, and first responders are directing you away from the site. You tell them you are a nurse and offer to help. At this moment, your help is not wanted but you are directed to a "holding" area. Your children, ages 7 and 10 are crying and asking questions. What is your emotional response right now? How will you answer and calm your children? After a few minutes, the police accept your

offer to help the wounded. Your children become hysterical at you leaving the vehicle, yet you feel responsible to help. What do you do? What stages of crisis are you experiencing?

5. Using the suggested nursing diagnoses shown here (or others you can think of), complete a nursing process for a patient being treated for a mental health alteration.

SUGGESTED NURSING DIAGNOSES

1. *Hopelessness*
2. *Thought Processes, Altered*
3. *Spiritual Distress (Distress of the Human Spirit)*

ASSESSMENT/ DATA COLLECTION	NURSING DIAGNOSIS	PLAN/ GOAL	INTERVENTIONS/ NURSING ACTIONS	EVALUATION CRITERIA

TEST QUESTIONS ■ ■ ■

MULTIPLE CHOICE QUESTIONS

1. Which of the following is *not* a behavior noted in the *crisis* phase of crisis?
   A. Denial
   B. Feeling of well-being
   C. Use of projection
   D. Rationalization

2. One of the first statements a nurse might make to a person who has been abused might be:
   A. "Why didn't you leave the first time you were attacked?"
   B. "Do you want to prosecute or not?"
   C. "What do you think made that person hit you?"
   D. "You're safe here. I would like to help you."

3. A therapeutic environment (milieu) is *best* defined as:
    A. An environment in which a patient is under a 72-hour hold
    B. An environment that is locked and supervised
    C. An environment that is structured to decrease stress and encourage learning new behavior
    D. An environment that is designed to be homelike for persons who are hospitalized for life

4. Which of the following *does not* state a goal of psychotherapy?
    A. Decrease emotional pain or discomfort.
    B. Increase social functioning.
    C. Increase ability to behave appropriately.
    D. Allow patient to avoid or deny uncomfortable situations.

5. Which of the following is *false* regarding ECT?
    A. It is used to treat depression and schizophrenia.
    B. It is used to stop convulsive seizures.
    C. Fatigue and disorientation are immediate side effects.
    D. Memory will gradually return.

6. Psychopharmacology (psychotropic drug therapy) is used:
    A. As a cure for mental illness
    B. Only to control violent behavior
    C. To alter the pain receptors in the brain
    D. To decrease symptoms and facilitate other therapies

7. Mrs. Henderson has been started on Thorazine. As her nurse, you are teaching her about the possible side effects of this antipsychotic drug. Which of the following will you include in your teaching?
    A. Photosensitivity
    B. Weight loss
    C. Elevated blood pressure
    D. Hypoglycemia

8. Avoiding such foods as bananas, cheese, and yogurt should be emphasized to patients who are taking:
    A. Prozac
    B. Lithium
    C. MAOIs
    D. Tricyclic antidepressants

9. The goals of crisis intervention include all of the following *except:*
    A. Safety
    B. Increasing anxiety
    C. Taking care of the precipitating event
    D. Return to precrisis or better level of functioning

10. In order for psychotherapy to be effective, it is necessary to do all of the following *except:*

A. Encourage the patient to repress feelings.
B. Reinforce appropriate behavior.
C. Establish a therapeutic patient-staff relationship.
D. Assist patient to gain insight into problem.

11. When forming a nursing diagnosis for a mental illness/behavior problem, you:

A. Look only at physical symptoms.
B. Focus on psychological needs but include physical needs.
C. Realize that goals will be met quickly.
D. Evaluate the plan.

12. Mr. Douglas is being treated with Haldol (an antipsychotic agent) for organic dementia. He is at first hard to arouse, then stays sleepy after the next three doses. You know sedation may occur with this drug. As his nurse, your first nursing action would be to:

A. Notify your supervisor; call the physician.
B. Realize that tolerance will occur and continue giving the drug.
C. Discontinue the drug immediately.
D. Administer an antidote.

13. It is 8 days later. You enter Mr. Douglas' room and observe tremors of his face and hands, drooling, and flat affect. You are *probably* observing signs of:

A. Acute dystonia
B. Parkinsonism
C. Acute drug toxicity
D. Withdrawal

14. If an EPSE such as tardive dyskinesia occurs, the treatment of choice is to:

A. Administer anticholinergic drugs as ordered.
B. Discontinue the drugs per order.
C. Increase the dose per order.
D. Administer antianxiety drugs per order.

15. Your patient, Mrs. L, is on your unit for bowel resection. She is exhibiting signs of nervousness and anxiety, which she attributes to the upcoming surgery. You note from her record that she has a history of ethyl alcohol (ETOH) abuse. Which of the following classifications of drugs would be potentially addictive for her?

A. Lithium salts
B. Antianxiety drugs
C. Antipsychotic drugs
D. Anticholinergics

16. James is a 13-year old who has been transferred to your medical-surgical unit after being stabilized in the ED. He slit both wrists and took an overdose of his Wellbutrin. You know medications such as Wellbutrin:

A. Are antidepressants and should have stopped his suicidal impulse
B. Have no particular nursing considerations for children and adolescents

C. Are antidepressants and may have an increase in the suicidal ideation for children and adolescents

D. Are not effective as antidepressants for children or adolescents

MATCHING QUESTIONS
Directions
Match the treatment on the left with the definition or technique on the right. There is one "best" definition or technique per treatment. There is one definition or technique that does not match with any of the treatments listed.

TREATMENT
1. Catharsis
2. Group Therapy
3. Tricyclic Antidepressants
4. ECT
5. Crisis Intervention
6. Antipsychotics
7. Behavior Modification

DEFINITION OR TECHNIQUE

A. Used when other therapies have not been helpful. Usually reserved for severe or long-term depression and certain types of schizophrenia.

B. Act on the central nervous system (CNS). Main action is to block the dopamine receptors

C. Signal for help. *Do not* leave the patient unless danger to yourself is imminent. Take care of your own safety; then take care of the patient's safety.

D. Purpose is to eliminate or greatly decrease the frequency of identified negative behaviors. One of the basic beliefs and techniques is whenever a behavior is removed, it must be replaced by another behavior.

E. Prevents the metabolism of monoamine oxidase.

F. Increase the level of serotonin and norepinephrine.

G. Therapists and counselors are tools; patient heals himself or herself. Patients must take the suggestions given by the therapist, try them, and see what works for them.

H. Therapist helps the person see the root of the problem and then, by talking or some other means, allows the patient to learn to evacuate this problem from the psyche.

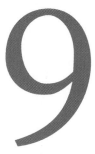
Alternative and Complementary Treatment Modalities

Robin A. Spidle, RN, PhD, CHT, CNLPM

Learning Objectives ■ ■ ■

1. Differentiate between alternative and complementary medicine.
2. Identify integrative medicine.
3. Identify the concept of the mind-body connection.
4. Identify support for patient beliefs and models.
5. Identify three alternative and complementary treatment modalities.
6. Identify three types of massage.
7. Differentiate between trance and sleep.
8. Identify the three primary channels of experience.
9. Define key terms.

Key Terms ■ ■ ■

- Alternative medicine
- Aromatherapy
- Beliefs
- Biofeedback
- Complementary medicine
- Hypnotherapy
- Integrative medicine
- Massage
- Mind-body connection
- Models
- Neurolinguistic Programming
- Placebo
- Presupposition
- Rapport
- Reflexology
- Reiki
- Trance

Medicine is a rapidly evolving field, and sometimes it is tempting for the nurse to assume that every patient he or she comes into contact with is knowledgeable about the current state of the art. For some patients, however, conventional western medicine is not the only course open to treat illness. Many factors might affect a patient's choice of treatment modalities: education, experience, economic status, belief system, and culture are but a few considerations.

There are many other means of treating illness and promoting good health that are collectively known as **alternative** and

159

complementary medicine. These systems, modalities, and practices exist apart from conventional medicine. Often these methods differ considerably from what is acceptable medical care in our culture. Alternative or complementary methods may lack extensive scientific research to prove their effectiveness or even their safety to the standards of conventional medicine. For those practices that do have at least some research validating that they are safe and do work, **integrative medicine,** which combines conventional and less traditional methods, provides the best of both worlds.

In general, alternative practices **replace** those of conventional medicine, while complementary methods are used **with** traditional treatments. An alternative practice, for example, would be to use an herbal preparation to combat depression instead of physician-ordered prescription medication. A complementary treatment might consist of using biofeedback to lessen the symptoms of anxiety associated with mental illness. Both approaches address a key concept in alternative and complementary medicine: the **mind-body connection.**

■ MIND, BODY, AND BELIEF

The ways in which our minds and bodies are interconnected stretch beyond the obvious physical world in which we live. First there is the *brain,* an organ directly connected to the body by tissue such as nerves and blood vessels. The brain is contained within the bony cavity of the skull, which constitutes its protection and support. The *mind,* on the other hand, represents the cognitive, emotional, and logical seat of all that makes us individual human beings. The mind is clearly more than just the brain, the sum of its cells, chemicals, electrical activity, and connections.

It may seem strange to think that there was ever a question about the interconnectedness of the mind and the body. It has long been known that disease affects the

mind, but conventional medicine has only recently started to accept that the reverse is also true. Our thoughts and emotions impact the way our bodies function, even on a cellular level. This **holistic** view makes alternative and complementary medicine increasingly popular choices for the treatment of all types of illness, including mental disorders.

Important to the effectiveness of any type of treatment are the patient's **beliefs.** Nursing requires respect for the beliefs and values of other people and cultures as fundamental to good practice. It is useful to remember that everyone has a different way of viewing the world around them. We all form **models** of the world around us based on beliefs, values, education, and experience. Models are pictures or ideas that we form in our minds to explain how things work. They help us understand and interact with other people and our environment, and they help us to formulate beliefs.

To a large extent, a person's beliefs will determine the success of a given treatment. This can be plainly seen when a **placebo** medication is given and is effective in relieving symptoms like severe pain, even though the placebo is no more than a harmless sugar pill. This illustrates that what the patient believes and expects the placebo to do can be more important than the actual composition of the tablet.

While the nurse might not be directly involved in the application of an alternative or complementary treatment, supporting the client's cultural and belief systems is an important role in helping him or her forward on a path to wellness. Much of the success of the healing process is up to the client; the nurse can ease that process by remaining nonjudgmental, open, and accepting of different ideas.

As always, the boundaries of legal and acceptable nursing practice vary from state to state. Be sure to check with your state Board of Nursing or other regulating agencies to determine acceptable standards of practice in regard to using alternative, integrative, and complementary therapies.

■ COMMON ALTERNATIVE AND COMPLEMENTARY TREATMENTS

BIOFEEDBACK

Stress-related **anxiety** is the common element of disorders relating to mental illness. It is known that the direct effects of sustained stress can be devastating. In a critical moment or progressively over time, the biological response to stress can impair the cognitive function of the mind, clouding a person's thinking. Prolonged stress can lead to emotional anguish that is experienced as fear, anxiety, anger, and depression. Anxiety contributes to physical symptoms as well, many of which can be reduced or controlled by **biofeedback** techniques. While biofeedback only recently has become a complementary medical therapy, it has been widely accepted by traditionalists in the west because of its use of scientific measuring devices and proven techniques.

The primary purpose of biofeedback training is to teach patients to recognize tension within the body and to respond with relaxation (Fig. 9-1). Typically, training for patients takes place in a series of one-hour sessions, sometimes spaced a week apart. The client is taught to obtain a deep level of relaxation as a means to control a light, buzzer, image, or a video game, to which they are attached by electrodes and cables. The machine is then gradually adjusted to greater sensitivity, and the client learns improved control. When training is completed, all that is needed to obtain relaxation and symptom resolution at any time or place is recall of the particular thought and feeling that worked in the clinic.

Biofeedback is being used with good results for conditions including insomnia, some types of seizures, functional nausea and vomiting, tinnitus, and phantom limb pain. As with other forms of therapy, biofeedback practitioners must be aware of functional or even psychological symptoms that are actually caused by organic problems and require different treatment. It may not be appropriate to use biofeedback to treat extreme or acute states of mental illness, like severe depression, mania, agitation, schizophrenia, paranoia obsessive-compulsive disorder (OCD), delirium, and identity or dissociative disorders. Critics have pointed out that the major effects achieved from biofeedback can be more economically and easily obtained through relaxation training, which does not require costly electronic monitoring equipment.

Patients with strong faith that they can influence their own health are the most likely to be successful at mastering biofeedback.

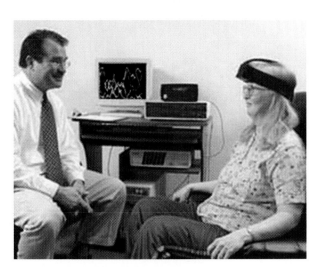

FIGURE 9-1. Biofeedback training teaches patients to recognize tension and respond with relaxation. (Courtesy of Santé Rehabilitation Group, Euless, TX.)

The experience of gaining control of one's physical reactions can have a tremendous effect on how the person will view stressful situations in the future. As an educational tool for more skeptical patients, learning biofeedback can demonstrate that they have a great deal more control over their responses and symptoms than they first expected.

AROMATHERAPY

Aromatherapy may well be one of the oldest methods used to treat illness in human beings. Related to herbal therapy, aromatherapy provides treatment by both the direct pharmacologic effects of aromatic plant substances and the indirect effects of certain smells on mood and affect. All through the history of mankind and in many different cultures there are accounts of the use of aromatics to treat varying forms of illness. Applied in salves or ointments, used in incense, reduced to essential oils for topical application, or even ingested, these substances often appeal to clients who are seeking a "natural" approach to healing (Fig. 9-2).

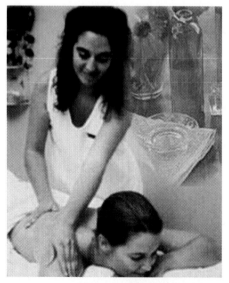

FIGURE 9-2. Aromatherapy can be applied in a variety of ways. Here the therapist uses it in the form of a massage oil. (Courtesy of stressbusters.co.uk)

Our response to the sense of smell has strong significance in our lives. We associate certain smells with certain situations, conditions, and emotional states. Many people are able to relive particularly strong memories when exposed to an aroma that was present when the remembered event occurred. For example, when presented with the fragrance of baking cookies or apple pie, it is not uncommon to be reminded of being at home and even experiencing some of the emotions connected to that memory. The ability for a particular smell to create positive alterations in mood makes aromatherapy attractive to many people and has created a large market in everyday products designed to evoke calm and well-being. Scented candles and personal care products like bath oils, shampoos, and body lotions are especially popular.

Treatment for anxiety-based mental illness and depression using aromatics like lavender, thyme, gardenia, and other botanicals is becoming a more acceptable adjunct to conventional methods. It is important to be aware that the oils and plant matter used in aromatherapy can be toxic if improperly administered and should be kept out of the reach of children and the cognitively impaired. Applied to skin, many plant oils are caustic or can trigger an allergic reaction. The nurse should observe and assess to determine if the products used are effective and if there are any side effects noted. As with all alternative treatment, it is advisable to find a competent and knowledgeable practitioner to benefit fully from the potential of aromatherapy.

HERBAL AND NUTRITIONAL THERAPY

Growing steadily in the United States today is the use of herbal compounds and nutritional supplements to treat illness. The popularity of self-treatment with herbs is in large part due to the desire of many people to return to a simpler lifestyle and as a means to avoid costly prescription medications. Most herbal products are considered to be **nutritional supplements** rather than medications, so these products avoid regulation by the Food and Drug Administration (FDA). They are also perceived by the public to be better, or safer, because they can be purchased over the counter and do not require a trip to the doctor's office.

There are literally hundreds of products available to consumers seeking relief through herbal and nutritional means. Once again, belief plays a considerable role in the acceptance and use of these products. With rapid changes in society since World War II has come the awareness that our lives are no longer as pastoral, calm, and idyllic as we would like to remember them to be. In a world full of processed food the quality of modern nutrition has come into ques-tion, and there is growing conviction that artificial additives lack the ability to provide us with the basics needed for good health.

Daily, we are assured in the popular press and the news media that the solution to many of our problems can be found in nutritional and herbal supplements. Lack of cortisol has been blamed for weight gain, and taking compounds rich in HGH (human growth hormone) have been credited with reversing aging. Infomercials tout the benefits of taking coral calcium and even improving sexual performance with herb-based preparations! The Internet is flooded with supplements (you can even buy them on eBay!) that promise to improve your life by making you healthier and stronger.

Some herbs have been researched and proven in their effectiveness in treating disease conditions. This should not be surprising, for many modern medications were developed from herbal and other botanical origins. Native Americans well knew the value of the inner bark of the willow tree, gathered and used for its ability to reduce fever and ease pain. They also used foxglove in their sweat lodges to energize the frail and restore vitality to the elderly. Little did they know that the salicylate in willow bark and digitalis in foxglove were the reasons for their effectiveness.

There is a tradition in Europe of using herbal medications and nutritional supplements to treat disease. Some herbal preparations are available there only by doctor's prescription, and others can only be obtained through a licensed pharmacist. People in Germany routinely plant and harvest herbs in their garden plots to create remedies for common ailments. In the United States, the use of fresh or garden-grown herbs is discouraged because of the difficulty in determining the strength of the active compounds produced by plants under different growing conditions. Europeans are guided by generations of experience and practice to safely use available botanicals.

Unfortunately, the belief in the relative safety of herbs is a misunderstanding that has caused much concern among health care providers. Deciding on an appropriate dose is difficult, because herbal preparations do not have to conform to any specific guidelines regulating strength or purity. People tend to think that if a small amount of the product is effective, more is better still. Some herbs are very toxic, particularly in pure form. Many will interact negatively with prescription medication. Nurses need to be able to teach their patients the importance of consulting with a physician before beginning any sort of herbal therapy. Table 9-1 describes the five most often used herbal medications and nutritional supplements in the treatment of mental illness in this country.

MASSAGE, ENERGY, AND TOUCH

Widespread among complementary and alternative treatment methods are modalities centered on manipulating the body's energy fields. **Massage** in one form or another has probably been known to man since before the dawn of history. Touch and movement are essential to life and well-being in both physical and psychological ways. We are shaped, almost literally, by our childhood experiences of touching. An infant has limited sensory discrimination, but will react positively to being cuddled and held and even to the feel of a snugly wrapped blanket.

TABLE 9-1 ■ *Common Herbal and Dietary Therapies*

SPECIFIC	ACTIVE INGREDIENTS	USUAL DOSE	USES	SIDE EFFECTS	CONTRAIN-DICATIONS	DRUG/FOOD INTERACTIONS	PATIENT TEACHING
GINKGO BILOBA	Ginkgentin, Ginkolic acid	120–140 mg PO daily, depending on what is treated; divide into 2–3 equal doses	Depression, combat short-term memory loss	Bleeding, contact dermatitis, nausea, vomiting, diarrhea, headache; rarely, subdural hematoma, seizures (especially in children)	Pregnant or breastfeeding, children; use cautiously for patient taking anticoagulants, MAOI medications as can act as a MAOI	May increase the effects of anti-coagulant and antiplatelet drugs. Avoid foods containing large amounts of tyramine: aged meat and cheese, red wine, pickled herring, yogurt, raisins, sour cream and other foods high in tyramine; also OTC cold and flu preparations.	Do not use if on Coumadin or aspirin. Works well for people over 50 as well as younger adults. May take 6–8 weeks to experience benefits. Use with some fruits and nuts can cause a poison ivy-like reaction.
KAVA KAVA	Kavapyrones, pypermethys-tine	10–110 mg PO dried kava extract three times daily, or freshly pre-pared kava beverages, 400–900 Gm *weekly*	Antidepressant, antianxiety, antipsychotic	Drowsiness, changes in reflex and judgment, nausea, muscle weakness, blurred vision,	Pregnancy, breastfeeding Skin yellowing from accumulation of plant pigment can occur in chronic use	*Do not use with:* Alcohol: increases risk of kava toxicity. Aprazolam: risk for coma exists. CNS depressants: kava potentiates these.	Symptom relief may occur in as little as 1 week. Potential for significant adverse reactions when using kava.

(continued)

KAVA KAVA *(cont'd)*				decreased platelet counts, decreased urea and bilirubin levels, dry skin, is a dopamine antagonist	Levodopa: can increase Parkinson-like symptoms. Phenobarbital: can increase effects.	Alcohol and CNS medications are enhanced with kava.
ST. JOHN'S WORT	Hypericum perforatum	300 mg PO three times daily for 4–6 weeks	Antidepressant	Severe photosensitivity, dry mouth, constipation, GI upset, sleep disturbances, restlessness	Pregnant or breastfeeding, children; use cautiously for patient taking anticoagulants, MAOI medications	MAOIs Avoid foods containing large amounts of tyramine: aged meat and cheese, red wine, pickled herring, yogurt, raisins, sour cream and other foods high in tyramine; also OTC cold and flu preparations. Alcohol. · Avoid prolonged exposure to sunlight. May increase the effects of MAOIs, OTC flu and cold medications, alcohol; do not use with these types of chemicals.
OMEGA 3 FATTY ACIDS (DIETARY SUPPLEMENT)	Alpha-linolenic acid (ALA), docosahexaenoic acid (DHA), and eicosapentanoic acid (EPA) 3:2 EPA to DHA (fish oil)	1–2 Gm PO daily for health, cognitive enhancement; clinical dose 2–5 Gm PO daily	Depression, postpartum depression, bipolar disorder, schizophrenia	Loose stools with higher doses; "fishy" reflux	Use cautiously for patients taking anticoagulants	May increase effects of anticoagulants · If taking anti-coagulant drugs or high doses of aspirin, practice good safety. The oils may increase clotting time

(continued)

TABLE 9-1   ■   *Common Herbal and Dietary Therapies (Continued)*

SPECIFIC	ACTIVE INGREDIENTS	USUAL DOSE	USES	SIDE EFFECTS	CONTRAIN-DICATIONS	DRUG/FOOD INTERACTIONS	PATIENT TEACHING
SAM-E (SUPPLE-MENT FOR NATURALLY PRODUCED BODY SUBSTANCE	s-adenosylme-thionine	See manu-facturer's specifications and use as directed by a physician	Depression	Mild and transient anxiety, insomnia, heartburn, loose bowels	Can cause mania in patients with bipolar disorder; rule out before beginning treatment		Patients with bipolar disorder should not use except under supervision of physician. Enteric coated preparations may reduce gastric upset.

Massage has evolved many variations as a result of its success (Fig. 9-3). Use of touch is common to many different treatment approaches, but there can be great variation in philosophical, theoretical, and practical ideas about how touch is applied. Western variations of massage include **Swedish,** which was developed in the early nineteenth century and is the type most people are familiar with. It is characterized by long, smooth strokes that go toward the direction of the heart.

The manipulation of specific body sites to relax muscle groups is known as **trigger point** massage. Conventional medical science has generated a similar trigger point therapy in which injections of steroids are applied at these key areas in place of massage to both relax the muscle group and reduce local inflammation. Of course there are also other means of more traditional massage available. **Rolfing,** for example, is a vigorous form of bodywork that is finding increasing acceptance.

Eastern massage traditions have followed a different path. It is widely believed among Eastern practitioners that the body is governed by energy paths, called **meridians.** This energy is perceived as the life force, or *chi*, *ki*, or *prana.* When the life force is obstructed, emotional and physical illnesses

result. Various types of pressure, massage, and other techniques are employed along these meridians to release the flow of chi, restore balance, and improve health. **Shiatsu** is a Japanese form of acupressure that uses pressure from the fingers to free energy flow. **Reflexology** is also based upon the belief that energy pathways and zones cross the body, connecting vital organs and body parts. Reflexologists use massage of the feet to act upon these pathways, unblocking and renewing the energy flow.

Therapeutic touch also deserves mention; **Reiki** is representative of methods of touch healing that are often associated with massage. Reiki is a term that means "universal life energy" and refers to the process whereby this energy is drawn along the body's meridians. Unlike methods that use physical movement, pressure, or massage to unblock these channels, Reiki uses the flow of life energy itself to accomplish the task. Practitioners are "attuned" to the energy channels and can manipulate them hands-on, hands just above the body, or even at a distance. Reiki techniques can even be employed as part of a more traditional massage session to enhance the physical benefits of the massage. Reiki has been demonstrated to increase warmth in the areas being treated and also to produce relaxation in the subject.

HYPNOTHERAPY

Hypnotherapy is one of the most controversial alternative and complementary modalities. Hypnosis is a means for entering an altered state of consciousness, and in this state, using visualization and suggestion to bring about desired changes in behavior and thinking. Called **trance,** people enter this state of focused attention every day. Our language even contains references to this common experience of "zoning out." Trance is not sleep, but rather describes a state of mind wherein a person is less aware of what is going on around him or her and instead is very focused on an internal experience, like a memory or an imagined event.

Everyone responds to **suggestion** to

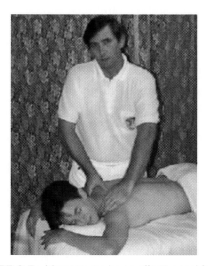
FIGURE 9-3. Massage can be an effective tool for relieving tension. (Courtesy of everything-jersey.com)

some extent. If you've ever been watching television and wanted a snack after seeing commercials for your favorite fast food restaurant, you have had an experience of suggestibility. Fortunately, our minds filter out suggestions that are unacceptably dangerous, or many more of us could be persuaded to imitate some of the more unsafe things we see on TV! A hypnotherapist uses suggestion, both direct and indirect, to help the patient create change.

The general public has been subjected to an enormous amount of misinformation about hypnosis by stage hypnotists, movies, and books. As a result, hypnotherapy is widely misunderstood and wrongly feared by many people. Watching a stage hypnotist appear to make a volunteer cluck like a chicken or dance on a table like Pee Wee Herman certainly does not inspire confidence in hypnosis as a therapeutic tool! It is very hard to overcome these fears, especially the stubborn belief in the myth that hypnosis is somehow "mind control" exercised for evil (or entertainment) purposes by the therapist.

While some researchers and practitioners contend that hypnosis cannot stand on its own as a treatment modality, others are equally convinced that even lay practitioners can deliver effective therapy with a minimum of training and practice. No doubt this controversy will continue, as there are at present few regulations governing the use of hypnosis. In some states a therapist must be certified or licensed, but in others no one but a psychologist, psychiatrist, medical doctor, or other professional may practice the techniques.

Milton H. Erickson, M.D. (1901–1980) was one of the best-known figures in the development of hypnosis for modern therapeutic purposes. Dr. Erickson was a victim of polio, which left him partially paralyzed. He had little strength in his arms and upper body and was confined to a wheelchair. As if that were not enough, he was dyslexic, tone-deaf, color-blind, and had heart problems. Left alone during long periods of illness, Erickson became a master of observation

and learned that subtle changes in facial expression, skin color, nuance of voice, and physical posture could tell him much about a person's inner state.

Dr. Erickson structured his therapeutic approach to patients in a new way. He refused to allow his own past disabilities ruin his living of life to its fullest and therefore refused to let old problems get in the way of his patients' enjoyment of living. Erickson ignored the past history of presenting patients, preferring instead to focus on present and future outcomes. In one classic case, Erickson gave the task of tending violets to a woman with depression. Combined with other therapeutic suggestions, she was kept too busy and involved in her community to remain depressed.

Traditional hypnotherapy and psychotherapy center on diagnosing problems and treating symptoms. Erickson promoted well-being, and study of his methods has challenged a whole new generation of hypnotherapists to do the same. Later, John Grinder and Richard Bandler would develop the field of neurolinguistic programming (NLP), based in large part upon their study of the extraordinary sensory acuity of Milton Erickson.

NEUROLINGUISTIC PROGRAMMING

Investigating the techniques and methods of many successful therapists, Bandler and Grinder searched for ways to make psychotherapy more consistently effective. It was through these explorations that they realized that language cues could be used to understand how an individual experiences his or her world. Using those cues, a practitioner can help patients change their experiences and respond to problems in a different way. Unlike traditional hypnosis, NLP does not use lengthy trance sessions and instead depends upon patients to take an active part in their treatment. When John Grinder and Richard Bandler began developing NLP, they based this extraordinary new type of therapy on a basic set of ideas, or **presuppositions**.

Presuppositions are the assumptions we make when forming communication. They are most often not spoken or written, but understood within the context of what is being communicated. For example, if the statement "I am so happy today!" is made, the presupposition, or unspoken assumption, is that the speaker is not normally happy. Our daily communications are filled with such assumptions, things that we take for granted. NLP differs from other therapies in that there is no presupposition that the patient is somehow "broken" and requires "fixing." Instead, practitioners are taught that patients are whole individuals who already possess the internal resources they need to recover from their illness. All that is required is to direct the patient to those resources and enable their use.

People observe their world through distinct **channels** of experience, tending to prefer one channel over another, but eventually using them all for important cues and sensory information about their environment and other people. The three primary methods of sensory representation are the **visual**, **auditory,** and **kinesthetic** channels (seeing, hearing, and touching). Of course, we also use taste and smell to gather information, but these paths are rarely the most important channel, and they are generally ignored.

Paying attention to speech patterns gives the practitioner a starting point for meaningful communication with the patient. The most obvious way to do this is to listen to the predicates a person uses while describing thoughts and ideas. The practitioner can then determine if the person favors sight, hearing, or touch and match those predicates, using the same language patterns to create positive **rapport**. As a nurse, recognizing these patterns can help improve your own communication with patients. Table 9-2 illustrates types of word patterns people use.

TABLE 9-2	*Representational System Predicates*	
VISUAL (SEEING)	**AUDITORY (HEARING)**	**KINESTHETIC (FEELING)**
an eyeful	clear as a bell	all washed up
appears to me	clearly expressed	boils down to
beyond the shadow of a doubt	call on	chip off the old block
bird's eye view	describe in detail	come to grips with
catch a glimpse of	earful	control yourself
clear cut	express yourself	cool, calm, collected
dim view	give an account of	firm foundations
eye to eye	give me your ear	get a handle on
get a perspective on	grant an audience	get in touch with
scope out	heard voices	hand in hand
hazy idea	hidden message	hang in there
horse of a different color	hold your tongue	hold on
in light of	idle talk	hold it
in view of	inquire into	keep your shirt on
make a scene	keynote speaker	know how
mental image	loud and clear	lightheaded
mind's eye	manner of speaking	moment of panic
naked eye	pay attention to	pain in the neck
paint a picture photographic	power of speech	pull some strings
memory	outspoken	sharp as a tack
plainly seen	rings a bell	slipped my mind
pretty as a picture	to tell the truth	start from scratch
sight for sore eyes	unheard of	underhanded
	word for word	under pressure

Of course, just about everyone uses all three forms of predicates at one time or another. The most important thing to remember is to **match** the dominant, or most used form.

EXAMPLES

(Visual)
Mary: "I can't picture myself getting any better."
Nurse: "In light of your progress, see yourself going back to school. How does that look to you?"
(Auditory)
James: "I've heard that the doctor is tuned in to the newest treatments."
Nurse: "He can describe those in detail to you. I'll tell him you want to hear about them."
(Kinesthetic)
Diane: "I couldn't come to grips with the situation. I was under too much pressure all the time."

Nurse: "It is hard to get in touch with what's important when you feel that way."

These exchanges demonstrate communication on more than one level. By using the same language used by the patient, the nurse can establish that she or he is listening closely to the message that is being sent. This is a powerful tool in creating and maintaining rapport, the foundation to a therapeutic relationship.

Nursing practice is evolving and is incorporating "alternative" or "complementary" therapies into traditional care delivery systems. State boards of nursing can determine at what level and scope of practice nurses provide the alternative therapy. In 2003, for example, the Minnesota Board of Nursing adopted guidelines and statements for appropriate use of complementary therapy in Minnesota. Those guidelines can be found at www.nursingboard.state.mn.us.

Key Concepts ▪ ▪ ▪

1. Alternative and complementary treatments provide options for patients other than those offered by conventional (Western) medicine. Alternative modalities are used instead of, and complementary are used in addition to, conventional practices.
2. The mind-body connection is an important concept in all types of medical treatment. Disease and wellness affect a whole person. Holistic treatments address both the illness and the person.
3. An individual has beliefs, based upon his or her model of the world. These beliefs must be respected by the nurse.
4. Anxiety is common to disorders relating to mental illness. Prolonged stress and anxiety lead to physical as well as mental and emotional afflictions.
5. Biofeedback is a technique that teaches the patient to recognize and control stress responses in the body. It is widely accepted because of its use of scientific measuring devices to demonstrate the effectiveness of the treatment.
6. Aromatherapy uses our emotional response to smell as well as the pharmacologic effects of various fragrant botanical and other substances to treat illness.
7. Herbal and nutritional therapies are becoming more prevalent as the public embraces "natural" healing. Many modern medications have evolved from uncultivated botanical products. Relative safety and effectiveness is

still in question, as the industry is largely unregulated, with no set standards for these products.

8. Other types of alternative and complementary therapy focus on manipulation, strengthening, and removing blockage from the free flow of energy in the human body. Massage and therapeutic touch modalities are successful groups of both stand-alone and adjunctive treatment for disease.

9. Hypnotherapy and neurolinguistic programming are two prominent modalities that address mental and bodily illness by empowering change in the patient's thought patterns. Both tightly focus on communication patterns and the client-therapist relationship.

REFERENCE

F.Y.I.—A Publication of the Minnesota Board of Nursing (2003). *Complementary Therapies* Spring/Summer 2003 Issue, *19*(1), 7.

WEBSITES

National Center for Complementary and Alternative Medicine (NCCAM): www.nccam.nih.gov/

Association for Applied Psychophysiology & Biofeedback: www.aapb.org/

Biofeedback Certification Institute of America: www.bcia.org

Mind/Body Connection: How Your Emotions Affect Your Health: www.familydoctor.org

Health Psychology: The Mind-Body Connection: www.mental-health-matters.com/articles/article.php?artID=498

The National Association for Holistic Aromatherapy: www.naha.org/

American Massage Therapy Association: www.amtamassage.org

National Certification Board for Therapeutic Massage and Bodywork: www.ncbtmb.com

The Association of Reflexologists - Home of Reflexology: www.reflexology.org

International Institute of Reflexology: www.reflexology-usa.net

Reiki Home, What Is Reiki, History of Reiki, Whole-Body Reiki ...: www.holistic-online.com/Reiki/hol_Reiki_home.htm

IARP - International Association of Reiki Professionals: www.iarp.org

The Milton H. Erickson Foundation: www.erickson-foundation.org

American Society of Clinical Hypnosis: www.hypnosis-research.org/hypnosis

Society of Psychological Hypnosis: www.apa.org/divisions/div30/

Neurolinguistic Programming. How Does It Work?: www.holistic-online.com/hol_neurolinguistic.htm

Neurolinguistic Programming Resources: www.umdnj.edu/psyevnts/neuroling.html

CRITICAL THINKING EXERCISE ■ ■ ■

1. You are assigned to the care of Ramona, a 23-year-old female who is suffering from severe depression, has been admitted following a suicide attempt, and whose progress on antidepressant medication has been slow. Over the next few days, you begin to notice that she is becoming restless and more moody, sometimes reacting angrily to you and other staff members. One day, you enter her room to find her dressed and packing her personal belongings into a suitcase. She tells you that she is leaving to return home,

where she plans to seek the help of a local healer. When you attempt to talk to her, she becomes enraged and begins to talk about how "you people" don't understand her illness. Finally, a family member arrives and she leaves the facility, without discharge orders or planning! How do you feel about Ramona's decision? Do you think that she shares the same beliefs about health care that you do? Do you think she will recover from her depression? Why?

TEST QUESTIONS ■ ■ ■

MULTIPLE CHOICE QUESTIONS

1. Alternative therapy modalities are used:
   A. Infrequently, as they have no value to patients today.
   B. In combination with conventional therapies.
   C. In place of conventional therapies.
   D. Only when there is no hope for recovery.

2. A treatment modality used with conventional medical therapies is:
   A. A medical approach.
   B. A model approach.
   C. A holistic approach.
   D. A complementary approach.

3. When traditional medicine is combined with less traditional methods, it is:
   A. Integrative medicine.
   B. Exclusive medicine.
   C. Based on the physician's opinions.
   D. Biofeedback.

4. The mechanism that describes thought and expectation affecting health is:
   A. A complementary therapy.
   B. A misconception that is dangerous to the patient.
   C. An integrated therapy.
   D. The mind-body connection.

5. Mrs. Lucas is telling you about her ideas for curing her depression by taking herbal medication. She is convinced that because St. John's Wort is a natural product, it is better for her than her prescription therapy. You should:
   A. Quickly get the drug handbook and show her she is wrong.
   B. Remain open and supportive.
   C. Point out to her that herbal therapy is contraindicated.
   D. Suggest some available brands for her to use.

6. Of the following, which are either complementary or alternative modalities?
   A. ECT, Reiki, rolfing
   B. Hypnotherapy, shiatsu, antianxiety medications

    C. NLP, psychotherapy, SAM-e

    D. Aromatherapy, biofeedback, massage

7. Mr. Douglas wants to know more about massage therapy. Which one of the following is NOT a massage modality?

    A. Reiki

    B. Trigger point

    C. Rolfing

    D. Swedish

8. Which of the following is *false* about trance?

    A. It is an altered state of consciousness, just like sleep.

    B. Humans move in and out of trance states during the day.

    C. It is a state of relaxed awareness.

    D. Trance is a common experience even if you aren't aware of it.

9. Which of the following statements indicates a visual channel preference for information?

    A. "That really feels good! My gut feeling is that it will work!"

    B. "It sounds good to me; this idea is worth paying attention to."

    C. "I can see the solution, and clearly it will work."

    D. "I smell a rat. I think the whole thing stinks."

10. Which of the following should be *avoided* when communicating with a mentally ill patient?

    A. Having an expectation that the patient will get better.

    B. Making the presupposition that the patient will not improve.

    C. Taking the time to convey respect for the patient.

    D. Demonstrating through your expression and posture that you are listening.

2

Threats to Mental Health

10

Mental Health Alterations

Learning Objectives ■ ■ ■

1. Define mental health.
2. Define mental illness.
3. Define health-illness continuum.
4. Define *DSM-IV-TR*.
5. Identify several methods used in diagnosing mental health alterations.

Key Terms ■ ■ ■

- Continuum
- *DSM-IV-TR*
- Mental health
- Mental illness

Within the mental health community, opinions differ as to just exactly what mental health and mental illness are. The Alliance for the Mentally Ill, which has state branches, a national branch, and international branches, defines mental illness as "biologically based brain diseases that can severely disturb a person's ability to think, feel and relate to other people and the environment." The alliance does not generally encompass the psychoanalytic or behavioral theories relating to threats to mental integrity.

This text uses the more liberal definitions of mental health and mental illness. It gives brief explanations of the most common psychological and biologic causes of individual illnesses.

Nursing language usually speaks in terms of "threats to . . . ," and this text discusses certain threats to mental health. **Mental health** has been defined by many different criteria, such as:

- The ability to be flexible
- The ability to be successful
- The ability to form close relationships
- The ability to make appropriate judgments
- The ability to solve problems
- The ability to cope with daily stresses
- The ability to have a positive sense of self

Mental illness, or, in nursing terminology, "threats to mental health," is defined as:

- Impairment of a person's ability to think
- Impairment of a person's ability to feel
- Impairment of a person's ability to make sound judgments
- Difficulty or inability to cope with reality
- Difficulty or inability to form strong personal relationships

It is important to remember that mental health and mental illness run on a **continuum**—it changes somewhat from day to day. We live in a society that bombards us with stressful situations continuously. It is natural for individuals to ebb and flow emotionally in daily response to the degree of stress they are experiencing. Individuals who remain mentally healthy are able to find methods of dealing with their stress and keeping it in perspective. Others cannot do so and over time may develop physical or emotional illnesses as a result of the constant stress in their lives. Visualize the "Scales of Justice," the scales that balance from side to side. Mental health and mental illness are like that scale (Fig. 10-1). Most of the time the scale is balanced. Mentally healthy people keep themselves in a state of emotional balance. Sometimes, the scale tips just a little to one side or the other, but

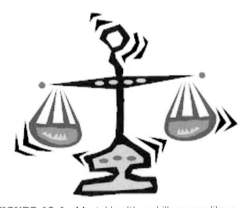

FIGURE 10-1. Mental health and illness are like a scale. Mentally healthy people are able to keep the scale mostly balanced, despite occasional fluctuations, but in mental illness, the scale tips way out of balance. (Courtesy of Washington State Department of Financial Institutions, Olympia, WA.)

mentally healthy people can cope with this fluctuation. When things become stressful or when bad (or good) things happen, people expect to see others expressing feelings of sadness, happiness, nervousness, or other emotions that reflect the event.

Sometimes, the scale tilts out of balance completely and one end goes way up while the other goes way down, and it stays where it is until someone alters the balance. Ultimately, it must be the patient who finds his or her own balance, and sometimes this takes help from an outside resource, such as a nurse or a physician. When people are way down or way up, they are not in emotional homeostasis. Patients may not see the depth of their situation and usually need help to learn ways to help themselves return to a state of balance. Most people strive to stay in balance most of the time. When we become out of balance, it is good to know that there are nurses, physicians, and other mental health professionals who are trained to help balance the weight of the stressors in our lives.

■ ETIOLOGIC THEORIES

The discussion of the etiology (causes) of mental illnesses continues to revolve around the "nature versus nurture" or "organic versus inorganic or functional" arguments. The connection between physical and emotional health is so closely intertwined that it is sometimes hard to decide if the emotional causes the physical or vice versa.

Experts have different opinions relating to the causes of mental illness, including the "nature" (organic or physical) causes and the "nurture" (inorganic or emotional) causes. These opinions are highly debated and, at this time, there are very few absolutes in psychiatric etiology. Nurses need to understand both general schools of thought on what causes alterations in mental health. You will also, no doubt, develop your own opinions about where the illnesses come from.

Explanations of mental illness include symptoms from both the psychoanalytic (or psychological) and the psycho-biologic (or biologic) theories. When pertinent, other theories (e.g., behavioral, environmental, and so on) are also presented. Brief descriptions of psychoanalytic and psycho-biologic theories follow.

PSYCHOANALYTIC THEORY

Psychoanalytic theory includes the "nurture," or inorganic or functional, rationales for mental illnesses.

Sigmund Freud believed completely that mental illness was a direct result of an ineffective parent-child relationship. The "nurture" issue implies that poor relationships with the significant people in a young person's life set the stage for a life of compensating. Freud believed this compensating occurs unconsciously. This theory postulates that the person with altered mental functioning endured a situation, often unknown, that happened early in life, over which the person had no control, and that he or she can't be held responsible for subsequent behaviors. This would cause the person's mental faculties to fail to function as they were intended to.

PSYCHOBIOLOGIC THEORY

The "nature," or organic, theory holds that, contrary to the psychoanalytic theory, altered mental status is a product of a genetic, physical, or neurochemical malfunction of the brain. Psychology and the study of mental illness are fairly new in relationship to the rest of the health-care field. Most mental illnesses have no definitive etiology. Some etiologic theories have stronger positive correlations to illnesses than others. When appropriate, this text gives the most popular or most accepted view of an etiology. At no time is an absolute etiology given for a condition because, truthfully, in most cases, absolute etiologies do not yet exist.

■ DIAGNOSING A MENTAL ILLNESS

The diagnostic tool used most frequently by psychiatrists and psychologists, the *Diagnostic and Statistical Manual of Mental Disorders-IV-Text Revision,* or **DSM-IV-TR,** offers a complex method of classifying criteria from different standpoints, or axes, ranking them by severity. The writers of *DSM-IV-TR* have made every attempt to build in cultural, ethnic, and religious considerations to avoid labeling a behavior that would be considered "normal" or acceptable in those defined groups. Applying them to an individual to arrive at an accurate diagnosis is no simple task, as most diagnoses require a stated number of symptoms to be present for a specific amount of time.

Of course, physicians can use other diagnostic criteria to diagnose mental illness. Sometimes they do this by testing for other illnesses in an effort to "rule out" (R/O) that illness. This results in a process-of-elimination method of diagnosis. Then, when other possibilities have been ruled out, the physician may choose to refer the patient to a psychiatrist or psychologist for further testing and diagnosis.

In addition to the *DSM-IV-TR*, batteries of psychological tests, or inventories, can be administered to individuals. These are administered and interpreted by psychiatrists or psychologists. Some of the more frequently used diagnostic inventories or tests are listed in Table 10-1.

Age, hand tremors, vision, language barriers, educational background, and the interpretation of the psychiatrist or psychologist could influence these tests. Any of these or other factors have the possibility of either positively or negatively influencing the results.

Besides the *DSM-IV-TR* and the many psychological testing inventories, other tests that may be performed to either confirm or rule out a diagnosis of a mental illness include:

TABLE 10-1	*Diagnostic Tests or Inventories Used in Diagnosing Alterations in Mental Health*	
TEST NAME	**DESCRIPTION OF TEST**	**WHAT THE TEST ASSESSES**
MINNESOTA MULTIPHASIC PERSONALITY INVENTORY (MMPI) (FOR CHILDREN AND ADOLESCENTS)	550 statements that must be answered "yes," "no," or "cannot say." Statements relate to emotions, attitudes, motor disturbances, psychosomatic symptoms. Nine "scales" exist, all looking for specific indications. Scales are built in for "faking" and "corrections" of hostile responses.	Depression, psychopathic/ antisocial tendencies, paranoia, schizophrenia, hypochondriasis, hysteria, social introversion, anxiety, phobia.
MMPI-2 (REVISED FORM FOR ADULTS)	104 new questions have been added, directed at adults.	Also measures tendency for eating disorders, drug abuse, and type A personality.
RORSCHACH INKBLOT	A series of 10 symmetrical inkblots. Patient answers questions about different parts of the "picture." Tester records the associations made by the patient.	*Projective:* Supposed to reveal patient's underlying feelings, traits, attitudes.
THEMATIC APPERCEPTION TEST (TAT)	A series of 30 photographs; the patient is asked to look at and explain the "story" in the pictures.	*Projective:* The "theme" told in the story reveals the thoughts and feelings of the patient, the current situation, what led to the situation, the potential outcome.
BENDER-GESTALT	Set of 9 pictures that the patient is asked to draw or reproduce as best as he or she can.	*Screener:* Used to diagnose intellectual ability, emotional problems, brain damage. Healthy or "intact" people see the "whole" picture.

Data from Aiken L.R.: Psychological Testing and Assessment, 8th ed. Copyright © 1994 by Allyn and Bacon, Needham Heights, MA. Adapted by permission.

■ Blood work (to R/O electrolyte imbalances, dehydration, drug toxicity, and so on)

■ Computed tomography (CT) or magnetic resonance imaging (MRI) scans (to R/O tumors, lesions, and so on)

■ Positron emission tomography (PET) scans (to identify how parts of the brain are functioning by showing chemical activity or metabolism)

■ CLASSIFICATIONS OF MENTAL ILLNESS

Classifications of mental illness according to *DSM-IV-TR* are listed in Appendix D. The *DSM-IV-TR* uses a system of five axes for grouping illnesses into categories. Axis I lists clinical disorders and includes delirium, dementia, mood disorders, mental disorders as the result of a general medical condition, and others. Axis II lists personality disorders/mental retardation. Mental retardation is not the same kind of mental disorder as other mental illnesses from a nursing standpoint and therefore is not discussed here. Axis III lists general medical conditions, which include diseases of the other body systems, neoplasms, and infectious diseases. Axis IV considers psychosocial and environmental problems, including educational, social, economic, and other social concerns. Axis V is the global assessment of functioning (GAF) scale, a numbering system for ranking the severity of symptoms.

This system is a very complex diagnostic tool, which you will not need to memorize. However, it is interesting for nurses to know how the mental health diagnoses are made and how easy it is to make incorrect diagnoses.

Key Concepts ▪ ▪ ▪

1. The definition and focus of mental health and mental illness are somewhat different from those of other organizations and disciplines within the health-care system. Nursing uses a more liberal, holistic focus in defining and caring for people with mental illnesses.
2. Mental health and illness run on a continuum that changes somewhat daily, which tends to keep stress in perspective and balance.
3. There are theories to support both the "nature" (organic/physical) and the "nurture" (inorganic/emotional) causes for mental illnesses.
4. Many tests and measuring tools are available to aid psychiatrists and psychologists in diagnosing mental illnesses. The *DSM-IV-TR* is a major tool used in these disorders.

REFERENCE

American Psychiatric Association. (2000). *Diagnostic and Statistical Manual of Mental Disorders—Text Revision.* American Psychiatric Association, Washington, DC.

WEBSITE

www.psych.org

CRITICAL THINKING EXERCISES ▪ ▪ ▪

1. Think about a patient you suspect might have one or more of the following threats to his or her mental health: depression, generalized anxiety disorder, schizophrenia.

   Obtain a copy of the *DSM-IV-TR* from the library. Look up the diagnostic criteria for the person you are studying. Compare the *DSM-IV-TR* criteria with the signs and symptoms you observe in the person you are considering. Would you be able to make a positive diagnosis? Why or why not? What information do you need to be able to make a positive diagnosis?

2. Using the suggested nursing diagnoses listed here (or others you can think of), complete a nursing process for a patient with a suspected mental health alteration.

SUGGESTED NURSING DIAGNOSES

1. *Self-Esteem Disturbance*
2. *Thought Processes, Altered*
3. *Ineffective Family Coping: Compromised*

ASSESSMENT/ DATA COLLECTION	NURSING DIAGNOSIS	PLAN/ GOAL	INTERVENTIONS/ NURSING ACTIONS	EVALUATION CRITERIA

3. Review the information on P.E.S. Attempt to write the same nursing process as you did in #2 above. Was your nursing diagnosis or outcome statement changed? In what way(s)?

TEST QUESTIONS ■ ■ ■

MULTIPLE CHOICE QUESTIONS

1. An LPN/LVN who is considering the possibility that a patient has a threat to mental health might base that assessment on the patient's:
   A. Intelligence only
   B. Behavior and its appropriateness to the situation
   C. Opinion of his or her physician
   D. Family members

2. Which of the following patients does not reflect mental health?
   A. Patient who is always happy and smiling
   B. Patient who can verbalize emotions
   C. Patient who is able to cope with "bad news"
   D. Patient who maintains some close, personal relationships

3. Nurses who are working with patients with mental illnesses understand that the illness is:
   A. Of biologic etiology only
   B. Of emotional etiology only
   C. Of environmental etiology only
   D. Of a complex etiology

4. List three terms to define the psychoanlaytic, or "nurture," theory:

   _____

   _____

   _____

5. List three terms to define the psychobiologic, or "nature," theory:

   _____

   _____

   _____

11

Anxiety Disorders

Learning Objectives ■ ■ ■

1. Define anxiety disorders.
2. Identify five specific anxiety disorders.
3. State physical and behavioral symptoms of five anxiety disorders.
4. Identify treatment modalities for five anxiety disorders.
5. Identify nursing care for five anxiety disorders.

Key Terms ■ ■ ■

- Anxiety
- Compulsion
- Eustress
- Free-floating anxiety
- Generalized anxiety
- Obsession
- Panic disorder
- Phobia
- Post-traumatic stress disorder
- Signal anxiety
- Stress
- Stressor

Stress produces **anxiety.** Stress is everywhere in our society. Most often, stress is associated with negative situations, but the good things that happen to us, such as weddings and job promotions, also produce stress. This stress from positive experiences, such as becoming newly married, promoted at work, or something similar, is called **eustress.** It can produce just as much anxiety as the negative stressors. A **stressor** is any person or situation that produces anxiety responses. Stress and stressors are different for each person; therefore, it is important that the nurse ask the patient what the stress producers are for that person. What is extremely stressful for one person (driving in rush hour traffic, for example) might be relaxing to someone else

(as a time to slow down and relax after a busy day).

Anxiety is the uncomfortable feeling of dread that is a response to extreme or prolonged periods of stress. The four commonly accepted levels of anxiety are mild, moderate, severe, and panic (Fig. 11-1). Hildegard Peplau teaches that a mild amount of anxiety is a normal part of being human and that it is necessary to change and develop new ways of coping with stress.

Anxiety may also be influenced by one's culture. It may be acceptable for some people to acknowledge and discuss stress, but others may believe that one should keep personal problems to oneself. This can be a challenge to the nurse during an assessment.

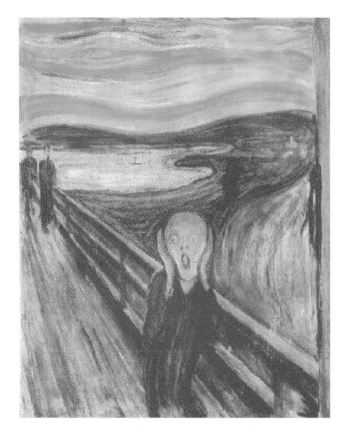

FIGURE 11-1. Anxiety ranges in severity from mild through panic. "The Scream," a famous painting by Norwegian artist Edvard Munch, depicts a person in a very high state of anxiety.

Anxiety is usually referred to in two ways: free-floating anxiety and signal anxiety. **Free-floating anxiety** is described as a feeling of impending doom. The person might say something like "I just know something bad is going to happen if I go on vacation," without knowing when or where the event might occur. **Signal anxiety,** on the other hand, is an uncomfortable response to a known stressor (e.g., "Finals are only a week away and I've got that nagging nausea again"). Both types of anxiety are involved in the various anxiety disorders.

Nurses working with children and teenage patients must also be aware that these patients experience anxiety and stress. They may not be able to verbalize their feelings, and they may display symptoms differently than adults.

Some indicators of stress and anxiety in these age groups include decline in school performance, changes in eating habits and sleeping patterns, and withdrawal from friends and usual activities.

There is a positive correlation between juvenile offenders and incarcerated young people. On average, more than 50 percent of juveniles who are in trouble with the law also have a mental illness, including drug/alcohol use, disruptive behaviors, anxiety, and/or suicide attempts.

Nurses can be instrumental in screening children and adolescents for signs of anxiety.

■ ETIOLOGIC THEORIES

Psychoanalytic theory says that there is a conflict between the id and the superego, which causes anxiety. At some time in the individual's development this conflict was repressed but emerged again in adulthood.

When conflict emerges, patients realize they have "failed," and the manifestations of anxiety are once again felt.

The biologic theory sees this situation differently. It considers the sympathoadrenal ("fight or flight") responses to stress and observes that the blood vessels constrict because epinephrine and norepinephrine have been released. Blood pressure rises. If the body adapts to the stress, hormone levels adjust to compensate for the epinephrine-norepinephrine release, and the body functions return to homeostasis. If the body does not adapt to the stress, then the immune system becomes challenged, lymph nodes increase in size, chances for heart and kidney failure increase, and death may occur.

Studies are continually being conducted trying to correlate the condition of stress to physical illness. In 2002, researchers at Carnegie Mellon University in Pittsburgh studied 334 paid individuals. They introduced a rhinovirus into the participants' noses. Then they placed the participants into individual, private hotel rooms. Several days later, they tested the individuals for symptoms. People who had described themselves as happier, contented type of personalities demonstrated cold/flu symptoms only one third as often as the individuals who did not use those kinds of words to describe themselves and their stress level. This is one study. We do not know all of the variables, but it does make a fairly strong argument for a positive correlation between emotional stress and physical illness.

Anger, especially the type of anger that nears rage level but is suppressed, may also have an effect on physical health. This condition may lead patients to experience chronic headache.

The LPN/LVN will frequently experience mental illness in conjunction with medical-surgical patients. Physical and emotional symptoms can interrelate. It is important for nurses to recognize the relationship between physical and emotional responses to stress. Nurses can be instrumental in gaining accurate diagnosis and treatment for their patients by providing accurate assessment and documentation of the patient's symptoms as his or her body adapts to stress. Table 11-1 gives some examples of medical conditions and the effects of the body's adaptation response to stress.

■ DIFFERENTIAL DIAGNOSIS

Because so many symptoms are associated with anxiety disorders, it is important for people to have a complete physical workup before being checked for these disorders. The symptoms of anxiety disorders are listed with each of the specific disorders. Symptoms of anxiety disorders can mimic those seen in diabetes, cardiac problems, medication side effects, electrolyte imbalances, or physical trauma. The physician must rule out a systemic infection or an allergy that might be related to chills or swallowing difficulty. Hot flashes, which can occur in some anxiety states, could be related to a fever or to menopause. The physician must always consider the possibility of drug or alcohol abuse as partial causes for the symptoms. Certainly, more than one condition can occur simultaneously.

■ TYPES

GENERALIZED ANXIETY DISORDER (GAD)

In **generalized anxiety disorder**, the anxiety (also referred to as "excessive worry" or "severe stress") itself is the expressed symptom. The *DSM-IV-TR* requires that this excessive worry be related to two or more things and last 6 months or longer.

Patients who have GAD may display any number of symptoms. The *DSM-IV-TR* lists 18 symptoms of anxiety, and the patient must show six or more in order to be con-

TABLE 11-1 ■ *Adaptation Responses to Stress*		
STRESS-RELATED MEDICAL CONDITION	**BODY'S ADAPTATION TO THE STRESS**	**OUTCOME OF STRESS ON THE BODY**
LOWERED IMMUNITY	Interferes with effectiveness of the body's antibodies; possibly related to interactions among the hypothalamus, pituitary gland, adrenal glands, and the immune system.	Increased susceptibility to colds, viruses, and other illnesses
BURNOUT	Associated with stress-related depression.	Emotional detachment
MIGRAINE, CLUSTER, AND TENSION HEADACHES	Tightening skeletal muscles, dilating of cranial artery.	Nausea, vomiting, tight feeling in or around head and shoulders, tinnitus, inability to tolerate light, weakness of a limb
STRESS (PEPTIC) ULCERS	Stress contributes to the formation of ulcers by stimulating the vagus nerve and ultimately leading to hypersecretion of hydrochloric acid.	Nausea, vomiting, gastrointestinal bleeding, perforation of intestinal walls
HYPERTENSION	Role of stress is not positively known but is thought to contribute to hypertension by negatively interacting with the kidneys and endocrine system.	Resistance to blood flow through the cardiovascular system, causing pressure on the arteries; can lead to stroke, heart attack, and kidney failure
CORONARY ARTERY DISEASE	Stressor increases the amount of epinephrine and norepinephrine.	Dilated coronary vessels, increased pulse and respirations
CANCER	Same mechanisms that lower immunity.	Lowered immunity may allow for overcolonization of opportunistic cancer cells
ASTHMA	Automatic nervous system stimulates mucus, increases blood flow, and constricts bronchial tubes; may be associated with other stress-related conditions such as allergy and viral infection.	Wheezing, coughing, dyspnea, apprehension; may lead to respiratory infections, respiratory failure, and/or pneumothorax

sidered "anxious." Some behaviors that may be present in the anxious person include restlessness, fatigue, feeling "on edge," or frightening very easily. Patients may have sleep disturbances also.

Symptoms may include:
■ Muscle aches
■ Shakes
■ Palpitations
■ Dry mouth

■ Nausea
■ Vomiting
■ Hot flashes
■ Chills
■ Polyuria
■ Difficulty swallowing

Several more potential symptoms of anxiety exist, but the ones listed here seem to be the most frequently seen. They are also, however, common symptoms of many other conditions. It is easy to see how mistakes in diagnosing can happen!

PANIC DISORDER

Panic is a state of extreme fear that cannot be controlled. It is also referred to as "panic attack," and people may not consider it to be a serious disorder. In more advanced classes, **panic disorder** may be differentiated into the categories "with agoraphobia" (fear of open places) or "without agoraphobia." For our purposes, these categories will not be elaborated on. General discussion of phobias continues in the next section.

Panic episodes present quickly. *DSM-IV-TR* criteria for panic disorder require at least 4 of a list of 12 possible symptoms, some of which are identified here. Some of the behaviors that may be observed in panic disorder include:

■ Fear (usually of dying, losing control of oneself, or of "going crazy")
■ Dissociation (a feeling that it is happening to someone else or not happening at all)
■ Nausea
■ Diaphoresis
■ Chest pain
■ Increased pulse
■ Shaking
■ Unsteadiness

PHOBIA

This is the most common of the anxiety disorders. **Phobia** is defined as an "irrational fear." The person is very aware of the fear and even of the fact that it is irrational, but the fear continues.

People develop phobias to many different things—approximately 700 different things, in fact! Snakes, spiders, enclosed spaces, and the number 13 are some of the more common phobias (Fig. 11-2). People also develop phobias of things such as caring for

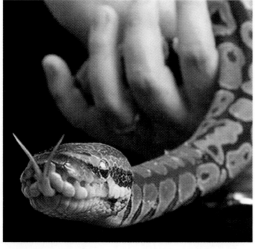
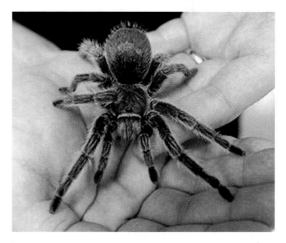

A   B

FIGURE 11-2. A, Fear of snakes (ophidiophobia) and, B, spiders (arachnophobia) are two of the most common phobias. (Courtesy of University of Texas, Austin, TX.)

their children (because they might hurt them) and eating in places other than their own home.

The psychoanalytic view implies that the fear is not from the object itself necessarily but rather a fear of the defense mechanism displacement. For example, the person with a phobia of snakes may have seen a frightening movie in which someone died from a snake bite. This person's fear of snakes, then, may result not from the snake itself, but from fear of dying from the venom of a bite. The stated object of the phobia would be interpreted as a symbol for the underlying cause of the fear.

Phobias have three subcategories: agoraphobia, social phobia, and simple phobia. Agoraphobia is the irrational fear of being in open spaces and being unable to leave or being very embarrassed if leaving is required. For example, people who fear shopping in large malls or who fear going to sporting events may actually fear the possibility of being unable to escape in the event of an accident. Social phobias are those in which people avoid social situations as a result of fear of humiliation. There are correlations between people with this type of phobia and people who misuse or abuse alcohol. The fear of speaking in public and the fear of using public facilities such as bathrooms or laundromats are examples of social phobias. Simple phobia is having an irrational fear of a specific object or situation, and these are the ones we hear most about. Examples of simple phobias are claustrophobia (fear of enclosed places), hematophobia (fear of blood), and acrophobia (fear of heights).

OBSESSIVE-COMPULSIVE DISORDER (OCD)

This type of anxiety disorder consists of two parts: the **obsession** (repetitive thought, urge, or emotion) and the **compulsion** (repetitive act that may appear purposeful). An example of OCD is the need to check numerous times that doors are locked before

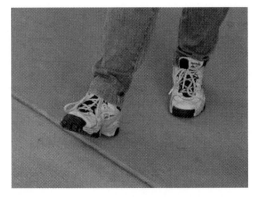

FIGURE 11-3. Compulsive behaviors include refusing to step on a crack in the sidewalk. The behavior is very ritualistic, and performing the action reduces the person's anxiety. (Courtesy of the National Institute of Mental Health, Bethesda, MD.)

one is able to sleep or leave the house. In reality, this need to repetitively check the locks may prevent the person from sleeping or leaving at all. The person with this kind of anxiety disorder is unable to stop the thought or the action. Behaviors become very ritualistic (Fig. 11-3). It is the thought or the action that reduces the anxiety.

Defense mechanisms that have been associated as possible contributors to OCD are repression, reaction-formation, and undoing. A genetic link among families who display OCD has been suggested. In 1987, the APA released a study saying that OCD is more common among first-degree biologic relatives of persons with this disorder than among the general population.

Behaviors in patients with OCD vary. Each person performs the thought or action that is the substitute for the anxiety producer. Some people wash their hands unceasingly. Others have a strict ritual that, if interrupted, requires starting over from the beginning. Some people have to check something or clean something over and over. People with this disorder tend to be perfectionistic and very rule-oriented.

Physical symptoms also vary. If the person is prevented from performing the obsession or compulsion, the anxiety converts itself into somatic (body-related) symptoms.

Note: DSM-IV-TR and some nursing textbooks recognize a disorder called "obsessive-compulsive personality disorder." Although there are some similar traits, it is separate and different from the disorder discussed here, which is classified as an anxiety disorder in *DSM-IV-TR*.

POST-TRAUMATIC STRESS DISORDER (PTSD)

This disorder is developed in response to an unexpected emotional or physical trauma that could not be controlled. *DSM-IV-TR* includes the words "actual or threatened" in describing the traumatic events that may trigger PTSD. People who have fought in wars, who have been raped, or who have survived violent storms or violent acts are examples of those who are susceptible to suffering from this disorder. Police, fire, and rescue personnel are at risk for PTSD when they see victims of violence and destruction whom they cannot help. The assault on the United States during the attacks on the World Trade Center towers, the Pentagon, and the passengers and crew on the ill-fated flight in Pennsylvania on September 11, 2001, has brought new attention to the condition of post-traumatic stress disorder. The horror of witnessing tragedy such as this now reaches anyone with a television or internet. People countries away are able to experience tragedy in "real time." Certainly those citizens who were on the scene and attempting to save lives saw destruction the likes of which most of us, hopefully, will never experience directly. They and their families are dealing with the post-traumatic effects of that day for some time to come. Think for a moment where you and your families were on that day. Think about the things you felt and shared with each other at that time. Magnify that as you think about "what if I was the one standing on that sidewalk watching people die or jump from those buildings, wanting to help and knowing I couldn't?" Dramatic? Maybe. Realistic? Yes. And just a very slight taste of the intensity of the fears and flashbacks people with PTSD experience.

A term associated with PTSD is "survivor guilt," the feeling of guilt expressed by survivors of a traumatic event. A Vietnam veteran may say, "Why me? Why did that lady and her kids get blown away and I lived? They didn't deserve that."

Symptoms may appear immediately or be repressed until years later. *DSM-IV-TR* requires that symptoms be present for at least 1 month. Family members and significant others such as spouses can develop certain behaviors also. Often, these people experience the same trauma, even though they were not present for the original event. This is a strange phenomenon, similar to men's experiencing "sympathetic labor" with their spouses. Symptoms include:

- "Flashbacks," in which the person may relive and act out the traumatic event
- Social withdrawal
- Feelings of low self-esteem as a result of the event
- Changes in relationship with significant other and difficulty forming new relationships
- Irritability and outbursts of anger toward another person or situation, seemingly for no obvious reason
- Depression
- Chemical dependency, as a physical or behavioral response to the traumatic experience

Trust and communication and listening skills are very important tools for nurses who have patients with PTSD. Encouraging expression of thoughts and feelings surrounding the experience and the survivor guilt is an important first step in the patient's ability to identify the source of the problem and begin the process of healing (Fig. 11-4). It is important to validate the patient's feelings regarding the situation. Honesty and genuineness in communicating with these patients will help to build a working rapport.

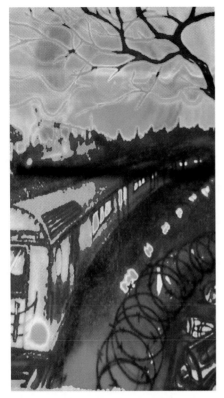

FIGURE 11-4. Encouraging the patient's expression of thoughts and feelings about the traumatic experience, as in this painting, is an important first step in identifying the problem and beginning the healing process. (Courtesy of the National Institute of Mental Health, Bethesda, MD.)

■ MEDICAL TREATMENT FOR PEOPLE WITH ANXIETY DISORDERS

Treatment is individualized to the patient and may include one or more of the following: psychopharmacology, individual psychotherapy, group therapy, systematic desensitization, hypnosis, imagery, relaxation exercises, and biofeedback.

Psychopharmacology involves the antianxiety classification of medications. The benzodiazepines are commonly used and are effective in most cases. Use of the antianxiety drugs is short term whenever possible because of the strong potential for dependency. Individuals with anxiety dis-orders who are chemically dependent are managed with other medications having calming qualities but not the same high potential for addiction as the antianxiety drugs. Hydroxyzine hydrochloride (Atarax), clonidine (Catapres), and sertraline (Zoloft) are common alternatives in this situation.

Antidepressants and antipsychotics are effective for some people. If these medications are not effective in treating the symptoms, monoamine oxidase inhibitors (MAOIs) or lithium carbonate may be prescribed.

The SSRI classification of drugs, specifically Luvox (fluvoxamine), seem to be emerging as the medication of choice for obsessive-compulsive disorder. Also used are Effexor (venlaxofine), Wellbutrin (bupropion), and Anafranil (clomiprimine); however, the side effects may be greater with these medications. Current evidence-based treatment is encouraging the use of the SSRIs as the first choice of medication for this disorder.

Counseling will be individually suited to the patient. Psychotherapy includes individual treatment, group therapy, and systematic desensitization techniques to help the patient experience the anxiety-producing situation in a controlled environment and integrate the painful feelings associated with the anxiety. Patients concentrate on esteem needs and reality. Hypnosis, imagery, relaxation exercises, and biofeedback are a few techniques that can be taught. Teaching these techniques provides the patients with the opportunity to manage their anxiety independently.

■ ALTERNATIVE INTERVENTIONS FOR PEOPLE WITH ANXIETY DISORDERS

AROMATHERAPY

Essential oils such as peppermint or eucalyptus are popular aids in relaxation.

Methods of application include using diffusers (machines that turn the oil into droplets that diffuse into the air), placing a drop on a piece of clothing, or actually applying directly to the skin, such as the temple area. Patients can purchase these essential oils and equipment at specialty stores, some bath oil supply stores, or even in some pharmacies. There are online resources as well. Prescriptions are not needed, but patients should be cautioned to use essential oils in very small amounts (drops at a time) and that some individuals may experience allergic responses, especially if applied directly to the skin.

BIOFEEDBACK

Biofeedback is a form of behavior modification. It is a system of progressive relaxation. There are many tapes and products on the market to assist patients in this "do-it-yourself" method of relaxation. Biofeedback done effectively alters the brain to a slower wave frequency and can actually increase the immune response for humans. The patient should discuss with the doctor if biofeedback is appropriate. The nurse may assist with providing information and resources.

HYPNOSIS

Hypnosis, done by a qualified, licensed therapist may be helpful. It will assist the person in relaxation. Some people joke about "going to my happy place," but there is validity in finding that pleasure or light-hearted memory. Patients will have to continue to take time to do the relaxation as directed by the therapist. Hypnosis is not a "one-time" therapy. It, like biofeedback, needs to be done routinely to be effective. The nurse's role may be as simple as to remind the patient to find quiet time for this, or if the patient is being seen as an outpatient, the nurse may ask the patient how frequently she or he has been able to do the hypnosis and what kind of results the patient has experienced thus far.

■ NURSING INTERVENTIONS FOR PEOPLE WITH ANXIETY DISORDERS

1. *Maintain a calm milieu:* Patients who have anxiety disorders need to have their treatment area calm and safe. Minimizing the stimuli helps the patient to keep centered and focused.
2. *Maintain open communication:* Encourage the patient to verbalize all thoughts and feelings. Honesty in dealing with patients helps them learn to trust others and increases their self-esteem. Patients will feel the value that nurses have in that relationship. Observe the patient's nonverbal communication. As previously stated, affect and body language often reveal more about a patient's thoughts and feelings than the words that are spoken.
3. *Observe for signs of suicidal thoughts:* Patients with anxiety disorders, especially those suffering with PTSD, are at risk for suicide as a result of feelings of low self-esteem or decreased self-worth. Nurses must be alert to this possibility and should observe and confront the patient and document any suspicions or statements the patient expresses.
4. *Document any changes in behavior:* Any change, no matter how small, can be significant to the patient's care. Positive or negative alterations in the way a patient responds to the nurse, to the treatment plan, or to other people and situations should be documented.
5. *Encourage activities:* Activities that are enjoyable and non-stressful help the patient in several ways. Activities provide a diversion, give the patient time to concentrate on something other than the anxiety-producing situation, and give an opportunity to provide positive feedback to the patient about the progress he or she is making.

These activities should be purposeful, not just "busy work." The patient should not be put in a situation of competition as a result of activities. Competition could increase the anxiety and be counterproductive to treatment.

Table 11-2 summarizes the types of anxiety disorders, the general symptoms, and common nursing actions for them.

TABLE 11-2 ■ *Anxiety Disorders*		
ANXIETY DISORDER	**SYMPTOMS**	**NURSING ACTIONS**
GENERALIZED PANIC DISORDER	Muscle aches, shakes, palpitations, dry mouth, nausea, chills, vomiting, hot flashes, polyuria, difficulty swallowing	Provide calm milieu, open communication, suicide precautions; document behavior changes; encourage activities
PANIC DISORDER	Fear, dissociation, nausea, diaphoresis, chest pain, increased pulse, shaking, unsteadiness	Same as above Stay with patient during attack
PHOBIA	Irrational fear of a particular object or situation	Same as above
OBSESSIVE-COMPULSIVE DISORDER	Repeated thoughts and/or repeated actions	Same as above Allow patient to express the anxiety Explore alternative methods of anxiety reduction
POST-TRAUMATIC STRESS DISORDER	"Flashbacks," social withdrawal, low self-esteem, relationships that may change or be difficult to form, irritability, anger seemingly for no reason, depression, chemical dependency	Same as above Keep patient oriented to the present Encourage patient and significant others to attend groups for patients with PTSD

Key Concepts ■ ■ ■

1. Anxiety disorders have many common characteristics. Psychoanalytic theories propose that it is important to find the underlying cause of the anxiety. Biologic theories postulate that the causes are not the primary concern, but rather the physical reasons may result in the anxiety.
2. Medications and therapies should be individualized for the patient.
3. Trust and communication techniques are important tools for the nurse caring for a patient with an anxiety disorder. Maintaining a calm milieu is also essential.

COMMONLY USED MEDICATIONS ■ *Anxiety Disorders*		
Alprazolam (Xanax)	**Clonidine** (Catapres)	**Oxazepam** (Serax)
Bupropion (Wellbutrin)	**Diazepam** (Valium)	**Prazepam** (Centrax)
Buspirone (BuSpar)	**Fluvoxamine** (Luvox)	**Sertraline** (Zoloft)
Clomipramine (Anafranil)	**Hydroxyzine** (Atarax)	**Venlafaxine** (Effexor)
Clonazepam (Klonopin)	**Lorazepam** (Ativan)	**Zolpidem** (Ambien)

CASE STUDY ■ ■ ■

A patient comes for his scheduled appointment with Dr. Sneeze. The patient is a well-known politician. He has been the subject of negative press in recent months. His main symptoms are general malaise, sneezing, chronic head-ache, and "like I have a constant cold." Dr. Sneeze orders blood work and chest x-ray and does a complete physical for the patient. You have collected vital signs and the health history when you roomed him. The patient does not have a young family at home but is on the road campaigning and meeting his constituents almost daily. He believes he has become infected with something serious, since his symptoms do not seem to subside. Dr. Sneeze delivers the news to the patient that he is "healthy." His examination and lab work do not show any physical illness, and he suggests perhaps the symptoms are "most likely viral in nature and probably stress and anxiety related." Dr. Sneeze suggests the patient take over-the-counter medications for his symptoms and find methods to reduce his stress. Dr. Sneeze leaves the room. The patient expresses his extreme disappointment at not being given "something to take" and asks you to explain to him how stress can give one a cold.

1. How will you respond to the patient's request for education?
2. What are your thoughts about the patient's expectation for receiving medications? How will you discuss that with him?
3. What alternatives (for example, dietary, herbal, etc.) can you discuss with him or ask the doctor to discuss with him?

REFERENCES

Anderson, R.A. (2001). *Clinician's Guide to Holistic Medicine.* McGraw-Hill, New York.

American Psychiatric Association. (2000). *Diagnostic and Statistical Manual of Diagnostic Disorders—IV-Text Revision.* Author, Washington, DC.

Braiker, H. (2002) *September 11 Syndrome.* McGraw-Hill, New York.

Cohen, S. et al. (2003). *Sociability and Susceptibility to the Common Cold.* Carnegie Mellon University (copyright American Psychological Society), *14* (5) September 2003, Washington, DC.

Nicholson, R.A. (2003). *Chill Out: Anger Can Give You A Headache.* Saint Louis University, St. Louis, MO.

Shives, L. and Isaacs, A. (2002). *Basic Concepts of Psychiatric-Mental Health Nursing,* 5th ed. JB Lippincott, Philadelphia.

Sierpina, V.S. (2001). *Integrative Health Care—Complementary and Alternative Therapies for the Whole Person.* F.A. Davis, Philadelphia.

WEBSITES

www.adaa.org
www.psych.org
www.ncptsd.org

CRITICAL THINKING EXERCISES ■ ■ ■

1. Tommy has come to your clinic with numerous cracks on his hands, which are bleeding and very sore. Tommy tells you that he just has to wash his hands all the time. His mother says he will wash for 2 to 3 hours at a time and he won't stop when she tells him to. The physician has diagnosed Tommy with OCD and has explained the illness to Tommy and his mother. When the physician leaves the room, Tommy's mother begins to cry: "What did he just say? What am I supposed to do? What did I do wrong that Tommy got this illness?" What will you tell her? What areas will you explore with her?

2. Jeanne is a 21-year-old single woman admitted for pneumonia. Her social history indicates that she survived a house fire when she was 10 years old and that her twin sister died in that fire. Today is the day for the monthly fire drill at the hospital. You note that Jeanne is not in her bed. You are unable to find her during the drill. After the drill, you search her room and find her sitting on the floor of the closet. She is wrapped in a blanket and is crying. She does not respond to your verbal cues. What do you think is happening to her? What illness might she have? How will you get her out of the closet? What can you do to help her?

3. Using the suggested nursing diagnoses shown here (or others you can think of), complete a nursing process for Tommy, in exercise 1.

SUGGESTED NURSING DIAGNOSES

1. *Thought Processes, Altered*
2. *Trauma, Risk for*
3. *Anxiety*

ASSESSMENT/ DATA COLLECTION	NURSING DIAGNOSIS	PLAN/ GOAL	INTERVENTIONS/ NURSING ACTIONS	EVALUATION CRITERIA

4. Using the suggested nursing diagnoses shown here (or others you can think of), complete a nursing process for Jeanne, in exercise 2.

SUGGESTED NURSING DIAGNOSES

1. *Post-Trauma Syndrome*
2. *Fear*
3. *Grieving, Dysfunctional*

ASSESSMENT/ DATA COLLECTION	NURSING DIAGNOSIS	PLAN/ GOAL	INTERVENTIONS/ NURSING ACTIONS	EVALUATION CRITERIA

TEST QUESTIONS ■ ■ ■

MULTIPLE CHOICE QUESTIONS

1. Your significant other is a veteran of the war in Iraq. It is very difficult for him or her to drive through a parking ramp because "There are people hiding behind the pillars! They have guns! Be careful!" This person is most likely experiencing:

   A. Auditory hallucinations
   B. Flashbacks
   C. Delusions of grandeur
   D. Free-floating anxiety

2. The foregoing situation would indicate what type of anxiety disorder?

   A. Generalized anxiety disorder
   B. Phobia
   C. Post-traumatic stress disorder
   D. Obsessive-compulsive disorder

3. Ms. T cannot leave her home without checking the coffee pot numerous times. This makes her late to many functions, and she misses engagements on occasion because of it. Ms. T probably is suffering from what kind of anxiety disorder?

   A. Generalized anxiety disorder
   B. Phobia

C. Post-traumatic stress disorder
D. Obsessive-compulsive disorder

4. Mr. L has a severe fear of needles. He is hospitalized on your medical unit. The lab technician enters to draw blood for the routine CBC and Mr. L begins to cry out, "Get away from me! I can't breathe! I'm having a heart attack!" Your first response to Mr. L would be:

A. "I'll take your vital signs and call my supervisor."
B. "Why do you think you're having a heart attack, Mr. L?"
C. "Don't worry. She's done this many times before!"
D. "Mr. L, relax. Take a few deep breaths. I'll stay with you."

5. Which of the following is *not* an anxiety disorder?

A. Panic disorder
B. Obsessive-compulsive disorder
C. Multiple personality disorder
D. Post-traumatic stress disorder

6. Mr. Uneasy states, "I never feel at ease. I always have a feeling of dread. I just know something is going to go wrong." He is experiencing:

A. Signal anxiety
B. Free-floating anxiety
C. Test anxiety
D. Atypical anxiety

7. A patient with an obsessive-compulsive disorder is:

A. Suspicious and hostile
B. Flexible and adaptable to change
C. Extremely frightened of something
D. Rigid in thought and inflexible with routines and rituals

8. Which of the following is *true* regarding a phobic disorder?

A. It involves repetitive actions.
B. It involves a loss of identity.
C. It results in sociopathic behavior.
D. It is an irrational fear that is not changed by logic.

9. Nursing interventions for anxiety disorders include all of the following *except:*

A. Encourage patient to verbalize thoughts and feelings.
B. Inform patient of expected behaviors and consequences.
C. Withhold information from patient to lessen stress.
D. Allow patient to control as much of his or her care as possible.

10. In obsessive-compulsive disorder, a compulsion is:

A. A repetitive thought
B. A repetitive action
C. A repetitive fear
D. A repetitive illusion

11. An example of a NANDA nursing diagnosis for a patient with signal anxiety disorder is:
    A. Risk for violence: self-directed
    B. Fear
    C. Chronic low self-esteem
    D. Noncompliance

12. The medication of choice for the treatment of OCD is:
    A. Paxil (paroxetine)
    B. Prozac (fluoxetine)
    C. Luvox (fluvoxamine)
    D. Effexor (venlaxofine)

13. Avoiding driving through a tunnel such as a mountain or freeway tunnel is _____ (identify the disorder)

14. Which of the following are NOT nursing interventions for people with anxiety disorders?
    A. Maximize stimuli to create diversion from the anxiety.
    B. Encourage the patient to verbalize all thoughts and feelings.
    C. Observe the patient's nonverbal communication for data on a patient's thoughts and feelings.
    D. Observe for signs of suicidal thoughts.
    E. Document only positive changes in behavior.
    F. Discourage activities: activities might only increase a patient's anxiety level.

■ ■ ■ ■ ■ ■ ■

CHAPTER

12

Mood Disorders

Learning Objectives ■ ■ ■

1. Define mood disorder.
2. Identify four types of mood disorders.
3. State physical and behavioral symptoms of four mood disorders.
4. Identify treatment modalities for four mood disorders.
5. Identify nursing care for four mood disorders.

Key Terms ■ ■ ■

- Affect
- Bipolar
- Cycles
- Dysthymia
- Hypomania
- Mania
- Mood

Mood disorders (also called affective disorders) are disorders in which people experience extreme changes in **mood** (emotions) and **affect** (the outward expression of the mood). Moods of extreme depression to extreme elation are observed in mood disorders, and sometimes both extremes can be observed in the same person. Changes in mood occur either frequently, as is the case with bipolar depression, or for prolonged periods, as in major depression or dysthymia. These kinds of disorders are considered to be clinical depression. Clinical depression is much more severe than normal depression, which is caused by low points in life that people experience as part of their mental health, and sadness becomes depression when it lasts a very long time (generally 2 years or more) or when it begins to interfere with normal day-to-day functioning (Fig. 12-1).

People of all age groups develop depressive disorders. Very young children display signs of depression. Nurses also care for older adults who are depressed and for people of every age in between. People of both sexes and all ethnic and socioeconomic groups experience mood disorders. See Box 12-1 for statistics on various mood disorders in the United States.

■ ETIOLOGIC THEORIES

Psychoanalytic theory indicates that people who have suffered loss in their lives are those who will develop depressions. This loss can be a result of ineffective developmental stages (see Chapter 4), which then leave the patient unconsciously unable to succeed. This includes people who have

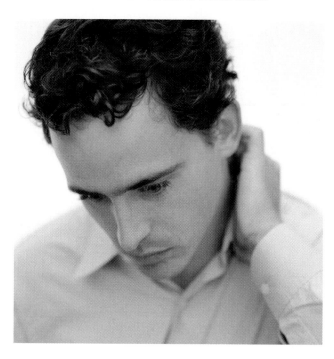

FIGURE 12-1. Sadness becomes depression when it lasts a very long time (generally 2 years or more) or when it begins to interfere with normal day-to-day functioning.

been divorced, single parents, and people with chronic physical illness. People who fail financially, socially, and professionally probably will find some underlying emotional scar that is manifesting itself as an inappropriate or extreme expression of mood. Theorists who believe that depressions have their roots in adolescence think it has a connection with the way boys and girls are socialized in the United States. These same theorists think that young women are more dissatisfied with their looks than young men are, which leads to their generally lower self-esteem. Depression is also associated with unresolved anger. It has been explained to the lay community as "anger turned inward." In other words, people who cannot or do not deal appropriately with things that anger them tend to repress that anger (turn or "stuff" it inside) and become depressed as a result of that repression.

The cognitive theorists (who think differently than the psychoanalytic and the biologic theorists) believe that the way people perceive events and situations leads to depression. Instead of thinking about failing an exam as being unfortunate and disappointing, some people with tendencies toward depression will "awfulize" (see Ellis, Chapter 8) and turn the situation into something much deeper than it is. This, according to the cognitive theorists, is maladaptive thinking.

Biologic theories offer more options: chemical imbalances and genetic links. The neurochemicals serotonin and norepinephrine have an effect on mood; if these neurochemicals are elevated, mood is elevated, but if they are low, mood will also be low.

Studies of families and identical twins offer some possible answers. Organizations such as the National Institutes of Health, American Psychiatric Association, and others indicate that disorders such as depression do run in families and are almost always genetic in origin.

Approximately twice as many women as men report feeling depressed. This might be a flaw in reporting (men may not discuss the depressed feelings as readily with their physicians or may discuss them in different

BOX 12-1	*Statistics on Mood Disorders in the United States*

General Facts About Depression

- Common not only in the United States but also internationally.
- Nearly twice as many women as men are affected by a depressive disorder annually.
- Depressive disorders are being diagnosed earlier in life than they were in previous generations.

Major Depressive Disorder

- Affects approximately 5% of the U.S. population age 18 and older annually.
- Average age of onset in the mid-twenties

Dysthymic Depression (Dysthymia)

- Affects approximately 5–6 percent of the U.S. population age 18 and older at some point in their lifetimes.
- About 40% of adults with dysthymic disorder also meet criteria for major depressive disorder or bipolar disorder.
- Often begins in childhood, adolescence, or early adulthood.

Bipolar Disorder

- Affects approximately 15–20 percent of the U.S. population age 18 and older annually.
- More than 2 million Americans have manic-depressive illness.
- Affects males and females at approximately the same rate.
- There is strong evidence for a genetic/inherited link, but a specific genetic defect has not yet been identified.
- Has been diagnosed in children under age 12, although it is not common in this group. At this age, symptoms can be confused with attention-deficit/hyperactivity disorder. Careful diagnosis is crucial for correct treatment.

Sources: *http://www.nimh.nih.gov/publicat/depression.cfm#ptdep2;*
http://12.31.13.40/HealthTopics/Depression.htm (Memorial Care Health System, Southern California);
health.msn.com (Depressions Health Center)

terms). Biologic theorists, however, believe a connection exists between the female hormones and the neurochemicals mentioned earlier. The processes of menstruation, pregnancy, childbirth, and menopause are major hormonal stresses in a woman's life. Because men do not undergo such stresses, these experiences may account for the 2:1 balance of female-to-male diagnoses of depression.

Symptoms of the specific illnesses are presented here with their definitions. Some of the frequently occurring general symptoms are low or depressed mood, high or manic mood, flat affect, sleep disturbances, constipation, irritability (especially in children and adolescents), fluctuations in weight in either direction, and withdrawal from usual friends and activities.

■ DIFFERENTIAL DIAGNOSIS

Symptoms of depression may occur as a result of other disorders, such as schizophrenia and drug side effects or overuse. Symptoms can mimic congestive heart failure, nutritional deficiencies, fluid and electrolyte imbalances, infections, or diabetes.

In young children as well as adults, symptoms of depression may manifest themselves as conditions of compromised immunity. Frequent "colds" and other viral infections may be among the first signs of depression.

In addition, nurses working with patients in isolation for a medical condition must be aware that patients in isolation may be at risk for depression. Studies show that nurses and others are less likely to visit patients requiring precautions due to the increased time required to gown and glove. Nurses should include adequate visits for patients in isolation precautions when planning their time management for their shifts.

■ TYPES

MAJOR DEPRESSION (UNIPOLAR DEPRESSION)

People who develop major depression exhibit a vast array of symptoms. These symptoms may be the same behaviors everyone displays while progressing through the "normal" ups and downs of life. People who have major depression just show these symptoms more strongly and longer than people who are not clinically depressed. Behavioral and physical symptoms include:

- Sad mood
- Loss of pleasure in usually pleasurable things
- No hallucinations or delusions and four of the following for at least 2 consecutive weeks:
  - Weight loss or gain resulting from increased or decreased appetite
  - Sleep pattern disturbances
  - Increased fatigue
  - Increased agitation
  - Increase or decrease in normal activity; lowered pleasure for life, including sexual activity

- Feelings of guilt or worthlessness
- Decreased ability to think, remember, or concentrate
- Suicidal thoughts

DYSTHYMIC DEPRESSION (DYSTHYMIA)

Dysthymia is defined as severe depression for at least 2 years for adults and at least 1 year for adolescents and younger children.

Dysthymic depression is not considered as severe as major depression, however. Symptoms of dysthymia include:

- A low or depressed mood that lasts the greater part of every day for a 2-year period
- No mania
- No major depression
- No other psychotic disorders (conditions of disorganized personality and impairment in perceptions of reality)
- No organic findings
- Seeming to have little or no interest in surroundings
- Anhedonia (inability to feel pleasure)

According to the *DSM-IV-TR*, symptoms include at least two of the following:

- Overeating or undereating
- Insomnia or hypersomnia
- Low energy or low self-esteem
- Difficulty making decisions
- Feelings of hopelessness

BIPOLAR DEPRESSION

At least 2 million Americans suffer from **bipolar** depression (manic-depressive illness, or bipolar disorder, as it is also sometimes called). This is the type of depression in which both extreme **mania** (extreme elation or extreme agitation) and extreme depression exist. The mania is part of the depression. There exists actually Bipolar I and Bipolar II disorders. Bipolar I is the more commonly recognized, and for purposes of this text, it will be the Bipolar I that is discussed.

Do not mistakenly think that when the person is in the manic phase, he or she is truly happy. Think of a color you like. Now think of all of the shades of that color from the very palest shade to the brightest, most intense shade. Both extremes of your color choice are very different, but both are still part of the same color. That is one way to remember that the mania and the depression are just opposite poles of the same illness.

It takes only one episode of mania to actually be diagnosed with bipolar disorder, but it is more common to see the patient alternating or "cycling" from one "pole" to the other. The periods of mania and depression do not necessarily last for the same amounts of time. Usually the depressive period lasts longer than the manic period, and a span of "normal" behavior exists between the episodes of depression and mania. People who are in manic phase are out of control but usually feel "on top of the world" or "unbeatable."

The changes in behavior from the depressed pole to the manic pole are usually very obvious, dramatic changes. One nursing home resident was known to alternate between extreme happiness and excitement in which she would tell tales about being personal friends with Amelia Earhart. She would recount tales about waving to her friend as Amelia flew over the patient's house. Then, just as quickly, the patient would revert to such extreme depression that staff members could not get her out of bed for baths, meals, or activities. Food would be brought to her room, and she would eat only small amounts of it. She would allow partial baths but would not participate. These **cycles** lasted approximately 3 weeks.

Hypomania is behavior that is similar to that of mania but not as severe. It is very hard to describe this, but it may be analogous to how someone might feel about winning the lottery: Winning $100 million would leave one feeling ecstatic, but $35 million would still make one really happy. The person who is experiencing the ecstasy of the $100 million would be comparable to the patient who is manic; the person who won the $35 million is comparable to the patient who is hypomanic. It is the degree of severity that defines this disorder. The physician will assess the extremes of mood changes, length of time in each mood, frequency of the cycling, and other symptoms exhibited by the patient in an effort to accurately distinguish hypomania from mania. Hypomania can be very difficult to diagnose and may even go unnoticed for years in some patients. The U.S. Department of Health and Human Services, Alcohol, Drug Abuse and Mental Health Administration (Hendrix, 1993) lists the following signs of mania and depression. Signs of mania include:

- Excessive highs or feelings of euphoria
- Sustained period of behavior that is different from usual
- Increased energy, activity, restlessness, racing thoughts, and rapid talking
- Decreased need for sleep
- Unrealistic beliefs in one's abilities and powers
- Extreme irritability and distractibility
- Uncharacteristically poor judgment
- Increased sexual drive
- Abuse of drugs, particularly cocaine, alcohol, and sleeping medications
- Obnoxious, provocative, or intrusive behavior
- Denial that anything is wrong

Signs of depression include:

- Persistent sad, anxious, or empty mood
- Feelings of hopelessness or pessimism
- Feelings of guilt, worthlessness, or hopelessness
- Loss of interest or pleasure in ordinary activities, including sex

- Decreased energy, a feeling of fatigue or being slowed down
- Difficulty concentrating, remembering, making decisions
- Restlessness or irritability
- Sleep disturbances
- Loss of appetite and weight loss or weight gain
- Chronic pain or other persistent bodily symptoms that are not caused by physical disease
- Thoughts of death or suicide, suicide attempts

The *DSM-IV-TR* (which actually differentiates bipolar disorder into four individual conditions) agrees with these symptoms but adds that symptoms may be present for days to months in the case of the manic phase or up to years for the depressive phase.

INVOLUTIONAL DEPRESSION/ MELANCHOLIA

This type of depression is somewhat different from the others presented here. Involutional depression or melancholia generally affects people over age 45. It, too, seems to affect women more frequently than men and has been nicknamed "empty nest syndrome" because symptoms generally appear or become pronounced after the last child leaves home. Symptoms are more somatic than the other depressions. Anorexia and sleep disturbances are common. Hypochondriasis (abnormally high anxiety or fear related to one's health) may occur. The unfortunate part of this type of depression is that people not only are not "cured" from this disorder but also rarely get any relief from the depression.

■ MEDICAL TREATMENT FOR PEOPLE WITH DEPRESSIVE DISORDERS

Depression often goes untreated. Effective treatments are available, but only one in three people with depression seeks help. With treatment, approximately 80 percent of people with serious depression can be helped in a matter of a few weeks. Some of the common medical treatments for depression are:

- Lithium
- Antidepressants
- Psychotherapy
- Electroconvulsive therapy (ECT)

Lithium is the drug of choice, in most instances, for the treatment of bipolar depression. Lithium, an electrolyte in our bodies, is inert and is present in very small concentrations. It does have the potential for many side effects, including dehydration as a result of electrolyte imbalance (particularly sodium).

Antidepressants such as Elavil (amitriptyline), Prozac (fluoxetine hydrochloride), and Desyrel (trazodone hydrochloride) may also be used.

Psychotherapy for the patient and family may be helpful in understanding the illness and learning problem solving and other new adaptive coping behaviors. For young children, play therapy is the most frequent and effective form of therapy. Children act out emotions and concerns as they interact with their toys. Children's drawings have pictured feelings that children do not know how to express. The therapist (and the nurse) is aware that "child's play" is often much more than that. Documenting the child's actions and responses to play will help sort out issues that the child needs help to identify and resolve.

ECT is an option when other therapy is not effective. It is also used in conjunction with other modalities for severe depression. People may have a therapeutic session of 6–10 treatments over 4–8 weeks. Usually, patients are also given a sedative prior to the actual treatment. Estimates are that it is helpful for approximately 80 percent of those who undergo the treatment.

■ ALTERNATIVE TREATMENT FOR PEOPLE WITH DEPRESSIVE DISORDERS

LIGHT THERAPY

Light therapy is being prescribed and used successfully with some individuals. It consists of special lights to be used for certain amounts of time during the day. It is used with some success in people with seasonal affective disorder (SAD).

HERBAL AND NUTRITIONAL THERAPY

Working with a nutritionist in addition to a physician, nurses may assist patients in choosing diets that will help change the chemical balance to improve a patient's mental state. Actions as simple as avoiding caffeine, sugar, and alcohol or adding servings of whole grains and vegetables may help a person step out of depression. Herbs such as St. John's Wort and SAMe have been documented to provide antidepressant effects in some patients with mild depression.

ACUPUNCTURE

Acupuncture must be performed by specially credentialed practitioners. Some patients may benefit and experience a lifting of depression from certain stimulation points.

BIOFEEDBACK AND HYPNOSIS

Benefits of biofeedback and hypnosis have been discussed in the previous chapter.

NEUROLINGUISTIC PROGRAMMING (NLP)

Nurses trained in this technique and who are allowed to do so by their state's nurse practice act can assist patients to "reframe" their self-messages and assist in helping people help themselves out of some depressive moments. See Chapter 9 for further information on NLP.

■ NURSING INTERVENTIONS FOR PEOPLE WITH DEPRESSIVE DISORDERS

1. *Patience, patience, patience!*
2. *Monitor lithium levels:* Normal range of lithium is 1.0 to 1.5 mEq/L while loading and 0.6 to 1.2 mEq/L on maintenance. Notify your supervisor and the physician immediately if the patient shows any abnormality in lab results or any other signs of lithium side effects.
3. *Honesty*
4. *Consistency*
5. *Activity:* This must be planned carefully. Activities that include small groups can be helpful for esteem building. Activities that can be undertaken alone are helpful when it is necessary to decrease stimulation. Activities should be age appropriate.
6. *Nutrition*
7. *Communication:* This is not a time for false reassurance. Do not use phrases like "Cheer up!" or "It could be worse!" People who are depressed need more concrete reinforcement. Effective therapeutic questioning and problem solving are very important for the nurse-patient interaction. Making an observation such as "I like the way you look in that blue outfit. Is it new?" may go further in helping the person improve self-esteem than "Cheer up!"
8. *Nurse-led therapeutic or support-type groups:* These are not the same as psychotherapy groups; rather, they encourage communication between patients with similar concerns and may help patients to identify problem solving strategies. Nurses function as facilitators.

Table 12-1 summarizes the symptoms and nursing interventions for four mood disorders.

TABLE 12-1 ■ *Mood Disorders*		
TYPE	**SYMPTOMS**	**NURSING INTERVENTIONS**
MAJOR DEPRESSION	Sad mood; loss of pleasure including sexual activity; weight loss or gain; sleep pattern disturbances; increased fatigue; increased agitation; increase or decrease in normal activity; feelings of guilt or worthlessness; decreased ability to think, remember, or concentrate; suicidal thoughts.	■ Patience ■ Honesty ■ Consistency ■ Meaningful activity ■ Nutrition teaching ■ Effective communication ■ Monitor for suicidal ideation
DYSTHYMIC DEPRESSION	Low or depressed mood that lasts the greater part of every day for a 2-year period, no other psychotic disorders, no organic findings, little or no interest in surroundings, anhedonia (inability to feel pleasure); according to the *DSM*, at least two of the following: overeating or undereating, insomnia or hypersomnia, low energy or low self-esteem, difficulty in making decisions, feelings of hopelessness.	■ Patience ■ Honesty ■ Consistency ■ Meaningful activity ■ Nutrition teaching ■ Effective communication ■ Monitor for suicidal ideation ■ Implement suicide precautions as needed
INVOLUTIONAL (MELANCHOLIA)	Generally affects people over age 45; seems to affect women more frequently than men. Symptoms generally appear after the last child leaves home; anorexia, sleep disturbances, hypochondriasis.	■ Patience ■ Honesty ■ Consistency ■ Meaningful activity ■ Nutrition teaching ■ Effective communication
BIPOLAR DISORDER	*Mania:* Excessive highs or euphoria; sustained period of behavior that is different from usual; increased energy, activity, restlessness; racing thoughts and rapid talking, decreased need for sleep, unrealistic beliefs in one's abilities and powers, extreme irritability and distractibility, uncharacteristically poor judgment, increased sexual drive, abuse of drugs, obnoxious behavior, denial. *Depression*: see Major Depression and Dysthymic Depression.	■ Patience ■ Monitor lithium levels ■ Honesty ■ Consistency ■ Meaningful activity ■ Nutrition teaching ■ Effective communication ■ Assist patient with basic daily needs ■ Monitor intake and output

Key Concepts ▣ ▪ ▪

1. Depressive disorders are common threats to mental health in the American population.
2. Signs and symptoms of depressive disorders are similar to the behaviors common in all people experiencing the usual ups and downs of daily life.
3. It is often the degree of severity and length of time the symptoms are present that determine the type of depression.
4. Some forms of depressive disorders are easier to treat than others. Patients may need to be on medications for long periods or perhaps for the rest of their lives. People who develop melancholia may never improve.

COMMONLY USED MEDICATIONS ■ *Mood Disorders*

Amitriptyline (Elavil)	**Nortriptyline** (Pamelor)
Bupropion (Wellbutrin)	**Paroxetine** (Paxil)
Carbamazepine (Tegretol)	**Phenelzine** (Nardil)
Doxepin (Sinequan, Adapin)	**Sertraline** (Zoloft)
Fluoxetine (Prozac)	**Tranylcypromine** (Parnate)
Isocarboxazid (Marplan)	**Trazodone** (Desyrel)
Lithium (Lithobid, Eskalith)	**Valproate** (Depakote)

REFERENCES

Anderson, Robert A. (2001). *Clinician's Guide to Holistic Medicine.* McGraw-Hill, New York.

BiPolar Disorder (author not cited) (2004). National Institute of Mental Health (NIMH), Bethesda, MD.

Depression (author not cited) (2004). National Institute of Mental Health (NIMH), Bethesda, MD. http://www.nimh.nih.gov/healthinformation/depressionmenu.cfm 08/17/2004.

Hendrix, M.L. (1993). *Bipolar Disorder—Decade of the Brain.* NIH Pub. No. 93-3679. U.S. Department of Health and Human Services, Alcohol, Drug Abuse and Mental Health Administration, Washington, DC.

National Institutes of Health. (1994). *Helpful Facts About Depressive Illnesses.* DHHS-NIH Pub. No. 94-3875. National Institutes of Health, Bethesda, MD.

Sierpina, V.S. (2001). *Integrative Health Care—Complementary and Alternative Therapies for the Whole Person.* F.A. Davis, Philadelphia.

Sullivan, P.F., Neale, M.C., and Kendler, K.S. (2000). Genetic epidemiology of major depression: review and meta-analysis. *Am J Psychiatry, 157,* 1552–1562.

WEBSITES

http://www.depression-guide.com/depression-statistics.htm

www. encarta.msn.com

www.nami.org

http://www.nimh.nih.gov

CRITICAL THINKING EXERCISES ■ ■ ■

1. You are one of the team of school nurses in your local high school. You notice that Maria, a 17-year-old student, is behaving oddly. She has always been rather loud and even has been referred to as "obnoxious" by several of her peers. Lately, you have observed her sitting alone, as if waiting for someone, but when you approach her, she barely greets you and then leaves. What are your concerns about Maria? What are some of the possibilities that might be affecting her? How will you approach her more effectively the next time you see her?

2. Your sister-in-law calls you at home one day to talk about your brother. You have all been concerned about Marcus since he lost his job last year. He has been unable to find adequate employment. Your sister-in-law has had to get two part-time jobs so that Marcus could continue to interview. He has been in a very low mood, has quit the bowling team, and has been sleeping 10 to 12 hours daily. Today, however, your sister-in-law is excited. "Marcus is a new man! I don't know what happened, but he just got a burst of energy. He told me not to worry about a thing, because he was first in line for the position of president at the local bank. He said I can quit my job! He went out and bought a new car and everything. Isn't that great?" What will you think about your brother? What questions will you ask your sister-in-law? What actions will you take when talking to Marcus?

3. J. R. is a single parent who has been on leave from his construction job for almost a year due to a work-related injury. J. R. is in today for a follow-up appointment for his workers' compensation, but today he seems different. He is short-tempered and critical of the care he is receiving. To date, he has stated satisfaction with the way things are progressing. J. R. states that he is losing his friends from work and that they think he is "faking it to get some free money." His benefits have not been meeting his expenses, and he is beginning to experience financial difficulties. His children will soon be starting Little League, but his upper-extremity injuries will not allow him to help coach the children. The doctor prescribed Prozac for J. R. during his last visit, but the pharmacy didn't fill it because "workers' compensation won't pay for it." How can you assist J. R.? What will you suggest as a potential nursing diagnosis for him? How will your state's workers' compensation laws affect the course of treatment for J. R.?

4. Using the suggested nursing diagnoses shown here (or others you can think of), complete a nursing process for Maria, in exercise 1.

SUGGESTED NURSING DIAGNOSES

1. *Thought Processes, Altered*
2. *Hopelessness*
3. *Self-Esteem, Chronic Low*
4. *Denial, Ineffective*

ASSESSMENT/ DATA COLLECTION	NURSING DIAGNOSIS	PLAN/ GOAL	INTERVENTIONS/ NURSING ACTIONS	EVALUATION CRITERIA

5. Using the suggested nursing diagnoses shown here (or others you can think of), complete a nursing process for Marcus in exercise 2 or for J. R. in exercise 3.

SUGGESTED NURSING DIAGNOSES

1. *Individual Coping, Ineffective*
2. *Social Interaction, Impaired*
3. *Adjustment, Impaired*

ASSESSMENT/ DATA COLLECTION	NURSING DIAGNOSIS	PLAN/ GOAL	INTERVENTIONS/ NURSING ACTIONS	EVALUATION CRITERIA

TEST QUESTIONS ■ ■ ■

MULTIPLE CHOICE QUESTIONS

1. You admit Mr. N to your unit. He is 49 years old, pleasant, and compliant. He admits to being "a little down. My last son left for college 1000 miles away. I feel so empty, especially since his mother died last year." The physician ordered Prozac for Mr. N, but you observe no change in his behavior, and on a scale of 1 to 5, Mr. N describes his mood as "somewhere below that 5." You suspect Mr. N is suffering from what type of depressive disorder?

   A. Major depression
   B. Bipolar depression
   C. Dysthymic disorder
   D. Melancholia

2. Ms. S is admitted to your medical unit with a diagnosis of dehydration and a history of depression. She tells you, "I just can't eat. I'm not hungry." Your best therapeutic response would be:

   A. "You aren't hungry?"
   B. "If you can't eat, what is that candy bar wrapper doing in your bed?"
   C. "Why aren't you hungry?"
   D. "You really should try to eat some real food."

3. Janey, a 7-year-old, is hospitalized in your unit for treatment of depression. Among other forms of treatment, you would expect to be involved in what type of therapy with Janey?

   A. Rational-emotive
   B. Play
   C. Transactional analysis
   D. Work

4. Mrs. Outofsync is admitted to your medical/surgical unit with a diagnosis of dehydration and pneumonia. She has a history of bipolar disorder and is controlled on medication. As her nurse, you know you must:

   A. Treat her carefully because she may become catatonic.
   B. Observe for signs of lithium toxicity from dehydration.
   C. Alert the other staff of the "psycho" on the unit.
   D. Treat the medical illness only.

5. Mr. Quiet is describing the fire that destroyed his home 2 weeks ago. His wife and son were critically injured and they lost all of their material possessions. He is burned over 70 percent of his body. His voice is dull, and he has no change in facial expression. This *outward display* of emotion is called:

   A. Ambivalence
   B. Flight of ideas
   C. Mood
   D. Affect

6. To communicate well with Mr. Quiet, you do all of the following *except:*
   A. Develop a trust.
   B. Show acceptance.
   C. Be judgmental.
   D. Be honest.

7. Mr. Quiet tells you he feels responsible for his family's injuries and does not know if he can face the family. He states, "I think it would be better if I would die." After leaving his room, your next action(s) is/are:
   A. Document the conversation, inform the charge nurse and physician, and observe the patient.
   B. Document the conversation, but omit the part about his dying, because he probably didn't mean it.
   C. Keep the information to yourself because it was confidential.
   D. Tell his wife so that she can reassure him.

8. From the previous information, which of the following is the best problem or focus to use in forming a nursing diagnosis for Mr. Quiet?
   A. Noncompliance
   B. Manipulation
   C. Ritualistic behavior
   D. Guilt

9. The nurse who is assessing a patient with major depression (unipolar depression) would expect to observe which of the following symptoms?
   A. Euphoria
   B. Extreme fear
   C. Extreme sadness
   D. Positive thinking

10. The nursing interventions for this patient with major depression would include all of the following *except:*
   A. Active listening skills
   B. Maintaining safe milieu
   C. Encouraging adequate nutrition
   D. Reassuring the patient everything will be "just fine"

11. Mrs. Dry has an appointment with the doctor. She began taking Eskalith one month ago as prescribed. She now states her mouth and lips are constantly dry and she states she sometimes feels confused and states, "I stagger like I'm drunk sometimes when I walk." You suspect:
   A. She is drinking to combat her depression.
   B. She is making it up to get different medications.
   C. She took too much lithium.
   D. She is dehydrated.

12. Mrs. Inshock was just admitted for observation. Three weeks ago, three of her four children were killed instantly in a motor vehicle accident. She has been crying and unable to function. You have completed the intake

questionnaire with her and are staying with her and her husband until the doctor arrives. What would your best nursing action be at this time?

A. Continue asking questions to obtain more details for the doctor.

B. Convey your sympathy and desire to help any way you can.

C. Tell her how you almost had a bad accident on that same curve in the road yourself.

D. Change the subject and begin discussing Sunday's big football game.

13. From what information you have, what would the most likely diagnosis for Mrs. Inshock be?

A. Involutional depression

B. Catatonia

C. Bipolar disorder

D. Dysthymic depression

14. Imbalances of which two neurochomicals frequently are associated with depression? _____

_____

If a person is depressed, will these levels most likely be HIGHER or LOWER? (Choose one.)

13

Personality Disorders

Learning Objectives ■ ■ ■

1. Define personality.
2. Identify seven types of personality disorders.
3. State physical and behavioral symptoms of seven personality disorders.
4. Identify treatment modalities for people with personality disorders.
5. Identify nursing care for people with personality disorders.

Key Terms ■ ■ ■

- Antisocial/sociopathic
- Borderline
- Dependent
- Narcissistic
- Paranoid
- Passive-aggressive
- Personality
- Personality disorder
- Schizoid

Personality is defined as "… the complex of characteristics that distinguishes an individual or a nation or group; *especially:* the totality of an individual's behavioral and emotional characteristics" (Webster Online). Personalities include the thoughts, feelings, and attitudes of each individual.

Personality disorder is a maladaptive behavior that results from ineffective personality development. Defects in personality affect the way humans interpret and respond to the world in which they live. People in these categories fit someplace between the labels "mentally healthy" and "mentally ill." Unfortunately, people with personality disorders are seldom seen in treatment for the disorder because they either do not see a need for treatment or are not always taken seriously by the medical community.

■ ETIOLOGIC THEORIES

Most of the major theorists believe that personality disorders originate in early childhood. This is one group of mental illnesses that most professionals believe is a result of overuse of defense mechanisms, which are learned at a very young age.

The biologic theorists and geneticists are not quite in agreement with the behaviorists and psychoanalytic theorists, however. Again, largely because of tests performed with identical twins, organizations such as the National Mental Health Organization and others believe that certain people may be genetically predisposed to personality disorders. Genetics combined with environmental conditions may also lead to this group of mental illnesses.

■ TYPES

BORDERLINE PERSONALITY DISORDER

Borderline personality disorder (BPD) is quite common and is seen more frequently in females. People with BPD display erratic behavior. Nurses are never sure how to approach these patients because it is not certain how they will interpret the interaction or what the response will be. The various behavioral responses are quite unpredictable.

Behavioral and Physical Presentation

In borderline personality, moods are very unstable and changeable. People may display uncertainty regarding their self-concept and their sexual orientation. These individuals may have substance abuse problems and attempt self-hurtful behaviors including multiple suicide attempts. Anhedonia (inability to feel pleasure) is often present and may interfere with a patient's ability to handle any strong emotion with success. People who have BPD will speak of feeling bored and empty. One belief about the etiology of this disorder relates to ineffective nurturing by the patient's parents. The child then grows up with conflicts between love/hate, abandonment/domination, dependency/detachment—a whole series of opposite emotions.

Several defense mechanisms are used in borderline personality. Denial, projection, and splitting (inability to integrate positive and negative feelings at the same time) are among the common defense mechanisms (Shives and Isaacs, 2002).

PARANOID PERSONALITY

Individuals with **paranoid** personality present with behaviors of suspiciousness and mistrust of other people. These individuals may seem "normal" in their speech and activity, except for the fact that they feel people treat them unfairly. People with paranoid personality disorder are prone to filing lawsuits when they feel wronged in some way. They also seem to be hypersensitive to activity in their environment. They may have difficulty maintaining focused eye contact, for example, because they are so alert to other activity around them. People with paranoid personality disorder are not easily able to laugh at themselves; they take themselves very seriously. They may not show tender emotions and may seem cold and calculating in their relationships. They tend to take comments, events, and situations very personally. In short, they may not be people who endear themselves to nurses.

Paranoid personality disorder should not be confused with paranoid schizophrenia (see Chapter 14). Patients with paranoid personality disorder do not have hallucinations and delusions; they are, however, suspicious of other people and situations. The suspiciousness may cross into other areas of the person's life. For instance, it may be very challenging to enlist the cooperation of a person with this disorder when it comes to taking medications.

Paranoid personality seems to have a high incidence of occurrence within families, which supports the theories of the geneticists.

SCHIZOID PERSONALITY

People with **schizoid** personality do not want to be involved in interpersonal or social relationships. They have very few, if any, social interactions. It is believed that ineffective and unemotional parenting may lead to this type of personality. It is unusual to see patients hospitalized for this disorder because they are so quiet that the disorder often goes unnoticed. They often are described by others as "loners." It is common to see people with this type of personality become very engrossed in books. The books may be a substitute for human companionship. Partly because of this aversion to social interaction, people with schizoid personalities tend to be very intellectual and quite successful in their choice of career.

People with schizoid personalities may appear to be shy and introverted. They have trouble developing friendships. They tend to respond in a very serious, factual manner that is pleasant but not warm or inviting.

DEPENDENT PERSONALITY

The *Diagnostic and Statistical Manual of Mental Disorders-IV-Text Revision (DSM-IV-TR)* defines **dependent** personality as a "pervasive pattern of dependent and submissive behavior." People with dependent personality disorder want others to make decisions for them and tend to feel inferior and suggestible, with a sense of self-doubt. These individuals tend to appear helpless and to avoid responsibility. On the other hand, individuals with this disorder tend to take everything to heart and go out of their way to satisfy people they feel close to and try to change those personality traits that people criticize.

There seems to be an inordinate amount of fear among people who experience dependent personality disorder. It may be the fear of criticism that brings about the inability to make decisions. Inability to make decisions can be severe enough as to limit a person's ability to have meaningful social interactions. Nurses must be cautioned here because the behaviors that have been discussed as symptomatic of dependent personality disorder are behaviors and conditions that are expected in certain cultures, especially among females.

NARCISSISTIC PERSONALITY

People with **narcissistic** personality disorder present behaviors almost opposite to those of people with schizoid personality disorder. Those who have this disorder tend to display an exaggerated impression of themselves. It is not the same degree of grandiosity as the nurse sees with people who have bipolar depression, but the person with narcissistic personality will "blow his own horn." People with narcissistic personality disorder appear to be very self-centered and express the need to feel grand self-importance. An example of this type of "horn blowing" might be the person who says, "I am with the Mormon Tabernacle Choir." A nurse might naturally assume that the person had a magnificent singing voice when, in reality, the person displaying narcissistic personality might be the one who drives the tour bus. In that person's opinion it is much more glorious to be the "on-stage" part of the choir than the person responsible for getting them there!

People with this kind of disorder will seem to take criticism lightly. In reality, deep feelings of anger, resentment, and poor self-esteem are being repressed. Friends will be chosen according to how good they make the person with the narcissistic personality feel.

PASSIVE-AGGRESSIVE PERSONALITY

The individual with **passive-aggressive** personality disorder (also termed negativistic personality disorder) presents with passive-type behaviors. People with this type of disorder are procrastinators. "Never do today what you can put off until tomorrow" seems to be their motto. They become pouty and irritable when asked to perform a task they do not wish to do. Those with this type of personality disorder "forget" to do things they have been asked to do and feel unfairly treated when asked to do something. It is not uncommon for someone with this disorder to undermine the success of a group effort by not getting their part of the task completed. When it is not completed, however, people who have passive-aggressive disorder always have an excuse for their behavior. These patients give the impression of being incompetent.

Experts believe that this disorder is also the result of ineffective parenting. This time, however, it seems to be the result of parents who are overbearing and have expectations that are too high for the child to achieve successfully. These parents are probably authoritarian and quite inflexible in their demands. Thus, the child grows up resenting authority and compensates by being defiant as a way of controlling his or her environment.

ANTISOCIAL/SOCIOPATHIC PERSONALITY

This group of people probably causes the greatest amount of trouble for society. Because this type of personality requires immediate self-gratification, people who have **antisocial/sociopathic** disorder are often in trouble with the law and find themselves in prison. Individuals may have been diagnosed with conduct disorder before age 15. These individuals have difficulty handling frustration and anger, and they seldom feel affection, loyalty, guilt, or remorse, showing very little concern for the rights or feelings of anyone else. People who have this disorder are also at high risk for substance abuse.

It is widely believed that the roots of this disorder, again relating to parenting and family life, probably grow from a family life with few or inconsistent limits. This may be from a permissive or authoritarian parenting style that does not include guidelines for appropriate social behavior. The disorder seems to affect males more frequently than females.

In spite of the inability to feel or show affection, patients with antisocial/sociopathic personality disorder are usually gregarious, intelligent, and likable (Fig. 13-1). They will not, however, have many satisfying sexual relationships. This can lead to some very serious maladaptive behavior, which may be exhibited by such groups as "flashers," who expose themselves in public, or serial killers. Certainly, the numbers of people who have that extreme form of the

disorder are very few, whereas people with antisocial traits exist everywhere throughout society. Most people with this illness are able to control their behavior out of fear of punishment; only those with extreme cases are unable to do so.

Because people with antisocial/sociopathic personality disorder are frequently highly intelligent, they learn the "jargon" of psychology and know how to manipulate it. Those with antisocial/sociopathic personality disorder are difficult to treat.

■ MEDICAL TREATMENT FOR PATIENTS WITH PERSONALITY DISORDERS

Medical treatment can be very difficult because the patient doesn't perceive a problem. Patients are very rarely hospitalized for the personality disorder, although nurses may encounter it when the person is a med-

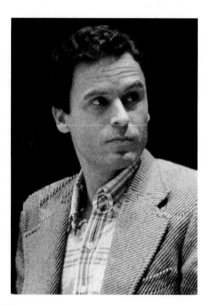

FIGURE 13-1. Handsome, charming, articulate, confident, and friendly are some of the words that have been used to describe Theodore Bundy, a serial killer who was executed after confessing to at least 28 murders throughout the United States. Fortunately, sociopaths as extreme as Bundy are rare. (Courtesy of rotten.com, Mountain View, CA.)

ical or surgical patient. When people with personality disorders do see the fact that help may be needed, misplaced anger is often directed at the therapist. Patients often leave treatment when confronted with their problem. The treatment program is designed specifically for the patient and may include psychotherapy, individual and group therapy, or cognitive therapy. Group therapy may be more effective than other forms because peer pressure can be very effective at getting the patient to see the need to modify certain behaviors. Therapy can be very long term, as the patient will start and stop therapy when things get uncomfortable. The hard truth is that people who have a personality disorder may not improve.

Medications are one option that may be used. Fluoxetine (Prozac) is being used with some success. Caution is given here: medications are frequently not effective. Patients who do not see they are ill, also see no need to medicate. They don't take the prescribed medications. It is very difficult to treat patients with disorders of personality.

■ ALTERNATIVE TREATMENTS FOR PATIENTS WITH PERSONALITY DISORDERS

Biofeedback and certain herbal and nutritional supplements may be helpful. However, as with prescribed medications, patients may not see the need to take a supplement or to discipline themselves enough to perform biofeedback and other relaxation techniques.

■ NURSING INTERVENTIONS FOR PATIENTS WITH PERSONALITY DISORDERS

The ultimate goal of nursing care for the person with a personality disorder is increased motivation and socialization. Nursing interventions must be designed to assist the

patient in learning new behaviors that will lead to improving social functioning.

1. *Unconditional positive regard:* It is important to display acceptance of the person, not the maladaptive behaviors.
2. *Trust:* People with personality disorders are difficult to work with. Trust and honesty are crucial, yet these people may be downright hostile toward the nurses and health-care team. Much patience is required from the nurse.
3. *Limit setting:* The patient needs consistent guidelines as to what is appropriate behavior and what is acceptable in certain situations. It is important to provide structure and parameters for behavior. Consequences for going beyond the established limit are set at the same time a limit is set. Do not get pulled in to patient behaviors designed to pit staff against staff.
4. *Communication:* Nurses must be aware of the possibility of being manipulated by patients with personality disorders. Power struggles may easily develop, and it is important for the nurse to recognize when this is happening. It may be necessary to use verbal communication techniques to calm the patient when he or she becomes agitated in an effort to set the limits of the situation.
5. *Role modeling:* Nurses will be working with the therapeutic plan of care through communication as well as through role modeling. The treatment plan dictates what is appropriate for each patient. For example, patients with dependent personality disorder need to have the nurse role-model ways of decision making.
6. *Safety/security:* Maintaining a calm atmosphere helps the patient with a personality disorder feel safe and trusting. This is no small task for the facility. Allowing flexibility with limits is a very vague description of the beginning of a safe milieu. The facility will be treating more than one patient, each of whom will have different

requirements. Starting with the color and style of furniture may be enough to promote a sense of calm.

Table 13-1 summarizes the symptoms and nursing interventions for personality disorders.

TABLE 13-1	*Personality Disorders*	
TYPE	**SYMPTOMS**	**NURSING INTERVENTIONS**
BORDERLINE	■ Moods unstable and changeable ■ Uncertainty regarding self-concept and sexual orientation ■ Substance abuse ■ Suicide attempts ■ Anhedonia ■ Difficulty handling strong emotion ■ Bored and empty feelings	■ Display unconditional positive regard for the person ■ Build trusting relationship ■ Set limits on behavior ■ Establish therapeutic communication ■ Demonstrate positive role modeling ■ Provide safety/security
PARANOID	■ Suspicious and mistrustful of other people ■ May seem "normal" in speech and activity ■ Believe that people treat them unfairly ■ Hypersensitive to activity in the environment ■ Difficult to maintain focused eye contact ■ Not easily able to laugh at themselves ■ Take themselves very seriously ■ May not show tender emotions ■ May seem cold and calculating in their relationships ■ Tend to take comments, events, situations personally ■ Few social interactions ■ Loners ■ Appear to be shy and introverted ■ Have trouble developing friendships ■ Tend to respond in a very serious, factual manner that is pleasant but not warm or inviting	■ Same as for borderline ■ Avoid situation that the patient may perceive as demeaning
DEPENDENT	■ Dependent and submissive ■ Want others to make decisions for them	■ Same as for borderline ■ Allow patient to make some decisions for his or her treatment

(continued)

TYPE	SYMPTOMS	NURSING INTERVENTIONS
DEPENDENT *(cont'd)*	■ Tend to feel inferior and suggestible and have a sense of self-doubt ■ Tend to appear helpless and avoid responsibility ■ Tend to take everything to heart—will go out of their way to satisfy people they feel close to and try to change those personality traits that people criticize ■ Inordinate amount of fear	■ Reinforce the patient's decisions ■ Encourage patient to make truthful, positive self-statements each shift
NARCISSISTIC	■ Exaggerated self-image ■ "Blow their own horn"—appear self-centered ■ Express need for self-importance ■ Take criticism lightly but in reality repress feelings of anger and resentment	■ Same as for borderline ■ Encourage patient to learn to accept limitations in self and others
PASSIVE-AGGRESSIVE OR NEGATIVISTIC PERSONALITY DISORDER	■ Procrastinators ■ Become irritable when asked to perform tasks they do not wish to do ■ "Forget" to do things they have been asked to do ■ Feel unfairly treated when asked to do something ■ May undermine group success by not completing their part in group activity ■ Consider their excuses good enough to pardon their behavior ■ Give the impression of being incompetent	■ Same as for borderline ■ Encourage patient to make one suggestion for improvement for each criticism ■ Teach/role-model the relationship between patient's "rights" and "responsibilities" ■ Encourage discussion of feelings
ANTISOCIAL/ SOCIOPATHIC	■ Require immediate self-gratification ■ Often in trouble with the law ■ Have difficulty handling frustration and anger ■ Seldom feel affection, loyalty, guilt, or remorse ■ Show very little concern for the rights or feelings of others ■ High risk for substance abuse ■ Usually gregarious, intelligent, and likable ■ Will not have many satisfying sexual relationships	■ Same as for borderline ■ Promote positive, healthy interpersonal relationships

Key Concepts ■ ■ ■

1. Personality disorders are maladaptive responses to personality development.
2. People with personality disorders are seldom hospitalized for them. They do not see a need for obtaining help and are not always taken seriously by the medical community.
3. When people with personality disorders are brought into treatment, they seldom stay for any length of time. Therefore, treatment is rarely successful.

COMMONLY USED MEDICATIONS ■ *Personality Disorders*

Note: A variety of medications may be prescribed, depending on a person's situation and willingness to comply with treatment. Just as most people with personality disorders stop attending therapy, they also quit taking their medications, making medications a secondary treatment choice in many cases.

Amitriptyline (Elavil)   **Fluoxetine** (Prozac)
Doxepin (Sinequan)

REFERENCES

Keltner, N.L., Schwecke, L.H., and Bostrom, C.E. (2003). *Psychiatric Nursing*, 4th ed. Mosby, Inc. St. Louis, MO.

Shives, L.R. and Isaacs, A. (2002). *Basic Concepts of Mental Health Nursing*, 5th ed. JB Lippincott, Philadelphia.

WEBSITES

www.mentalhealth.com
www.nlm.nih.gov/medlineplus
http://www.nmha.org

CRITICAL THINKING EXERCISES ■ ■ ■

1. You have just admitted Jonathan, a 40-year-old man, to your unit. Jonathan is an executive with a major auditing company. He is admitted for treatment of bleeding gastric ulcer. He is unmarried, 20 pounds overweight, and balding. Jonathan delights in telling the nursing staff about his sexual escapades. "Why give all of this magnificence to one person? No, I'll never commit to a monogamous relationship; not as good a catch as I am!" What personality disorder would you think Jonathan is displaying? How will you converse with him? What limits will you set on his behavior with you?

2. Using the suggested nursing diagnoses listed here (or others you can think of), complete a nursing process for Jonathan (narcissistic personality disorder).

SUGGESTED NURSING DIAGNOSES

1. *Verbal Communication, Impaired*
2. *Defensive Coping*
3. *Individual Coping, Ineffective*

ASSESSMENT/ DATA COLLECTION	NURSING DIAGNOSIS	PLAN/ GOAL	INTERVENTIONS/ NURSING ACTIONS	EVALUATION CRITERIA

3. Using the suggested nursing diagnoses listed here (or others you can think of), complete a nursing process for a person with antisocial/sociopathic personality disorder.

SUGGESTED NURSING DIAGNOSES

1. *Thought Processes, Altered*
2. *Individual Coping, Ineffective*
3. *Sexuality Patterns, Altered*

ASSESSMENT/ DATA COLLECTION	NURSING DIAGNOSIS	PLAN/ GOAL	INTERVENTIONS/ NURSING ACTIONS	EVALUATION CRITERIA

CASE STUDY: HORACE ◼ ◼ ◼

Horace is a 48-year-old professional male. He is in the clinic today to be evaluated by a counselor. You are rooming the patient and taking his information. Horace shares that he has just lost another job. He doesn't understand why, because he states, "I have a very good skill set on my resume." He tells you he was a star athlete in school. He lettered in basketball. He attributes the loss of this last job to jealous coworkers. Further investigation into Horace's history shows he was removed from the team his senior year because of poor grades and poor performance on the court. His work history, starting from the most current job, indicates he cannot perform even the simplest of his job duties and after his 3-month probation was let go, as he was taking too much time from other staff members who were trying to teach and train him in the essential functions of his job.

What personality disorder(s) might Horace be experiencing? What communication skills would be helpful when working with Horace? Using the NANDA nursing diagnoses listed or others you can think of, write a care plan for Horace.

1. Adjustment
2. Thought process
3. Spiritual distress

TEST QUESTIONS ◼ ◼ ◼

MULTIPLE CHOICE QUESTIONS

1. When setting limits with patients with personality disorders, the consequences to those limits should be set:
   A. When the behavior is done
   B. Just before the nurse anticipates the behavior
   C. When the staff or family complains about the behavior
   D. When the limit is set

2. David, 30 years old, comes to your unit for treatment of multiple broken bones following a car accident. He is friendly and flirtatious but very demanding. As you take your data from him, you learn he has had the police looking for him for petty theft. He laughs and says, "Like they don't have better things to do!" He states he has changed jobs three times in the past year and has just broken off his second engagement. His former fiancée is visiting and privately tells you that you need to be careful because "he doesn't always tell the truth." You suspect which of the following personality disorders?
   A. Paranoid
   B. Dependent
   C. Antisocial
   D. Schizoid

3. A primary mechanism used by people with personality disorders is:
   A. Manipulation
   B. Depression
   C. Projection
   D. Euphoria

4. Nurses understand that, for the person with a personality disorder, which of the following behaviors would be the most difficult for the patient to comply with?
   A. Listening to music
   B. Abiding by the rules in the hospital
   C. Playing volleyball
   D. Developing a friendship

5. The person who is in trouble with the law would probably have which of the following personality disorders?
   A. Narcissistic
   B. Schizoid
   C. Antisocial
   D. Borderline

6. People who display very erratic behavior most likely have which of the following types of personality disorder?
   A. Narcissistic
   B. Schizoid
   C. Antisocial
   D. Borderline

7. Characteristics of paranoid personality disorder include:
   A. Suspiciousness and mistrust
   B. Gregariousness and joviality
   C. Fear and withdrawal
   D. Hallucinations and seductiveness

8. Your patient has been admitted with a diagnosis of bilateral pneumonia. You have trouble communicating with this patient, who is pouty and seems to procrastinate and "forget" to do tasks you have requested. Besides the pneumonia, you ask the physician if there is a history of which of the following personality disorders?
   A. Schizoid
   B. Antisocial
   C. Passive-aggressive
   D. Borderline

9. Nursing care for people with personality disorders includes all of the following *except:*
   A. Unconditional positive regard
   B. Trust
   C. Limit setting
   D. Vague communication (to decrease feelings of inferiority)

10. You are caring for a 25-year-old male who has been admitted for infections that resulted from self-inflicted burns. This is not the first admission for this young man, but he is new to you as a new nurse on the unit. You have not read his entire chart, but you suspect he has a history of which one of the following personality disorders?

    A. Narcissistic
    B. Borderline
    C. Schizoid
    D. Passive-aggressive

11. He tells you that he also has been sexually active with a multitude of partners of both sexes. You are not certain yet if he is being truthful, but you use your gloves and handwashing techniques when working with his blood and body fluids because you are aware he may be at risk for:

    A. Hepatitis B
    B. Hepatitis C
    C. HIV
    D. All of the above

MATCHING QUESTIONS
Directions
Match the trait or definition in column B with the personality disorder in column A. There is one trait that will not be used. All other answers are to be used only once.

COLUMN A
1. Dependent
2. Borderline
3. Schizoid
4. Narcissistic
5. Passive-aggressive
6. Paranoid
7. Antisocial/sociopathic

COLUMN B
A. Tend to display an exaggerated impression of themselves
B. May undermine the success of a group effort by not getting their part of the task completed or give impression of being incompetent
C. Behaviors of suspiciousness and mistrust
D. Pervasive pattern of dependent and submissive behavior
E. Often in trouble with the law
F. More common in females; anhedonia; moods are unstable and changeable
G. "Loners"; very few, if any, social interactions
H. Results from effective personality development

14

Schizophrenia

Learning Objectives ▪ ▪ ▪

1. Define schizophrenia.
2. Identify three types of schizophrenia.
3. State physical and behavioral symptoms of three types of schizophrenia.
4. Identify possible psychoanalytic, genetic, environmental, and socioeconomic theories of causes of schizophrenia.
5. Define the 4 A's of Eugene Bleuler.
6. Identify treatment modalities for people with schizophrenia.
7. Identify nursing care for people with schizophrenia.

Key Terms ▪ ▪ ▪

- Catatonic schizophrenia
- Delusions
- Echolalia
- Echopraxia
- Hallucinations
- Illusions
- Paranoid schizophrenia
- Schizophrenia

Schizophrenia is becoming more widely viewed as a group of illnesses rather than a single condition. People with schizophrenia seem to be very distractible. It is difficult for them to focus on any one topic for any length of time. As with any "rule," however, there are exceptions. For example, some people with schizophrenia have worked with their illness and become famous, successful individuals (Fig. 14-1). Of note, Mary Todd Lincoln, wife of United States President Abraham Lincoln, Syd Barrett, of the band Pink Floyd, Lionel Aldridge, member of a football team that won the Superbowl, and Nobel Laureate in Economics, John Forbes

Nash, Jr., who was documented in the book and movie *A Beautiful Mind*. The list goes on!

Schizophrenia seems to strike adolescents and young adults between the ages of 16 and 35, with women tending to experience symptoms approximately 5 years later than males. Schizophrenia is rare in young children. Prevalence of people with schizophrenia is the same across race, gender, and culture. The National Institute of Mental Health (NIMH) estimates that nearly 3 million Americans will develop schizophrenia during the course of their lives. That is about 1 percent of the population (NIMH, 1999).

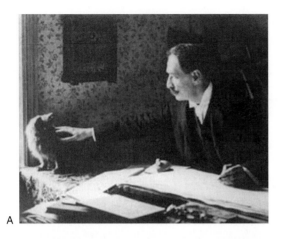

A

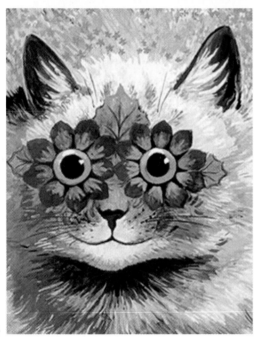

B

FIGURE 14-1. A, Louis Wain was an English artist who suffered from schizophrenia. He is famous for his wide variety of images of cats (B).

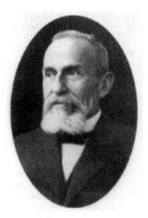

FIGURE 14-2. Eugene Bleuler (1857–1940) was a Swiss psychiatrist who coined the term *schizophrenia* and contributed to the understanding of the disorder. (Courtesy of Wikiverse.org.)

The term *schizophrenia* (which means "split mind") was first used by a Swiss psychiatrist, Eugene Bleuler (Fig. 14-2). Schizophrenia is a serious psychiatric disorder. People with schizophrenia have a "split" between their thoughts and their feelings and between their reality and society's reality. The person may have issues concerning confused gender identity. People who have schizophrenia may not be able to differentiate between what is theirs and what is everybody else's with respect to social functioning. Poor self-esteem is also an issue for patients with schizophrenia. It is a surprise to many students that these individuals are generally highly intelligent. Schizophrenia is *not* the same thing as multiple personality disorder (see Chapter 22).

Schizophrenia is said to have an insidious onset. The early symptoms of quietness and withdrawal in an adolescent may be shrugged off as "just a stage." It may easily be a school nurse or counselor who begins to notice these changes. School grades may begin to drop off. The adolescent may have a change in personality or a change in the way he or she relates to other people. It is easy to misinterpret these behaviors as part of the adolescent experience.

Several difficulties are associated with the diagnosis and long-term treatment of patients with schizophrenia. Signs and symptoms must be present for 6 months or more before a positive diagnosis can be made. Once released from the treatment facility into alternative or step-down types of housing, patients often find themselves at the mercy of society. The jobs they accept and the responsibility of paying bills and of taking their medications often prove too stressful and competitive for these individuals. They may lose the job and the ability to remain in the housing, be unable to secure other housing, and be unable to pay for their medications. For these reasons, a high percentage of homeless people are also schizophrenic.

Bleuler used a system of "4 A's" to define schizophrenia:

1. Associative disturbance: In associative disturbance, or "associative looseness," as it is also called, the patient typically exhibits three main behaviors:
   - Making up words ("neologisms")
   - Rambling from topic to topic
   - Using revolving words and syllables that may associate to a specific word but are out of context with the conversation. Bleuler tells the story of a woman who was asked to list her family members. She answered "father, son … and the Holy Ghost" (Bleuler, 1911, p. 26). Making up words that rhyme with other words is another behavior that is sometimes observed.

2. *Affect:* Affect, you will recall, is the outward expression of emotion. People with schizophrenia generally have what is called a flat, or blunted, affect. This means that they rarely show signs of any emotion. Looking at their faces and nonverbal forms of communicating, the nurse would not be able to guess at an emotion. In schizophrenia, however, there may also be inappropriate or incongruent affect, such as laughing when the patient states that he or she feels sad or depressed; the outward expression of the mood does not match the stated feeling. Exaggerations of affect are also present in some patients.

3. *Autism:* Autism is an emotional detachment. People who display autistic behavior are preoccupied with the self and show little concern for any reality outside their own world.

4. *Ambivalence:* Ambivalence means having opposite feelings about one person or situation at the same time. An example is the love/hate relationships sometimes seen in jobs or marriages. Be cautioned that not all people who have a love/hate relationship with their jobs are schizophrenics. The statistics for the numbers of people who have schizophrenia would take a steep turn upward if that were true.

In addition to the 4 A's, patients with schizophrenia display other common symptoms of delusions, hallucinations, and illusions. **Delusions** are fixed, false beliefs that cannot be changed by logic. Patients resist any factual proof that their beliefs do not exist. Typically, patients exhibit delusions of grandeur, persecution, or guilt. **Hallucinations** are false sensory perceptions that can affect any of the five senses. **Illusions** are mistaken perceptions of reality.

Students often confuse hallucinations and illusions. Anyone who has ever watched a magician or seen certain images in cloud formations has witnessed an illusion. In illusion, something is there; it is just perceived incorrectly: that card did not just magically appear; it was set up to appear when the magician wanted it to. In hallucination, there is nothing to misinterpret. The person who sees a lamb in a certain cloud formation is experiencing an illusion; the person who sees a lamb in a cloudless sky is experiencing a hallucination.

■ ETIOLOGIC THEORIES

Psychoanalytic and biologic theories of the causes of schizophrenia both exist. The schizophrenias are highly debated on both sides of the "nurture/nature" theory.

The psychoanalytic, or "nurture," theories revert to the anal stage of Freudian theory. The inability to meet the challenge of oral gratification leaves people in the adolescent and young adult years unable to handle their developing sexuality, according to Freud. Lack of oral gratification or nurturing mother-child relationships also would lead to personalities that are "cool" or aloof (or indifferent) in their relationships. Freud would also attribute the disruption of effective communication to failure to reach oral gratification. There seems to be less research to support this theory than there is to support the biologic theories.

Schizophrenia and its relationship to genetics has been observed in twin studies, family studies, and adoption studies for approximately 75 years. Studies on identical twins (the psychobiologic, or "nature," theory) show that if one twin has schizophrenia the other has a 50 percent chance of developing it. In fraternal twins, and patients with a parent having schizophrenia, that percentage drops to approximately 10 percent (Choure, Muzina 2002/2004). To date, the best reason for this probability decrease in fraternal twins seems to be in the amount or reaction to the neurochemical dopamine. Patients with schizophrenia may have elevated levels of dopamine or a brain that overreacts to the amount of dopamine that is present, which would account for their hyperexcitability and hallucinations.

As already indicated, however, the dopamine theory accounts for only about 50 percent of patients with schizophrenia. The other half of patients do not fit into that biologic theory. One question that is posed concerns the relationship between the neurochemical level and the increased hormone production that is also happening in the person's physical development. It is now suggested that viruses experienced by a woman during her pregnancy or complications during birth may contribute to a person having schizophrenia. Again, this is theory, but nurses working with pregnant women should be sure to stress healthy lifestyles and encourage proper prenatal care for all pregnant patients.

Another biologic possibility in the twin and family studies has to do with the genes themselves. Studies show that it may take more than one gene (monogenic theory) to cause the abnormalities of schizophrenia. Genes that collect at a particular place on a chromosome may accumulate to produce certain traits and tendencies. If this is the case, many people have a predisposition to developing schizophrenia. It is believed that the more schizophrenia-related genes twins or family members have in common, the greater the chance of their developing schizophrenia.

In adoption studies, researchers are looking for correlations between the children developing schizophrenia from the biologic parent who either does or does not have schizophrenia and those developing schizophrenia from the adoptive parent who either does or does not have schizophrenia. The research also looks at potential environmental factors that may contribute to the development of the disease in the adoptive home.

Studies also support the possibility that socioeconomic factors may play a role in the development of schizophrenia. More than 50 studies have been performed in several countries, including the United States and Canada, which indicate a higher number of diagnosed cases of schizophrenia among people of lower socioeconomic levels than among those of higher socioeconomic levels. Unfortunately, there is no explanation for this at present. Theories relating to stress and poor coping skills are being studied as possible explanations.

Students of psychology should remember that this group of disorders is very intricate and is still being researched extensively.

■ DIFFERENTIAL DIAGNOSIS

It is common for people with schizophrenia to display other thought disorders also. Extensive, careful screening for these disorders must be done to rule out those that are not applicable and to obtain accurate diagnoses for the patient.

Use of drugs such as methamphetamine, mescaline, and LSD can produce behaviors that very closely mimic those seen in patients with schizophrenia. These behaviors are usually short lived, but methamphetamine, mescaline, and LSD may produce permanent damage to the brain.

■ TYPES

PARANOID SCHIZOPHRENIA

Paranoid schizophrenia is schizophrenia in which the person exhibits unusual suspiciousness and fear. People with this disorder may also exhibit hostile and aggressive behavior. The main symptom of paranoid-type schizophrenia is suspiciousness. Some of the absent symptoms include catatonia, incongruent affect, and loose associations in speech.

Patients with this type of schizophrenia tend to have delusions of persecution and grandeur. In persecutory delusions, patients state that they feel tormented and followed by people. These people could be staff, relatives, or the announcer on the radio or television. The patient may state, "Everyone is out to get me," and will often accuse the nurses of being "part of it, too." As the nurse, however, you don't know what "it" is, and the patient will not tell you. The patient with delusions of grandeur may state that he or she is "God" or "the President of the United States" or may simply say something like "You will soon be receiving a new car and new house because you are such a great nurse."

Hallucinations almost always go along with delusions. The hallucinations can affect any of the five senses but are most frequently auditory or visual. Patients with paranoid schizophrenia will speak of "the voices." These voices are frightening and derogatory to the patient and are responsible for many of the actions performed by these individuals. The patient will experience increased fear and anxiety as a result of "the voices." These so-called voices, as well as some other types of hallucinations,

have led people to attempt suicide. It is entirely possible that "the voices" were responsible for the assassination of Senator Robert Kennedy on June 5, 1968. Sirhan B. Sirhan, the man who shot Senator Kennedy, was diagnosed with chronic paranoid schizophrenia. The nurse caring for a patient with paranoid schizophrenia may see or hear the patient arguing with what at first appears to be himself or herself. In actuality, the patient is arguing with the voices he or she hears, which seem very real. It is hard to explain what "the voices" sound like, but, if you can, imagine that you are in a room with six televisions or radios on different stations all at the same time.

DISORGANIZED (HEBEPHRENIC) SCHIZOPHRENIA

People with disorganized schizophrenia display unusual behavior and facial contortions. Speech may be very bizarre and incoherent. The person may use a random set of words that may make some sense to him or her but not to anyone else (referred to as "word salad"), and the person may express emotions inappropriate to the situation (e.g., patients may giggle, act silly or giddy, or behave in other inappropriate ways while watching a tragic news story on television). Auditory hallucinations are present but disorganized. These hallucinations do not necessarily pertain to the issue at hand for the patient at that moment. Disorganized schizophrenia is a more severe disorganization of personality than the other type of schizophrenia, and its prognosis is poor.

CATATONIC SCHIZOPHRENIA

Catatonic schizophrenia is seen less frequently than some other forms, largely as a result of effective medications. In catatonic schizophrenia, the motor activity of the patient is disturbed. People with catatonic schizophrenia vacillate between extreme muscle rigidity and agitation. The rigidity can affect the whole body or just certain limbs or muscle groups. The symptoms present quickly and can change quickly, especially if stimulated by a loud noise or a sudden movement in the environment.

In the rigid state (sometimes referred to as catatonic stupor), the person may not change position and may stare into space for hours or even days. People with catatonic schizophrenia may still be in touch with reality and may be very suggestible. They sometimes display echolalia and/or echopraxia. **Echolalia** is the repetition of words the patient may hear. For example, if the nurse is passing medications and tells Mrs. Brown that "It is time for your pills," a person experiencing echolalia may repeat, "your pills ... your pills ... your pills ..." over and over. **Echopraxia** is the same kind of repetition, except that the patient repeats an action. The patient with echopraxia may mimic the nurse's action of handing the medication to Mrs. Brown by pretending to hand a pill to someone who is probably not there.

There may be an element of negativism in patients who are catatonic. Even in their rigid state, attempts to move them may result in patients' setting even more firmly into their position. Nurses will be able to feel the resistance. The attempt to move the patient in catatonia may be enough to stimulate the agitation part of the disorder. The patient may flail around, strike out, or begin running up and down the hallway.

■ MEDICAL TREATMENT FOR PATIENTS WITH SCHIZOPHRENIA

Current opinion holds that schizophrenia is not curable (because no cause can be isolated) but that it is certainly treatable. Medications, electroconvulsive therapy (ECT), and psychotherapy are indicated for patients with schizophrenia. Among the classifications of medications prescribed for certain patients are the antipsychotics.

These create decreased dopamine levels, which in turn lead to extrapyramidal side effects. Some common antipsychotic medications are Risperidone (Risperdal), olanzapine (Zyprexa), clozapine (Clozaril), and older generations of antipsychotics such as haloperidol (Haldol) and chlorpromazine (Thorazine). Consult your drug reference book for more antipsychotic medications. Anticholinergic medications are used to combat these side effects because the anticholinergics help return balance among dopamine, acetylcholine, and other neurotransmitters.

It must be noted that some cultures may respond differently to medications. Some may be reluctant to take the medications based on religious beliefs while others, such as some Asian or African American patients frequently metabolize medications differently and may actually require a lower dose of medication. Nurses should always consult the best drug reference book or other drug resource available (for example, a pharmacist) and be comfortable asking the doctor if there are any questions about dosing of medications.

Psychotherapy includes individual, group, and family therapy. ECT is used in cases that are severe or difficult to treat and is not used until all other methods of therapy have failed.

■ ALTERNATIVE TREATMENT FOR PATIENTS WITH SCHIZOPHRENIA

Care must be taken with therapies that could enhance delusions, hallucinations, illusions, or hearing of voices. Certainly for patients with schizophrenia, it is encouraged that all therapy be closely monitored and that it be delivered by trained professionals. It will always depend on the individual and the type and severity of the schizophrenia. The following are some techniques that may be safe for nurses to use.

NUTRITIONAL SUPPLEMENTS

Some doctors and nutritionists suggest a dose of niacin (vitamin B3) may be helpful in some patients with schizophrenia. Niacin has an effect on the serotonin and tryptophan (remember your nutrition class?) in the brain, and increasing it may help lower the behaviors associated with schizophrenia in some patients. Niacin comes in oral pill form as well as in dietary sources such as turkey (yes, THAT tryptophan!), peanut butter, whole grains, salmon, beef, and other foods.

MASSAGE THERAPY

Relaxing back or shoulder massage may help the individual to relax. This should be used with caution, however, and always in compliance with a written care plan. Some individuals may respond negatively to the touch or amount of pressure used in a massage.

NEUROLINGUISTIC PROGRAMMING

Again, care must be taken to use appropriate framing for the type of schizophrenia the patient is experiencing. Using rapport techniques such as "I hear" or framing words into auditory terminology may have negative effects on the person who hears "voices."

■ NURSING INTERVENTIONS FOR PATIENTS WITH SCHIZOPHRENIA

The goals of nursing interventions include support, structure, consistency, and safety for the patient. Hildegard Peplau stated in 1962 that to help the patient is to remember and fully understand what is happening. Some suggested interventions follow.

1. *Never reinforce hallucinations, delusions, or illusions:* It is necessary to keep the patient in reality as the nurse knows it. Nurses must realize how frightening hallucinations are and must be prepared to spend time with the patient to help decrease the patient's anxiety level. Some examples of responses to patients who are hallucinating are listed in Table 14-1.
2. *Never whisper or laugh when the patient cannot hear the whole conversation:* It is important, especially with patients who have paranoid schizophrenia, to avoid any situation that might encourage the suspiciousness. Include the patient in the entire discussion, or withhold the discussion until the patient is out of the area. It is also a good idea to face the patient. Turning away may be interpreted as

TABLE 14-1	*Suggested Interventions for Patients with Schizophrenia Who Are Hallucinating*
SUGGESTED ACTION	**RATIONALE**
1. "Mr. R, I don't see any snakes. It is time for lunch. I will walk to the dining room with you."	1. This lets the patient know you heard him but brings him immediately into the reality of time of day and the need to go to the dining room.
2. "I see a crack in the wall, Mr. R. It is harmless; you are safe. Susan is here to take you down to Occupational Therapy now."	2. This is in response to a probable illusion. It lets the patient know that you see something. It validates his fear but tells him what you see and then moves him into the here and now.

(continued)

| TABLE 14-1 | *Suggested Interventions for Patients with Schizophrenia Who Are Hallucinating (Continued)* |

SUGGESTED ACTION	RATIONALE
3. "I know that your thoughts seem very real to you, Ms. C, but they do not seem logical to me. I would like you to come to your room and get dressed now, please."	3. Again, you are validating the patient's concern without exploring and focusing on the delusion.
4. "Ms. C, It appears to me that you are listening to someone. Are you hearing voices other than mine?"	4. This is a method of validating your impression of what you see. This is as far as you will go into exploring what she may be hearing.
5. "Thank you, Ms. C. I want to help you focus away from the other voices. I am real; they are not. Please come with me to the reading room."	5. In this statement, you respond to her in the present and reinforce her response to you. This response attempts to redirect her thinking.

rejection. Whispering, laughing, or turning away from the patient may be enough to cause his or her aggressive behavior. This behavior could be directed at the nurse, another patient, or the person who felt the rejection.

3. *Avoid placing the patient in situations of competition or embarrassment:* People with schizophrenia do not usually have the emotional stability to handle stressful situations. Patients may revert to former behaviors or refuse to participate in therapy if they feel embarrassed.

4. *Trust:* It is crucial for a trusting relationship to exist between the nurse and patient. Keep promises. Be honest and consistent in all aspects of the patient's treatment plan. Allow the patient to vent thoughts and feelings, but do this according to the appropriateness of the time and place. Relating with unconditional positive regard to people with schizophrenia will help validate them as people and will build their self-esteem. Whenever possible, it is suggested to assign the same nurse to the same patients to ensure the best possible consistency of care.

5. *Milieu:* The treatment setting must be calm and conducive to making progress. It must be structured in a way that helps promote healthy behaviors and minimize anxiety. Providing written instructions or information boards can help promote reality and self-responsible behavior. Furnishing the treatment area in colors that are considered calming, such as blues and greens, may be helpful. Setting limits on noise, physical activity, and types of music in the treatment area may help to provide a setting in which patients can focus on healing.

6. *Communication:* Keep communication simple. Be brief and clear with all instructions. State what is acceptable and give the rationale and consequences at the same time. Emphasizing behavior that is appropriate to the situation is important. Stating information in the positive rather than the negative is also helpful (e.g., say "Eat your food calmly" rather than "Do not throw your food").

Table 14-2 summarizes symptoms and nursing interventions for the types of schizophrenia discussed earlier.

TABLE 14-2 ■ *Schizophrenia*		
TYPE	**SYMPTOMS**	**NURSING INTERVENTIONS**
PARANOID	■ Suspiciousness ■ Hostility and aggression ■ Incongruent affect ■ Loose associations in speech ■ Delusions of grandeur and persecution ■ Hallucinations of any of the five senses, but usually visual or auditory ("the voices")	■ Never reinforce hallucinations, delusions, or illusion ■ Avoid whispering or laughing when the patient cannot hear the whole conversation ■ Avoid putting patient into situations that are competitive or embarrassing ■ Build trust ■ Establish calm milieu ■ Use therapeutic communication skills
DISORGANIZED (HEBEPHRENIC)	■ Unusual behavior and facial contortions ■ Bizarre, distorted speech ■ "Word salad" ■ Expression of emotions inappropriate to the situation ■ Disorganized auditory hallucinations	■ Use therapeutic communication ■ Stress reality ■ Observe for signs of regression or social withdrawal
CATATONIC	■ Motor activity disturbed ■ Vacillation between extreme muscle rigidity and agitation ■ Symptoms that present quickly and can change quickly, especially if stimulated by noise or sudden movement ■ Echolalia ■ Echopraxia	■ Provide for basic physical needs ■ Ensure adequate nutrition ■ Ensure safety

Key Concepts ■ ■ ■

1. Schizophrenia is best described as a group of disorders in which patients display unusual behaviors. There are viable arguments for both psychoanalytic and biologic causes of schizophrenia.
2. Onset of schizophrenia most often occurs in the adolescent or early adult years.
3. Schizophrenia is a challenging disorder to treat from a medical and a nursing standpoint.

COMMONLY USED MEDICATIONS ■ *Schizophrenia*	
Clozapine (Clozaril)	**Thioridazine** (Mellaril)
Risperidone (Risperdal)	**Haloperidol** (Haldol)
Olanzapine (Zyprexa)	**Benztropine** (Cogentin)
Chlorpromazine (Thorazine)	**Trihexyphenidyl** (Artane)

REFERENCES

American Psychiatric Association. (2000). *Diagnostic and Statistical Manual of Mental Disorders—Text Revision*, 4th ed. Author, Washington, DC.

Bleuler, E. (1911). *Dementia Praecox (Emil Kraepelin) or the Group of Schizophrenias.* International Press, New York (p. 26).

Chure, J. MD and Muzina, D. MD *Schizophrenia* The Cleveland Clinic Foundation. Published 10/21/2002, Revised 11/15/2004.

Hoffer, A. (1998). *Vitamin B-3 and Schizophrenia: Discovery, Recovery, Controversy.* Quarry Press, Kingston, Ontario, Canada.

Murray, B. (2004). *Psychiatric Nursing: Current Trends in Diagnosis and Treatment.* Western Schools, Brockton, MA.

NIMH from Internet (1999–2004). 1. When Someone Has Schizophrenia NIMH http://www.nimh.nih.gov/publicat/schizsoms.cfm. 2. Schizophrenia NIMH http://www.nimh.nih.gov/healthinformation/schizophreniamenu.cfm updated 4/21/2005.

Rubin, Z., Peplau, L., and Salovey, P. (1993). *Psychology.* Houghton Mifflin, Boston (pp. 479–480).

Shives, L.R. and Isaacs, A. (2002). *Basic Concepts of Psychiatric-Mental Health Nursing*, 5th ed. Lippincott, Philadelphia

Sierpina, V.S. (2001). *Integrative Health Care—Complementary and Alternative Therapies for the Whole Person.* F.A. Davis Company, Philadelphia.

WEBSITES

www.encarta.msn.com

http://www.islandnet.com/~hoffer/hofferhp.htm (Canadian)

www.nimh.nih.gov

www.schizophrenia.com

http://www.clevelandclinicmeded.com/diseasemanagement/psychiatry/schizophrenia/schizophrenia.htm

CRITICAL THINKING EXERCISES ■ ■ ■

1. Your 17-year-old nephew has always been an honor roll student, but he has been earning C and D grades the last 6 months. He quit the football team, stating that "all the other members were plotting against" him. When he saw the results of the high school game on a television sports show, he said, "See, they all know about me." His parents ask you if you think he is taking drugs. What will you say to them? What suggestions will you make? How will you approach your nephew?

2. You are answering the phone on the midnight shift. A young woman's voice on the other end of the telephone tells you that she has cut herself "just like they told me to. I had to do it; they made me do it. Why won't they leave me

alone? What else do they want from me?" What will you say to her? What is your priority? How will you get help to her?

3. You are at home preparing to go to work. There is a frantic knock at the door. Your neighbor begs you, "Please help! My brother went off again. Mom is not home. I don't know what to do." You arrive to find the 13-year-old male in a corner telling you to, "Stay away. Don't hurt me!" What are some possible causes for his behavior? What approaches will you take to help him and his very frightened sister? What other information will you try to obtain, both subjective and objective?

4. Using the suggested nursing diagnoses listed here (or others you can think of), complete a nursing process for paranoid schizophrenia.

SUGGESTED NURSING DIAGNOSES

1. *Injury, Risk for*
2. *Thought Processes, Altered*
3. *Violence, Risk for: Self-Directed or Directed at Others*

ASSESSMENT/ DATA COLLECTION	NURSING DIAGNOSIS	PLAN/ GOAL	INTERVENTIONS/ NURSING ACTIONS	EVALUATION CRITERIA

5. Using the suggested nursing diagnoses listed here (or others you can think of), complete a nursing process for catatonic schizophrenia.

SUGGESTED NURSING DIAGNOSES

1. *Physical Mobility, Impaired*
2. *Verbal Communication, Impaired*
3. *Thought Processes, Impaired*
4. *Sensory Perception, Disturbed*

ASSESSMENT/ DATA COLLECTION	NURSING DIAGNOSIS	PLAN/ GOAL	INTERVENTIONS/ NURSING ACTIONS	EVALUATION CRITERIA

TEST QUESTIONS ■ ■ ■

MULTIPLE CHOICE QUESTIONS

1. The main symptom of paranoid schizophrenia is:

   A. Stupor
   B. Associative looseness
   C. Suspicion
   D. Hyperexcitability

2. Brian, an 18-year-old with schizophrenia, has a negative attitude, is delusional, and is withdrawing from others. A nursing intervention that is appropriate for promoting activity for Brian is:

   A. Tell him "the voices" told you he should participate in the weekly party.
   B. Remind him that he does not want to get worse by sitting alone.
   C. Tell him he must join the party; it is part of his care plan.
   D. Invite him to join in the party.

3. Shawna is a 22-year-old woman who has episodes of extreme muscle rigidity and hyperexcitability. She sometimes repeats a word or a phrase over and over. Attempts to move her are met with even more muscle resistance. Shawna probably has what type of schizophrenia?

   A. Catatonic
   B. Disorganized
   C. Paranoid
   D. Schizotypal

4. Mr. Goodbody is calling out, "Nurse!" When you arrive in his room, he tells you to be careful of the snake in the corner. You do not see anything in the corner. Mr. Goodbody is experiencing a(an):

   A. Hallucination
   B. Attention-getting behavior
   C. Illusion
   D. Delusion

5. Of the following responses, which would be your *best* response to Mr. Goodbody regarding the snake?

   A. "Don't worry; I'll get rid of it" (you pretend to remove the snake)
   B. "I don't see a snake; what else do you see that isn't there?"
   C. "I don't see a snake. It is time for your group meeting. I'll walk with you to the meeting room."
   D. "Where is it? I hate snakes. Let's get out of here."

6. Which of the following is *not* a sign of untreated schizophrenia?

   A. Loss of reality
   B. Living in one's own world
   C. Functioning normally in society
   D. Delusions, hallucinations

7. A nursing intervention for a person with schizophrenia is to:

   A. Reinforce the hallucinations.
   B. Keep the person oriented to reality and to the present.
   C. Administer ECT as necessary.
   D. Encourage competitive activities.

8. Mr. S states, "Look at the snakes on the ceiling." You see some cracks in the plaster. Mr. S is experiencing a(an):

   A. Hallucination
   B. Illusion
   C. Delusion
   D. Flashback

9. Your best response to Mr. S might be:

   A. "How many snakes do you see, Mr. S?"
   B. "Yes, I see them, too. Let's go to the dayroom."
   C. "I see some cracks in the plaster, but I do not see snakes. Let's go to the day room."
   D. "I don't think your medication is working. I'll call the doctor."

10. Ms. Tight is on your unit for treatment of kidney stones. She suddenly walks to the side of the hallway and becomes rigid and immovable. She begins to repeat the same word over and over. You check her medical record and find she has a history of which of the following disorders?

    A. Paranoid schizophrenia
    B. Disorganized schizophrenia
    C. Schizoaffective schizophrenia
    D. Catatonic schizophrenia

11. A patient who repeats a word or part of a word over and over might be said to have which of the following symptoms of catatonic schizophrenia

    A. Echolalia
    B. Ecopraxia
    C. Ecocardia
    D. Word salad

12. Pha is a 32-year-old patient newly diagnosed with schizophrenia. Dr. Med has ordered Clozaril (clozapine) for this patient. Part of the discharge teaching for Pha includes informing the patient about medications. Your nursing knowledge reminds you to check the dose with Dr. Med because
    A. You are not sure if the Dr. wrote Clozapine or Clonazepam.
    B. Pha is of a cultural group that may require a lower than normal dose of medication.
    C. Pha is of a cultural group that may require a higher than normal dose of medication.
    D. Both A and B

13. Seeing the face of a famous performer in the coffee cup after pouring cream into it is an example of: _____

    _____

14. An individual stands on the train track with the train coming nearer. The person exclaims, "I am invincible! The train will not hurt me" is an example of: _____

    _____

Organic Mental Disorders (Delirium and Dementia)

Learning Objectives ▪ ▪ ▪

1. Define delirium.

2. Define dementia.

3. Identify characteristics of delirium.

4. Identify characteristics of dementia.

5. Identify medical treatments for patients with organic mental disorders.

6. Identify nursing interventions for patients with organic mental disorders.

Key Terms ▪ ▪ ▪

- ▪ Cognitive
- ▪ Delirium
- ▪ Dementia
- ▪ Organic

This chapter discusses two types of **cognitive** disorders called **delirium** and **dementia.** *Cognitive* means pertaining to thinking and the thought processes. These disorders either temporarily or permanently affect the patient's ability to think, remember, and make sound judgments.

Delirium and dementia are considered **organic**—that is, there is a known or presumed underlying cause. There are many potential causes, however. This category of disorders may be confusing to nursing students, because the *Diagnostic and Statistical Manual of Mental Disorders-IV (DSM-IV)* has divided organic illness into organic mental syndromes and organic mental disorders.

Many different kinds of organic mental *disorders* exist, including primary degenerative dementia of Alzheimer type, vascular dementia, also known as multi-infarct dementia (series of several small strokes or transient ischemic attacks), and drug-induced organic mental disorders. Vascular dementia is irreversible and requires other criteria such as hypertension and enlarged heart in order to make positive diagnosis. One cerebrovascular accident (stroke) does not generally earn a diagnosis of vascular or multi-infarct dementia.

Organic mental *syndromes* are further classified as acute or chronic. Acute organic mental syndromes are temporary, manifest quickly, and can affect any age group. They interfere with affect, memory, intelligence, and ability to make appropriate judgments. There are physical symptoms in some situations, which are related to the cause of the syndrome. Acute organic mental syndromes are generally reversible: patients usually get better.

Chronic organic mental syndromes are irreversible: patients are not going to get better. Onset is *insidious* (gradual, subtle, cumulative) and is seen typically in persons between the ages of 40 and 70. Symptoms include slurred speech or other speech difficulties, confusion, memory loss, and changes in affect and ability to make appropriate judgments. In addition to these symptoms, which seem similar to the acute form of this syndrome, the patient will display emotional symptoms of irritability, anger, depression, temper outbursts, and other behaviors that may have been uncharacteristic for the patient. Physical symptoms exist, which, again, are related to the underlying cause. Patients with chronic organic mental syndromes will continue to show decline in physical and intellectual ability.

It is very difficult to differentiate between acute and chronic organic mental syndromes at their onset. Time and the astute observation and documentation of the nurse caring for the patient are among the best sources of information about the type of mental problems the patient is experiencing.

Delirium and dementia are classified as organic mental syndromes, but Alzheimer's disease, which is primary degenerative dementia, is included with the organic mental disorders.

Dementia is a chronic, progressive deterioration of the brain usually characterized by severe memory loss, disorientation, and impairments associated with attention, judgment, and inability to take in and use new information. The symptoms are severe enough to interfere with the patient's activities of daily living (ADLs). Dementia is not a part of normal aging. It involves physical changes in the brain and damage at the cellular level that are usually irreversible.

Delirium is an acute condition; it develops quickly, often in response to prescription medications, alcohol, exposure to some toxic environmental substance, fever, or systemic illness. People in a state of delirium may feel frightened, anxious, and confused, and they may also experience hallucinations.

■ ETIOLOGIC THEORIES

Psychoanalytic theories about potential causes of organic mental disorders include effects of fear, depression, or anxiety; however, the various biologic theories have more research to support the validity of a nonpsychological cause.

Biologically, dementia can mimic treatable conditions, such as drug toxicity, depression, electrolyte imbalance, and nutritional complications. Biologic causes may also relate to aging, severe alterations in temperature (hypothermia or hyperthermia), systemic illness, physical trauma (anoxia), or chemical trauma (carbon monoxide poisoning, drug or alcohol overuse), which affects the brain.

■ DIFFERENTIAL DIAGNOSIS

Other medical or metabolic conditions have symptoms similar to those of delirium and dementia. It is important for physicians to work at ruling out other etiologies for the symptoms being observed and experienced. Graves' disease (hyperthyroidism), myxedema (hypothyroidism), Huntington's disease, and diabetes mellitus are some of the metabolic illnesses that may cause patients to exhibit behaviors that may be mistaken for delirium or dementia. Arteriosclerosis, which is a narrowing of the arteries to the brain, causes a decreased supply of oxygen to the brain. Lack of oxygen can lead to a patient's confusion. Systemic infections, nutritional abnormalities, and electrolyte imbalances are also capable of producing dementia-like symptoms in people. A complete physical examination and patient history are crucial to rule out some of these medical or metabolic disorders and assign the patient a true diagnosis of an organic mental disorder.

■ TYPES

DELIRIUM CAUSED BY A MEDICAL CONDITION

You may encounter a number of patients on your medical or surgical unit who suffer some symptoms of delirium. Anesthesia, medications, pain, or just unfamiliar surroundings may be enough to cause this temporary situation. This type of delirium may affect any age group, but it is sometimes more difficult for the very young or the older adult to recover from the disorientation.

Patients who are experiencing delirium may show any of the following symptoms:

- "Fogging" of consciousness (sometimes called mental "sluggishness")
- Incoherent or slurred speech
- Perceptual disturbances
- Sleep-cycle disturbances (this may be related to a person's normal routine, so be sure to find out if this is someone who works nights and sleeps days)
- Either an increase or a decrease in psychomotor activity
- Disorientation
- Memory impairment
- Symptoms that develop within a span of several hours to 2 days and then fluctuate in intensity during the day

ALZHEIMER'S DISEASE

Alzheimer's is one of a group of dementia disorders called "organic brain disorders." The symptoms were first noted in 1906 by Alois Alzheimer (Fig. 15-1). The American Psychiatric Association (APA) says these seem to be caused or in some way associated with impairment of brain tissue function. It is progressive and irreversible; in other words, it only worsens with time and at this point is not curable. Onset is usually in the 30s or 40s. The significant symptoms, which leave people incapable of caring for themselves, do not usually appear until approximately age 65, or 10 to 20 years after onset. It may start as a simple matter and then progress (e.g., forgetting where the car keys were placed in the house—who among us has not had that experience?). Gradually, these episodes become more frequent and involve more significant situations (e.g., going for a walk and forgetting how to get home, making decisions that are out of character for the individual, such as a wild spending spree).

The world watched as former President Ronald Reagan progressed through Alzheimer's-type dementia (Fig. 15-2). Many

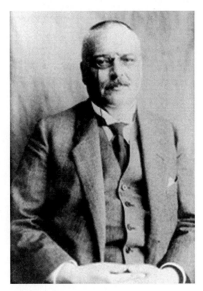

FIGURE 15-1. Alois Alzheimer (1864–1915) was a German neurologist who first identified Alzheimer's disease in 1906. (Courtesy of Wikipedia.org.)

are using the term "the long goodbye." Some excellent information is available about dementia of the Alzheimer's type. Researchers know that there are physical changes in the sulci (peaks and valleys) in the structure of the brain. Two main changes are seen in the plaques (chemical deposits made of degenerating nerve cells and a protein called "beta amyloid") and "tangles" (malformed nerve cells). All patients with Alzheimer's-type dementia show these changes, which can be observed only on autopsy (Alzheimers Disease Education and Referral Center, http://www.alzheimers.org/diagnosis.htm). Autopsy is currently the only method for positive diagnosis of the illness (Fig. 15-3).

The neurochemical acetylcholine also has an impact on the development of Alzheimer's-type dementia. There are also genetic markers on chromosomes 14, 19, and 21 that point to a potential for a higher incidence of Alzheimer's dementia in certain families.

Scanning techniques are also used to diagnose Alzheimer's-type dementia. Com-

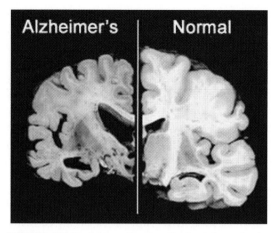

FIGURE 15-3. Autopsy is currently the only method for positive diagnosis of Alzheimer's disease. Note the atrophy of the brain caused by the disorder. (Courtesy of Neuropathology Program Service, Yale University School of Medicine, New Haven, CT.)

puterized axial tomography (CAT) scan, positron emission tomography (PET) scan, and magnetic resonance imaging (MRI) are all being used to gain information about the physical and chemical changes taking place in the brains of people who develop Alzheimer's dementia. These scans seem to be most helpful in the later stages of the disease, but as technology improves, it is expected that the scans will be helpful in identifying the earlier symptoms and diagnosing the illness as well.

The work of finding causes for dementia of the Alzheimer's type and ways to diagnose and treat it continue. Stem cell research is a hotly debated topic, but many researchers believe gains in diagnosing and treatment for Alzheimer's and other conditions may lie in stem cell research. Dietary factors continue to be considered as contributory in some way. In September of 2004, information was published indicating that researchers at Columbia University identified a component in triglycerides that increases the amount of beta-amyloid, which is thought to be a possible risk factor for acquiring Alzheimer's-type dementia. The industry is working continuously to unlock the mysteries surrounding this type of dementia.

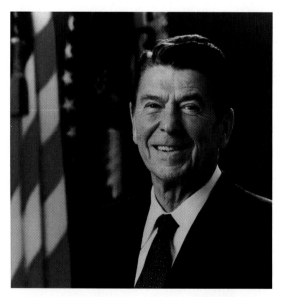

FIGURE 15-2. The world watched sadly as President Ronald Reagan passed through the stages of Alzheimer's disease before his death in 2004. According to a 2003 study by Hebert and others, the number of Americans with Alzheimer's disease has more than doubled since President Reagan was first elected in 1980.

Approximately 1 in 10 people over the age of 65 have Alzheimer's. The number of people with the disease doubles every 5 years beyond age 65. Age is identified as the most important known risk factor for Alzheimer's disease. Family history and genetics are also strong contributors to the illness.

Alzheimer's disease is frightening for the patients because of the realization that their memory is "slipping." Patients may make comments like "I'm just not as good as I used to be" or "I'm not myself" but cannot give specific information to support those feelings. Usually, the memory problems are more frequently associated with short-term memory. People might remember what happened 40 years ago, but they can't remember what they did 5 hours ago. In fact, when making the mental health assessment on this person, the nurse might find that the patient states, "It's 1950," when asked the year, which is actually 2001. It can be very unsettling for the individual to realize that he or she is not in complete control and yet not know why or how to fix it. These first symptoms are usually not severe enough to warrant seeing a physician. Patients often state, "They would just tell me I'm imagining it." This kind of statement is discouraging to patients because they know they are not imagining it. They are undergoing a change that maybe only they are aware of at this point.

Alzheimer's disease has four stages of progression. Table 15-1 gives some of the

TABLE 15-1	*Stages and Symptoms of Alzheimer's-Type Dementia*
STAGE	**SYMPTOMS**
First	■ Slight memory loss. ■ May wander and become lost. ■ Disoriented to time and place.
Second	■ Memory loss worsens. ■ Loses ability to make sound judgments or define simple proverbs such as "a stitch in time saves nine"—the person will give a very literal translation rather than understand the underlying message of such proverbs. ■ Neglects personal hygiene, grooming, and health. ■ May show antisocial behavior.
Third	■ "Forgetting" worsens. ■ May not be able to identify own name or recognize family and close friends. ■ May display inappropriate behaviors such as screaming. ■ May start to lose control of bowel and bladder. ■ May become unsteady walking.
Fourth	■ Unable to care for self. ■ Unable to walk well, if at all. ■ Incoherent. ■ Totally incontinent. ■ May have seizures.

Adapted with permission from Kalman, N (1993). *Mental Health Concepts*, 3rd ed. Albany, NY: Delmar Publishers, Copyright 1993.

signs and symptoms typically associated with each stage.

At this time there is no cure for Alzheimer's disease. Patients are susceptible to other diseases and infections as a result of decreased activity and diminished nutritional status. This is one reason why this disease is classified as a delirium *and* a dementia. The irreversible part of Alzheimer's disease is the dementia, which will not improve. Delirium that may result from infections or improper self-care may add to the illness. The delirium will disappear when the infection or nutritional deficit is under control. As the disease progresses, however, it will be increasingly more difficult to differentiate between the two syndromes.

■ DEMENTIA CAUSED BY HUMAN IMMUNODEFICIENCY VIRUS

Human immunodeficiency virus (HIV) is the virus that leads to the development of acquired immunodeficiency syndrome (AIDS). Neither of these conditions is a mental illness; they are both physical illnesses. AIDS, however, in its advanced stages, does present symptoms that require mental health knowledge.

AIDS is fatal. People live with the illness for varying amounts of time and in varying qualities of life. Medications are effective in many patients to control symptoms; they do not cure the illness.

Realizing that one has acquired an illness from which one cannot recover can lead to feelings of depression, anger, and frustration. Patients frequently receive antidepressants and other psychoactive medications to help with these feelings.

There are physical complications as well. Patients lose weight, in spite of eating voraciously. As time passes, other complications take over and the patient's appetite wanes. Patients become nauseous and have frequent emesis. Antiemetics such as prochlor-

perazine (Compazine), which is also an antipsychotic, are frequently required to control the nausea and emesis.

Opportunistic infections (infections that take advantage of an immunocompromised body) are frequent invaders of people with HIV/AIDS. Complications of these infections can cause delirium in persons with AIDS, just as they can in any other person.

As the nervous system becomes involved, people with AIDS may develop a neuropathy similar to the type seen in patients with diabetes mellitus. Some relief can be obtained in how one feels and functions through the use of medications such as amitriptyline (Elavil).

Knowledge of the psychotropic medication classifications is very important when working with patients with AIDS. However, nurses must also be aware that, as the disease advances, patients will exhibit many of the same symptoms and behaviors as patients with diseases that are organic mental disorders. Among these behaviors are forms of delirium (hallucinations, confusion, forgetting names of people close to them, and so on) and forms of dementia (forgetting common information, inability to answer questions or process information, and inability to care for personal needs). At this point in the illness, it is not important that AIDS is a medical illness as opposed to a mental illness; it is important that the nurse understand that the symptoms and behaviors are exactly the same as those of patients who have Alzheimer's dementia. The safety and mental well-being of the person who is ill is the major concern. The medical and nursing interventions are consistent with those for any patient who is diagnosed with an organic mental disorder.

■ DEMENTIA CAUSED BY HEAD INJURY

Head injuries, too, are medical disorders in which patients display many symptoms and behaviors associated with organic mental disorders.

Head injuries cause trauma to the brain that is sometimes reversible and sometimes irreversible. The patient who has sustained a head injury, then, may display signs of delirium or dementia, or both.

■ MEDICAL TREATMENT OF PATIENTS WITH DELIRIUM OR DEMENTIA

Finding the cause of the delirium and dementia is a key to finding the cure. If medication is suspected as the cause, stopping or changing the medication in question or administering an antipsychotic medication such as haloperidol (Haldol) may be helpful. Generally, the risk of the medication side effects is a deterrent to medicating for a short-term condition. Medications currently approved for treating Alzheimer's-type dementia include donepezil (Aricept), galantamine (Reminyl), and rivastigmine (Exelon). Their action is to raise acetylcholine levels in the brain. Since some of the symptoms and behaviors of Alzheimer's dementia are believed to be caused by a decrease of acetylcholine, these medications relieve some of the symptoms of Alzheimer's dementia in some patients. However, there is no proof at present that the drug actually reverses the progression of the dementia.

Aricept seems to be the early favorite among these new medications. Side effects include but are not limited to bradycardia, headache, depression, dizziness, drowsiness, insomnia, fatigue, syncope, hypertension, hypotension, vasodilation, diarrhea, nausea, anorexia, vomiting, ecchymoses, weight loss, arthritis, and muscle cramps.

Recently (October 2004), information began appearing from several sources indicating that the classification of medications known as ACE inhibitors (enalapril, captopril, etc.) are able to cross the blood-brain barrier and may be able to slow the progression of Alzheimer's-type dementia.

Nurses should monitor vital signs, especially heart rate, and should monitor memory, attention, reasoning, language, and ability to perform simple tasks periodically for as long as the patient remains on this medication.

Studies have been done to assess the effectiveness of estrogen therapy on women with Alzheimer's. To date, there is no proof that estrogen improves the symptoms of Alzheimer's disease. Studies continue to look at the possibility of delaying or preventing the onset of Alzheimer's if the treatment is started early. There is no evidence at this time that estrogen can affect the onset of Alzheimer's.

Also being studied are various nutritional or supplemental modalities. Studies currently are looking at the omega-3 fatty acids—found in fish and nuts—as nutrients possibly affecting the rate at which Alzheimer's progresses. Early studies are indicating a significant decrease (up to 60% in some studies) in males and females who eat fish at least once weekly. It is believed the omega-3 fatty acids have positive effects on protein building and on the coronary vessels as well as keeping the mind sharp. While this is certainly hopeful research being conducted worldwide, there is no definitive proof that this or any other food group can actually prevent Alzheimer's. To date, there is no absolute prevention and no cure.

Restraints for the safety of the patient may be required for the more active phases of either delirium or dementia. Restraints have become controversial in some areas due to the potential for injury to the patient. Nurses must know the state law and facility policy for use of physical or chemical restraints. Physicians or nurse practitioners will order the type of restraint and give the reason for the restraint.

Patients with dementia are followed closely, and treatment regimens change with the patient's condition. Treatment includes diet, medication, and ancillary therapies such as occupational therapy, physical therapy, and reality orientation.

■ ALTERNATIVE TREATMENT FOR PATIENTS WITH DELIRIUM OR DEMENTIA

NUTRITIONAL AND HERBAL SUPPLEMENTS (ESPECIALLY IN EARLY STAGES)

The use of nutritional and herbal supplements in treating delirium and dementia is controversial, although good nutrition is important for all people. In Alzheimer's-type dementia, there is some belief that supplementing with B-complex vitamins, elements such as zinc and selenium, and certain fatty acids may subdue the effects of memory loss for a time.

AROMATHERAPY

Essential oils such as rose or eucalyptus, or comfort smells such as bread or chocolate chip cookies baking may bring memories and comfort to patients with dementia. At some level of awareness, they may experience some peace and decreased anxiety.

■ NURSING CARE FOR PATIENTS WITH DELIRIUM OR DEMENTIA

1. *Data Collection:* Collect information on vital signs, medications used by the patient, circumstances immediately preceding symptoms, and any other information the patient or person who may be accompanying the individual can provide. Note also anything that is considered to be a change in the patient's condition.
2. *Stay calm:* Be ready for anything.

Patients with symptoms of delirium and/or dementia can be very changeable. No matter what the situation, nurses must diffuse the situation calmly, calm the people involved, and return the situation to safety. It is very important to make every attempt to maintain the patient's dignity during periods of excitability.

3. *Do not argue:* Patients with dementia and/or delirium have cognitive impairment. They do not have the capacity to make rational decisions during the delirium. Attempting to model the desired behavior or simply waiting a few minutes and attempting the verbal instruction again may prove to be successful techniques.
4. *Use clear, simple verbal communication:* Sensory overload is very possible for patients experiencing delirium and dementia. To avoid a behavioral "short circuit," it is a good idea to use simple communication and activity in the room. Keep the area quiet. Keep curtains drawn or partially open; keep televisions and radios off or at a very low volume. The stimulation can be adjusted according to the patient's tolerance.
5. *Allow time for patient to respond:* The ability to function cognitively and physically is diminished when a person is in delirium or dementia. Nurses and other health-care workers must remember to plan to allow more time for performing care. Patients suffering from delirium will eventually return to normal response times; those with dementia will continue to deteriorate.
6. *Use touch when appropriate:* It is impossible not to touch this group of patients. Nurses need to direct and assist with cares for people who are experiencing delirium and dementia. There is a danger for misinterpretation of that touch, however. People who have a threat to their ability to

process and understand information may not remember the situation as it actually happened. They may have forgotten the episode of incontinence and not understand why "that nurse had to touch me there!" Having a second person—another nurse or a family member—in the room can be a helpful protection for both the nurse and the patient. Documenting all actions and patient responses very carefully is also necessary.

7. *Restraints:* Patients in a state of delirium or dementia may wander. This is a major safety risk that frequently encourages nurses to request restraint orders from the physician. When the physician has ordered restraints, either chemical or physical, the nursing responsibilities include careful observation and documentation. For physical restraints, each state has guidelines for how often to check, release, and reposition or exercise the patient. Assessing for signs of dermal ulcers and stiffness of muscles helps to maintain skin integrity and full range of motion. For chemical restraints, the nurse must document the effect of the medication and any possible side effects. Many medications have side effects such as confusion, restlessness, and forgetfulness and may be counterproductive for people with dementia. Medications should not be used as a substitute for appropriate activities, programming, and personal interaction.

8. *Assist with ADLs as appropriate to the situation:* The nurse will be doing as much for the patient physically as the individual condition requires. For temporary delirium and early stages of dementia, the nurse may have to give only some verbal cues as to what the patient needs to do. For deeper delirium and later stages of dementia, performing total cares for the patient

may be necessary. Always maintain the patient's dignity and allow him or her to do as much independently as able.

9. *Provide adequate stimulation:* It is as detrimental to under-stimulate people with organic mental disorders as it is to overload them. The brain needs some encouragement to activate. Just as nursing students may need something to get brains firing again after a week of final exams, patients with delirium or dementia need some sort of stimulation to maximize their mental capabilities. This will be a "trial-and-error" situation between the nurse and the patient, and it will be different for every patient. Some success has been made with music or play therapy.

10. *Maintain appropriate milieu:* People living with irreversible, progressive dementia require special attention to the milieu. Acceptance is mandatory. Nurses should not emphasize "reality orientation." Changes in the brain will not allow the memory to function successfully and may, in fact, cause the patient to experience frustration, agitation, and increase acting-out behaviors if "reality orientation" is used. Color of the room, unit, or home should also be considered. For example, blue carpets may remind the person of water. Mirrors give the illusion of "other people" in the room. A patient with Alzheimer's-type dementia could react with fear, confusion, or any number of responses. Noise is also a factor. When possible, radios, televisions, and overhead pagers should be kept off or at a minimum.

Table 15-2 summarizes the symptoms and nursing interventions for the disorders of delirium and dementia discussed previously.

TABLE 15-2 ■ *Delirium and Dementia*		
TYPE	**SYMPTOMS**	**NURSING INTERVENTIONS**
DELIRIUM	■ "Fogging" of consciousness— incoherent or slurred speech ■ Perceptual disturbances ■ Sleep cycle disturbances ■ Increase or decrease in psychomotor activity ■ Disorientation ■ Memory impairment ■ Symptoms that develop within a span of several hours to 2 days and then fluctuate in intensity during the day	■ Stay calm. ■ Do not argue. ■ Use clear, simple verbal communication. ■ Allow time for patient to respond. ■ Use therapeutic touch when appropriate. ■ Use restraints for safety (with physician orders when required). ■ Assist with ADLs as appropriate. ■ Provide adequate and appropriate sensory stimulation.
HIV-RELATED DEMENTIA	■ Feelings of depression, anger, and frustration ■ Forms of delirium (hallucinations, confusion, forgetting names of people close to them, and so on) ■ Forms of dementia (forgetting common information, inability to answer questions or process information, and inability to care for personal needs)	■ See "Delirium" and "Alzheimer's-Type Dementia."
DEMENTIA RELATED TO HEAD INJURY	■ Trauma to the brain, which is sometimes reversible and sometimes irreversible ■ May display signs of delirium or dementia, or both	■ Teach patient to keep written lists (e.g., "to do," when to take medications) if patient is able. ■ See "Delirium" and "Alzheimer's-Type Dementia."
ALZHEIMER'S-TYPE DEMENTIA (ORGANIC MENTAL DISORDER)	■ Has memory loss that starts as slight and gradually worsens. ■ May wander and get lost. ■ Disoriented to time and place. ■ Loses ability to make sound judgments. ■ Neglects personal hygiene, grooming, and health. ■ May show antisocial behavior. ■ "Forgetting" worsens. ■ Has inability to identify own name or recognize family, friends.	■ Allow the patient as much independence as possible. ■ Address the patient by his or her given name (use of "nicknames" is discouraged). ■ Maintain a milieu of acceptance. ■ Allow patient to have as many personal, familiar items as possible. ■ DO NOT use reality orientation. ■ Lower stimulation (e.g., minimize noise from radios, paging, etc.). ■ Consider changing room or unit color if able.

(continued)

TYPE	SYMPTOMS	NURSING INTERVENTIONS
ALZHEIMER'S-TYPE DEMENTIA (ORGANIC MENTAL DISORDER) *(cont'd)*	■ Exhibits inappropriate behaviors (screaming). ■ Loses control of bowel and bladder. ■ Exhibits unsteady walking that gradually worsens. ■ Is unable to care for self. ■ Is incoherent. ■ May have seizures.	■ Remove mirrors as able. ■ All nursing interventions as listed with "Delirium." (Note: appropriateness of stimulation in "Dementia" is different from appropriate stimulation in "Delirium.") ■ Behaviors such as wandering may respond to environmental cues such as locks or signs such as "STOP" or "NO."

Key Concepts ■ ■ ■

1. Organic mental disorders are complex alterations to mental integrity. Dementia and delirium are the two most frequently occurring forms of organic mental disorders.
2. Delirium is usually reversible; dementia is usually irreversible.
3. Nursing care involves safety, honesty, and patience. Medical and nursing interventions are specific to the patient.
4. HIV/AIDS, head injuries, stroke, and other medical conditions are not mental health issues. The behaviors of delirium and dementia that may be a result of these medical illnesses require knowledge of mental health principles.
5. Medications often have side effects of confusion and should be chosen carefully in people with dementia. Medications are chosen to treat specific behaviors; they are not a substitute for more direct interventions.

COMMONLY USED MEDICATIONS ■ *Organic Mental Disorders*

Buspirone (BuSpar)	**Trazodone** (Desyrel)
Doxepin (Sinequan)	**Thioridazine** (Mellaril)
Haloperidol (Haldol)	**Diphenhydramine** (Benadryl)
Tacrine hydrochloride (Cognex)	**Temazepam** (Restoril)

REFERENCES

Bilanow, T. (reviewed by Samuel E. Gandy, MD, PhD, Chair of the Scientific Advisory Board) *Fish and Nuts May Ward Off Alzheimer's.* Fisher Center for Alzheimer's Research Foundation. www.alzinfo.org. July 23, 2003; *Fish Oil Shows Promise in Alzheimer's Fight.* March 28, 2005.

Boggs, W. (November 2004). Brain-penetrating ace inhibitors slow alzheimer's. *Neurology Online.* http://www.neurology.org. (Copyright 2004 by AAN Enterprises, Inc./Lippincott Williams & Wilkins, 351 West Camden Street, Baltimore).

Hebert, L.E., Scherr, P.A., Bienias, J.L., Bennett, D.A., and Evans, D.A. (2003). Alzheimer Disease in the U.S. Population: Prevalence Estimates Using the 2000 Census. *Archives of Neurology, 60*(8), 1119–1122.

Rubin, Z., Peplau, L., and Salovey, P. (1993). *Psychology.* Houghton-Mifflin, Boston.

WEBSITES

www.alzheimers.org
www.alz.org
http://www.neurology.org
www.stroke-site.org
www.strokefoundation.com

CRITICAL THINKING EXERCISES ■ ■ ■

1. Uncle J is 65 years old. He has been picked up by the local law enforcement, who found him wandering along the main thoroughfare in your city. He is combative and keeps calling you by his wife's name. Three hours later, Uncle J is reoriented to person, place, and time. What will you do for Uncle J? Develop a plan of care for Uncle J. What assessments will you make with Uncle J?

2. Using the suggested nursing diagnoses listed here (or others you can think of), complete a nursing process for a patient with Alzheimer's-type dementia.

SUGGESTED NURSING DIAGNOSES

1. *Incontinence, Total*
2. *Social Interaction, Impaired*
3. *Thought Processes, Altered*
4. *Self-Care Deficit, Dressing/Grooming*

ASSESSMENT/ DATA COLLECTION	NURSING DIAGNOSIS	PLAN/ GOAL	INTERVENTIONS/ NURSING ACTIONS	EVALUATION CRITERIA

CASE STUDY: "CC" ■ ■ ■

CC is a 30-year-old female sales person for a pharmaceutical company. She was involved in a work-related motor vehicle accident and sustained a closed head injury. She is one year post accident and is having memory problems. Periodically, she attempts to return to work, but she is unable to stay focused on even the simplest of office tasks.

She has been evaluated by a psychologist. Her Wechsler-Adult scores are below normal for her age. She claims memory loss and does get lost driving at times. Today, she waited in the parking lot for nearly 2 hours for her appointment. She tearfully tells you she was afraid she would get lost and be late for her appointment. She is afraid her employer will not hold a job open for her much longer. She also shares that her partner of 5 years has left her because he felt CC was "faking" her memory loss, stating, "You can act normal when you want to!"

From just the information presented here and your knowledge of delirium and dementia, which would you choose for the diagnosis? Defend your diagnosis.

What can you say to provide help and encouragement to CC?

Using one of the following NANDA nursing diagnoses, or one of your choosing, develop a care plan for CC.

1. Memory

2. Adjustment

3. Role conflict

4. Intracranial adaptive capacity

TEST QUESTIONS ■ ■ ■

MULTIPLE CHOICE QUESTIONS

1. You are working the night shift in your surgical unit. Ms. Y, 1 day postoperative for total hip replacement, is taking several medications for pain, along with an antibiotic. She is 70 years old and presented as alert and oriented prior to surgery. She lives independently. Ms. Y suddenly begins screaming and thrashing in bed, begging you to "Get the spiders out of my bed!" What is the best explanation for Ms. Y's behavior?

   A. Delusions
   B. Delirium
   C. Dementia
   D. Dilemma

2. The best nursing intervention for you, the LPN/LVN, to help Ms. Y is:

   A. Inform the charge nurse and doctor immediately.
   B. Turn on the light and ask her where the spiders are.
   C. Stop her pain medications.
   D. Check her medical record for a diagnosis of mental illness.

3. Mr. H has been admitted to your nursing home in third-stage Alzheimer's disease. Mrs. H is crying and says to you, "Nurse, when will he get better? I don't know what I will do without him home. Why can't the doctor fix him?" Your best response to Mrs. H is:

   A. "Don't worry, Mrs. H. Everything will be fine."
   B. "Relax and enjoy yourself, Mrs. H. You should go out to lunch with your friends and forget about this for a while!"
   C. "Why are you afraid to be home alone, Mrs. H?"
   D. "Mrs. H, your doctor has explained that Mr. H will not get better. How can I help you plan for your future?"

4. Aricept is a medication approved for the treatment of symptoms of Alzheimer's-type dementia. Nurses must be alert to which of the following side effects?

   A. Tachycardia
   B. Bradycardia
   C. Mania
   D. Weight gain

5. Which statement is *not* true about Alzheimer's disease?

   A. It is a dementia disorder.
   B. It may occur in middle to late life.
   C. It is a chronic disease.
   D. It is caused by aging and hardening of the arteries.

6. Which of the following would you expect to see in a patient who is diagnosed with an organic mental disorder?

   A. Intact memory
   B. Appropriate behavior
   C. Disorganization of thought
   D. Orientation to person, place, and time

7. Ms. P has been admitted to your unit with a diagnosis of right tibial fracture. Her emergency department notes say that she fell at home. She admits to having "a lot to drink" over the past week. She is disoriented to time, forgets where she is momentarily, is easily distracted, and has a short attention span. She does not answer questions appropriately. She is probably experiencing:

   A. Delusions
   B. Delirium
   C. Dementia
   D. Dilemma

8. Your patient, who is recovering from an exacerbation of an AIDS-related infection, is opting to be treated by family and friends at home. The family has expressed concern because they sense a change in the patient's cognitive abilities. Part of the discharge teaching for this family might include:

   A. "It's nothing, really. Patients sometimes get confused in the hospital."
   B. "Keep an eye on him. You don't want him to start wandering."

    C. "You're concerned about the change in his ability to rememb things? Let me call the doctor for you. This is something that y need to discuss together."

    D. "I thought something was strange!"

9. Mr. Forgetful is brought in by a family member who expresses concern over Mr. Forgetful's memory loss. The physician diagnosed Mr. Forgetful with vascular dementia (multi-infarct dementia). You realize this disorder

    A. Is irreversible

    B. Requires other conditions to be present for positive diagnosis

    C. Indicates the patient has most likely experienced more than one CVA

    D. All of the above

10. Choose ALL effective communication skills or nursing actions for caring for the patient with dementia:

    1. Document all changes in the patient's condition.

    2. To patient with dementia: "Mr. X. Remember you need to please sit quietly. You are disrupting the others in this room."

    3. To patient with delirium: "Yes, Mrs. P. We did talk about mealtimes, and you are correct: they are at 7:30 AM, 12:00 noon, and 5:30 PM."

    4. Keep televisions and radios on whenever possible to encourage patient interaction.

    5. Allow more time for performing cares.

    6. Document all nursing actions and patient responses very carefully to avoid misinterpretation of cares.

    7. Physically restrain all patients with dementia for their safety.

    8. Maintain the patient's dignity and allow him or her to do as much independently as able.

    9. Provide adequate stimulation: it is as detrimental to under-stimulate people with organic mental disorders as it is to overload them.

    10. Emphasize "reality orientation."

16

Somatoform Disorders

Learning Objectives ■ ■ ■

1. Define somatoform.
2. Identify signs and symptoms of somatoform disorders.
3. Identify possible underlying causes of somatoform disorders.
4. Identify medical treatments for people with somatoform disorders.
5. Identify nursing interventions for people with somatoform disorders.

Key Terms ■ ■ ■

- Conversion
- Dysmorphophobia
- Hypochondriasis
- "La belle indifference"
- Malingering
- Primary gain
- Secondary gain
- Somatization
- Somatoform
- Somatoform pain disorder

Somat/o, you will recall from your medical terminology class, is the combining form for *body.* The **somatoform** disorders are conditions in which there are physical symptoms with no known organic cause. It is believed that the physical symptoms are connected to a psychological conflict. Because these patients cannot control their symptoms, the symptoms are considered to be caused by some unconscious mechanism.

■ ETIOLOGIC THEORIES

Psychoanalytic theorists believe that the somatoform disorders are rooted in unconscious mechanisms that develop to deny, repress, and displace anxiety. Ineffective personality development in childhood predisposes certain individuals to handle their anxiety ineffectively.

Biologically, research has been conducted concerning the possibility of a genetic predisposition to somatic difficulties. At this point, this research is not conclusive or widely distributed, however.

■ DIFFERENTIAL DIAGNOSIS

Pathology of this group of illnesses is symptomatic. The patient will unconsciously choose the dysfunction according to the root of the anxiety. The symptoms the patient develops will determine the diagnosis. Nurses must be alert to physical illness

257

that may actually be causing the symptoms. Multiple sclerosis, for example, can present with many and varied symptoms that may be as yet undiagnosed. Discuss with the patient's medical doctor all possibilities for physical illness rather than a somatoform disorder.

■ TYPES

There are actually five separate illnesses within the category of somatoform disorders. This text gives brief explanations of all five disorders.

CONVERSION DISORDER

Conversion reaction, as defined in the defense mechanisms (see Chapter 6), is converting anxiety into a physical symptom. Conversion disorder is the illness that emerges from overuse of this mechanism. In conversion disorder, there is a loss or decrease in physical functioning that seems to have a neurologic connection. Paralysis and blindness are two of the more common examples of this disorder. It is common for the dysfunction to somehow be deeply connected to denial and to a prior negatively perceived experience (e.g., someone who loses the sense of vision after watching a pornographic movie). Age of onset is usually adolescence and young adulthood, but it can occur later in life as well.

The symptoms, although not supportive of organic disease, are very real to the patient. It should not be conveyed to these patients that the nurse thinks they are "faking" the illness; they are not. Patients are truly experiencing the symptoms. Even though the patient is concerned enough about the symptoms to consult a physician, he or she gives the impression of really not caring about the problem. **"La belle indifference"** is the clinical term used to describe this condition.

The belief about this disorder is that the symptom, the paralysis or blindness, is allowing the person to avoid a situation that is unacceptable to him or her. This unacceptable situation is the source of extreme anxiety, which is converted into the dysfunction. The dysfunction, then, is relieving the anxiety. This is called **primary gain** and is believed to be the function of the paralysis or blindness. **Secondary gain** is the extra benefits one may acquire as a result of staying ill. Secondary gain includes extra emotional support such as sympathy and love or financial benefits.

Malingering is a situation for achieving personal gain that differs from the others mentioned. Malingering is a conscious effort to avoid unpleasant situations. The patient "fakes" or pretends to have the symptoms.

HYPOCHONDRIASIS

These people are sometimes referred to as "professional patients." The person with **hypochondriasis** is worried about getting "it"—whatever "it" is. They have an intense fear that they will become seriously ill. People who have hypochondriasis are preoccupied with the idea that they are seriously ill and cannot be helped. Patients may also be concerned that they are not taken seriously and therefore sense that physicians are not evaluating them properly. The term *hypochondriac* has become a negative, stereotypical word socially, but hypochondriasis is a recognized, official term and illness according to the *Diagnostic and Statistical Manual of Mental Disorders-IV-Text Revision (DSM-IV-TR)*.

A major difference between hypochondriasis and conversion disorder is that the person with conversion disorder focuses on the symptoms of the illness, and the person with hypochondriasis is afraid they will *get* a serious disease.

DYSMORPHOPHOBIA/BODY DYSMORPHIC DISORDER

In **dysmorphophobia** the onset is generally in the teens through the 30s. Symptoms, which may be present for many years, include excessive preoccupation with an imagined defect in one's physical appearance (usually facial) and obsessive and/or compulsive behaviors.

SOMATIZATION DISORDER

The onset of symptoms is usually observed at approximately age 30. The *DSM-IV-TR* lists 35 symptoms that may be present in **somatization** disorder. For a positive diagnosis of this disorder to be made, 13 of the 35 symptoms must be present. Some of the more frequently seen symptoms of somatization disorder include

- Free-floating anxiety
- Emotional turmoil expressed in physical symptoms, usually resulting in a loss of physical functioning
- Pain that changes location frequently
- Depression
- Suicidal ideation

Nurses must remember that these behaviors may look very purposeful, but the patient is not able to control them voluntarily. Patients with somatization disorder often have medically unnecessary surgery in an effort to remove any possible physiologic cause for the illness.

SOMATOFORM PAIN DISORDER

Somatoform pain disorder can manifest itself at any age but seems to occur most often in adolescence and early adulthood. It also tends to affect women more frequently than men. Theories are emerging to suggest that the reason for this is a hormonal interaction with neurochemicals, but this has not yet been proved.

This disorder requires very good data collection on the part of the nurse. There may, in some cases, be a physical finding, but the level of pain the patient states is inconsistent with the physical condition. Some of the symptoms of somatoform pain disorder include

- Psychalgia (emotional pain that manifests as physical pain) as the main concern of the patient

- Pain that is usually not consistent with expected neural pathways
- Pain that does not change location, as in somatization disorder

Because symptoms may be very subtle, communication and documentation skills are very important. Nurses need to ask themselves questions as they take the history of patients with somatoform pain disorder, for example, "Is this person's pain related to some physical finding?" "Does the severity of pain expressed by the patient correspond with the physical findings?" and "What evidence is there for psychological etiology in this patient's pain?"

■ MEDICAL TREATMENT FOR PATIENTS WITH SOMATOFORM DISORDERS

Hospitalized patients are usually admitted to a medical unit rather than a psychiatric unit. Treatment focuses on the symptoms, which more than likely are medical in nature. The patient does not generally display unusual or unmanageable behavior that indicates the need for mental health unit admission. Patients with somatoform diagnoses are more frequently seen in medical-surgical hospital units or the medical clinic.

Treatment is, of course, individualized for each patient. Hypnosis and relaxation techniques are used with many patients. It is beneficial for the therapist to help the patient express the underlying cause of the anxiety; hypnosis can be very effective in making this determination.

Methods of stress management are also taught. Patients may resist accepting that their problem is psychological or emotional and therefore cannot understand how a paralyzed limb or blindness has anything to do with anxiety. People who have a somatoform disorder may feel insulted, become resistive to treatment, and search for other ways to explain the physical problem.

Behavior modification therapy may be effective for some patients. Because these are chronic disorders, treatment can take a long time, and some patients may become frustrated at the slowness of behavior modification. For those who are motivated and have strong support systems, however, behavior modification can be quite effective.

Medications are used sparingly because these patients typically have a history of overmedication. When medications are ordered for a patient, the classifications of choice are usually selected serotonin, selective serotonin reuptake inhibitors (SSRIs) (e.g., fluoxetine), or antidepressants, particularly the tricyclics such as Imipramine or antianxiety drugs, or both. At this time, if medications are considered, SSRIs are greatly preferred over the other classes of antidepressants and probably should be first-line agents.

■ ALTERNATIVE TREATMENTS FOR PATIENTS WITH SOMATOFORM DISORDERS

Alternative treatment of choice is related to the particular condition or symptom set. Choices may include the following treatments.

MASSAGE

Massage therapies are believed to not only relieve tensions and discomforts in the musculoskeletal system, but also may assist with blood and lymph flow. It may be effective, especially with medication, to assist the patient to overcome physical symptoms. Caution should be used, however, not to actually emphasize the body complaint and reinforce the illness.

HERBAL/NUTRITIONAL SUPPLEMENTS

It is possible that a patient is experiencing a nutritional deficiency or possibly a condition such as arthritis along with the somatoform disorder. Herbs or supplements geared to the specific pain issue may help the patient to experience less pain, either physically or psychologically.

■ NURSING MANAGEMENT FOR PATIENTS WITH SOMATOFORM DISORDERS

COMMUNICATION SKILLS

Honesty in dealing with the patient is very important. Gaining trust that will encourage the patient to verbalize thoughts and feelings about the physical and emotional aspects of this type of disorder is crucial. Do not discount the patient's disorder. An example of a way to be honest about the situation follows.

EXAMPLE

> Nurse: "Ms. P, your physician can find no physical or life-threatening conditions at this time. We will continue to observe and examine you. We will make every attempt to help you improve."

In this way, the patient understands that nothing is showing up in the tests that have been made to this point. The person hears that nothing life-threatening is causing the symptoms. You have said that the staff is attempting to help the person, but you have stopped short of promising improvement or of "curing" the patient.

THERAPY

Keeping the patient focused on other topics may help in the recovery. Nurses will involve the patient in the goal setting and interventions of the care plan. Aiding the patient in learning assertive communication skills can be helpful. Working with other health-care staff in occupational therapy, recreational therapy, and social activities can also act as a diversion to focus away from the dysfunction.

SUPPORT

It is important for the nurse caring for patients with somatoform disorders to remember to pay attention to the person but not to reinforce the symptom. Always make a thorough head-to-toe assessment. This shows patients you are concerned for their health but you will not be focusing on the area of dysfunction or reinforcing the problem. Document all findings in a matter-of-fact way. Patients need to know that they are being taken seriously, even though they may not agree with the medical findings of their illness.

Table 16-1 summarizes the symptoms and nursing interventions for the somatoform disorders discussed previously.

TABLE 16-1 ■ *Somatoform Disorders*		
TYPE	**SYMPTOMS**	**NURSING INTERVENTIONS**
CONVERSION DISORDER	■ Loss or decrease in physical functioning that seems to have a neurologic connection (paralysis, blindness) ■ Indifference to the loss of function ■ Primary and secondary gain	■ Use therapeutic communication skills. ■ Encourage therapy (occupational therapy, physical therapy, etc.) ■ Provide emotional support.
HYPOCHON-DRIASIS	■ "Professional patient" ■ Intense fear of becoming seriously ill ■ Preoccupation with the idea of being seriously ill and not being helped—may be concerned about not being taken seriously or evaluated properly	■ Do not reinforce the symptom. ■ Be nonjudgmental.
DYSMORPHO-PHOBIA/BODY DYSMORPHIC DISORDER	■ Onset is usually teens through 30s ■ Excessive preoccupation with an imagined defect in appearance (usually facial) ■ Obsessive and/or compulsive behaviors ■ Symptoms possibly present for several years	■ Take information in a matter-of-fact way. ■ Report all findings to the physician.
SOMATIZATION DISORDER	■ Onset of symptoms is usually observed at approximately age 30 ■ *DSM-IV-TR* lists 35 symptoms that may be present including: 1. Free-floating anxiety 2. Emotional turmoil expressed in physical symptoms 3. Pain changing location frequently 4. Depression and suicidal ideation	■ Treat symptoms. ■ Assess for underlying causes. ■ Maintain effective communication.

(continued)

TABLE 16-1 ■ *Somatoform Disorders (Continued)*		
TYPE	**SYMPTOMS**	**NURSING INTERVENTIONS**
SOMATOFORM PAIN DISORDER	■ Manifests at any age, but most often in adolescence and early adulthood ■ Tends to affect women more frequently than men ■ Psychalgia (emotional pain that manifests as physical pain) the main concern ■ Pain usually not consistent with expected neural pathways ■ Pain location unchanging	

Key Concepts ■ ■ ■

1. Somatoform disorders are conditions that present as chronic, physical dysfunctions that may include paralysis and blindness, among other dysfunctions. These body-related symptoms seem to be a result of a deeply rooted anxiety.
2. Somatoform disorders usually begin in adolescence and young adulthood.
3. Treatment and nursing care for patients with somatoform disorders may be difficult and long term, as these are chronic disorders. Patients use the defense mechanisms of denial and conversion reaction.

COMMONLY USED MEDICATIONS ■ *Somatoform Disorders*

Medications are ordered judiciously for these disorders. When a medication is used, it is generally an antidepressant or an antianxiety agent.

Amitriptyline (Elavil)	**Paroxetine** (Paxil)
Bupropion (Wellbutrin)	**Sertraline** (Zoloft)
Doxepin (Sinequan)	**Trazodone** (Desyrel)
Fluoxetine (Prozac)	

REFERENCES

American Psychiatric Association. (2000). *Diagnostic and Statistical Manual of Mental Disorders—Text Revision*, 4th ed. Author, Washington, DC.

Anderson, R.A. (2001). *Clinician's Guide to Holistic Medicine*. McGraw-Hill Publishing, New York.

(1999). *The Merck Manual*, 17th ed. Merck And Company, West Point, PA., Mark H. and Robert Berkow, M.D., eds.

Sierpina, V.S. (2001). *Integrative Health Care— Complementary and Alternative Therapies for the Whole Person.* F.A. Davis Company, Philadelphia.

WEBSITES

www.medicine.com
www.psyweb.com

CRITICAL THINKING EXERCISES ■ ■ ■

1. Penny is a 35-year-old married mother of three children, ages 2 years, 3 years, and 4 months. She works as a clerk in a large office. She has been visiting the clinic regularly since her last pregnancy. She is experiencing severe, intermittent pain in her right arm and left foot. The pain does not interfere with her life as a wife and mother, and she is not able to detect any kind of pattern to the pain. She tells you that she is not especially concerned about the pain. "When it gets too bad for me, my husband cooks and cleans the kitchen."

   Penny says that she thinks the source of her pain is related to "the day I banged my right hip real hard on the door of the copy machine." She also has begun expressing concern that things are going so well for her that she "just has the feeling that something terrible is about to happen." What is your preliminary idea of Penny's illness? What other information might you want to obtain from Penny?

2. Using the suggested nursing diagnoses listed here (or others you can think of), complete a nursing process for Penny.

   SUGGESTED NURSING DIAGNOSES

   1. Anxiety
   2. Pain, Chronic
   3. Individual Coping, Ineffective

ASSESSMENT/ DATA COLLECTION	NURSING DIAGNOSIS	PLAN/ GOAL	INTERVENTIONS/ NURSING ACTIONS	EVALUATION CRITERIA

TEST QUESTIONS ■ ■ ■

MULTIPLE CHOICE QUESTIONS

1. Nurses working with patients who have somatoform illnesses understand that the symptoms will be primarily:
   A. Body related
   B. Memory related
   C. Emotion related
   D. Chemically related

2. Somatoform disorders are those with:
   A. Physical symptoms with organic causes
   B. Physical symptoms that are confirmed with MRI
   C. Physical symptoms and hallucinations
   D. Physical symptoms with no organic cause

3. Mr. Icantdoit has lost functional use of his right arm. There is no confirmation of organic illness. He seems willing to help himself, except for his inability to move that arm. He may be experiencing a:
   A. Catatonic disorder
   B. Conversion disorder
   C. Chemical disorder
   D. Compensation disorder

4. In planning nursing interventions for Mr. Icantdoit, nurses would:
   A. Encourage use of the right arm at least twice daily (focus on right arm).
   B. Allow patient to eat meals only if he uses his right arm.
   C. Include patient in activities that require use of both arms (such as swimming, volleyball, and so on).
   D. Encourage patient to verbalize feelings about inability to use right hand.

5. Ms. H has very suddenly lost sight in both eyes. She states she has had some headaches lately but rates them as a 2 on a scale of 1 to 5. She is on your unit for a neurologic workup to rule out tumor. She tells you that the blindness is the reason she went to the physician but then states, "I'm not all that worried. It will either go away or it won't. I'll get by." Her apparent lack of concern for her symptoms is called:
   A. Primary gain
   B. Ambivalence
   C. Anhedonia
   D. "La belle indifference"

6. According to somatoform disorder theory, the blindness is the behavior that is alleviating Ms. H's anxiety. The act that alleviates anxiety is called:
   A. Primary gain
   B. Secondary gain

   C. Manipulation
   D. Behavior modification

7. A major symptom of hypochondriasis is:

   A. Pain that changes locations
   B. Belief that an illness exists for which the patient cannot be helped
   C. Anhedonia
   D. Blindness

8. The best nursing action for a patient with hypochondriasis is to:

   A. Assist the patient to focus on his or her abilities and strengths
   B. Provide reading material explaining why the patient is not ill
   C. Instruct the patient to go home, take the prescribed medications, and return to the clinic in one week if not better.
   D. Obtain an in-depth history of the patient's physical symptoms

9. The somatoform disorder that has the symptoms of psychalgia, pain that does not change location and that does not seem to follow the normal nerve pathways, is called: _____

   _____

10. The somatoform disorder that has the symptoms of free-floating anxiety and pain that changes location frequently is called: _____

   _____

17

Substance-Related Disorders

Learning Objectives ▪ ▪ ▪

1. Define substance abuse.

2. Define substance dependence.

3. Define codependency.

4. Identify common medical treatments for abuse disorders.

5. Identify nursing interventions for patients with abuse disorders.

Key Terms ▪ ▪ ▪

- Addiction
- Alcohol abuse
- Alcohol dependence
- Codependency
- Dysfunctional
- Methamphetamine
- Psychoactive Drugs
- Substance abuse
- Substance dependence
- Tolerance
- Withdrawal

Psychoactive drugs are chemicals that alter mood perception, mental functioning, and/or behavior. They include narcotic analgesics, alcohol, sedative/hypnotics, stimulants, hallucinogens, and psychotropic agents. Most of these categories of substances can be and are used legally and therapeutically. They all have the strong potential to be abused and to become addictive.

Alcoholism and chemical dependency are serious conditions in American society (Tables 17-1 and 17-2). Substance abuse disorders are certainly not new; in Sigmund Freud's time, the social drug of choice was cocaine. Western European men sat around

and smoked cocaine then in much the same way that people sit and have a beer today. Were the men of the 1800s addicted?

In the 1960s, the era of the "hippies," "free love," and "flower power" (see Chapter 5), a Harvard psychologist, Timothy Leary, was part of a team of psychologists and psychiatrists who studied the effects of drugs on the human brain. Leary's claim to fame was studying the lysergic acid diethylamide (LSD) "trip." LSD has not gone away. It is available in the form of small, hard candy that comes on pieces of paper, as well as other forms, making it very appealing to children. Timothy Leary was a cultural leader of the time; he continued for

TABLE 17-1 Trends in Percentage of Full-Time Workers, Ages 18–49, Reporting Drug Use, by Industry Categories, 1985–1993

INDUSTRY CATEGORY	CURRENT ILLICIT DRUG USE						PAST YEAR ILLICIT DRUG USE						HEAVY ALCOHOL USE					
	1985	1988	1990	1991	1992	1993	1985	1988	1990	1991	1992	1993	1985	1988	1990	1991	1992	1993
TOTAL	16.7	9.9	8.2	7.5	7.0	7.3	26.3	19.5	18.5	15.3	14.3	15.3	9.7	7.0	7.5	7.4	6.8	7.4
AGRICULTURE, FORESTRY & FISHERIES	9.0	8.9	14.5	6.3	4.7	7.8	15.9	*	*	19.1	10.1	*	11.0	*	*	8.1	6.5	9.9
MINING	*	*	*	*	*	*	*	*	*	*	*	*	*	*	19.9	12.8	11.3	22.8
CONSTRUCTION	23.1	18.5	16.9	12.7	12.2	11.6	34.7	33.7	31.9	20.5	19.6	21.8	18.4	20.7	21.5	15.2	11.8	13.6
MANUFACTURING, NONDURABLE GOODS	17.4	9.0	8.8	6.0	6.0	8.7	26.2	20.0	21.3	16.2	13.8	13.8	11.4	8.8	6.9	6.2	8.5	6.4
MANUFACTURING, DURABLE GOODS	N/A	8.3	5.2	7.1	6.3	6.7	N/A	17.9	16.7	17.2	14.0	12.8	N/A	4.5	5.9	7.7	9.4	6.1
TRANSPORTA-TION, COMMU-NICATION & OTHER UTILITIES	18.7	7.8	8.7	4.3	7.3	5.4	27.0	15.9	16.4	13.1	19.9	15.0	17.4	3.8	11.7	7.9	6.4	8.2
WHOLESALE TRADE, DURABLE GOODS	15.0	*	*	10.3	6.1	*	27.2	*	*	16.4	14.7	18.1	11.2	*	*	8.0	*	10.2
WHOLESALE TRADE, NON-DURABLE GOODS	N/A	*	*	7.3	10.4	3.7	N/A	*	*	13.5	18.1	13.1	N/A	*	*	10.5	11.1	13.8

(continued)

RETAIL TRADE	19.2	10.6	11.7	11.4	9.5	11.7	29.0	23.2	25.1	19.6	19.1	20.6	5.2	7.6	7.3	8.7	8.1	10.1
FINANCE, INSURANCE & REAL ESTATE	12.3	6.6	7.1	6.9	4.0	5.3	26.2	13.3	17.5	17.0	11.8	14.9	4.0	9.3	5.0	5.6	3.1	4.9
BUSINESS & REPAIR SERVICES	11.5	16.1	9.7	11.1	10.5	11.7	23.0	23.4	17.1	20.4	18.2	21.0	12.9	5.7	5.0	7.8	8.9	12.4
PERSONAL SERVICES	*	*	6.0	10.2	7.9	12.4	*	*	*	18.0	20.8	19.2	*	*	5.5	6.8	7.3	3.8
ENTERTAINMENT & RECREATION	*	*	*	18.3	9.7	*	*	*	*	*	16.4	*	*	*	*	8.7	4.4	7.1
PROFESSIONAL & RELATED SERVICES	12.8	8.6	5.3	4.4	4.7	3.6	21.0	16.8	12.4	9.7	10.4	11.0	3.9	3.0	4.7	4.1	2.9	2.8
PUBLIC ADMINISTRATION	*	7.3	4.6	5.3	3.1	2.1	*	12.5	12.8	9.3	7.9	8.3	10.7	5.2	5.9	7.0	4.6	9.0

Note: Heavy alcohol use is defined as drinking five or more drinks on five or more occasions during the previous 30 days.
*Low precision; no estimate reported.
N/A: Not Available
Adapted from Office of Applied Studies, Substance Abuse and Mental Health Services Administration: National Household Survey on Drug Abuse: 1985–1993, Rockville, MD.

TABLE 17-2 ■ *Industry Categories with the Highest and Lowest Rates of Heavy Alcohol Use, Full-Time Workers, Ages 18–49, 1991–1993*

TEN HIGHEST RATES OF HEAVY ALCOHOL USE			TEN LOWEST RATES OF HEAVY ALCOHOL USE		
RANK	INDUSTRY CATEGORY	PERCENTAGE REPORTING HEAVY ALCOHOL USE	RANK	INDUSTRY CATEGORY	PERCENTAGE REPORTING HEAVY ALCOHOL USE
1	Computer and Data Processing	16.2	1	Physicians, Dentists, Chiropractors, etc. Offices	0.1
2	Eating and Drinking Places	15.4	2	Professional and Related Services, misc.	0.6
3	Construction	13.4	3	Child Care Services	0.9
4	Auto Supply and Gas Stations	13.2	4	Apparel and Shoe Stores	1.5
5	Lumber and Wood Products	12.0	5	Hospitals	2.1
6	Automotive Service & Repair	11.4	6	Accounting and Bookkeeping	2.3
7	Horticultural	10.8	7	Electrical Machinery	2.7
8	Metal Industries	10.0	8	Elementary and Secondary Schools	2.7
9	Wholesale Trade, Groceries	9.8	9	Private Household	2.8
10	Hotel and Motel	9.6	10	Legal Services	3.0

Note: Heavy alcohol use is defined as drinking five or more drinks on five or more occasions during the previous 30 days.
Adapted from Office of Applied Studies, Substance Abuse and Mental Health Services Administration: National Household Survey on Drug Abuse, 1991–1993, Rockville, MD.

many years to study aspects of the mind, including the potential uses for and effects of cryogenics.

People start using alcohol and drugs for many reasons, but the main reason usually is to feel accepted by a peer group or to feel comfortable in a social situation. People mistake the temporary "high" as a stimulant. In reality, alcohol is a depressant. Other drugs can be either "uppers" or "downers." The desire for the high feeling people get from the drug may be another reason for developing misuse and dependence.

The United States is facing many debates about the legalization of "street drugs" such as marijuana, cocaine, and LSD. Proponents believe that legalizing these drugs will take the lucrative business away from the pushers and sellers, much as the legalization of alcohol did. Opponents believe it will only make access to the chemicals easier, thus encouraging a problem that already has an impact on many people in this country.

Some medical professionals argue that marijuana is not any more dangerous than alcohol and that it has therapeutic value for people who suffer chronic pain and chronic emesis (such as patients with cancer who receive chemotherapy). They refer to the many prescription drugs that can be as addictive as the street drugs but that are given out quite freely—and legally—by some physicians. Personally, the nurse will have his or her own ideas on this debate; professionally, nurses must understand that any chemical can be potentially dangerous. The study of alcohol and other mind-altering chemicals is of high priority because of their prevalence in our society.

The cost of abuse-related medical care to the employer as well as to the health-care industry is great. Illness and time lost from work are major expenditures for employers. Accidents inside and outside the home are also major medical costs. Approximately $85 billion is spent annually in the United States for alcohol-related conditions.

Addiction means physical dependence on a substance. **Tolerance** (the ability to endure the effects of a drug or the need for higher amounts of the drug to produce the high) and **withdrawal** (unpleasant physical, psychological, or cognitive effects that result from decreasing or stopping the use of the chemical after regular use) are characteristics of addiction. The general definitions of substance abuse and substance dependence apply to any substance. **Substance dependence** is a condition in which a person has had three or more of the following symptoms for 1 month or longer:

- Person needs more substance and at more frequent intervals.
- Person spends a lot of time obtaining the substance.
- Person gives up important social or professional functions in order to use the substance.
- Person has tried at least once to quit but still obsesses about the substance.
- Misuse or withdrawal symptoms interfere with job, family, or social activities.
- Person uses the substance regardless of the problems that ensue.
- Tolerance increases greatly (by approximately 50 percent).
- Person uses to avoid withdrawal symptoms.

Substance abuse differs from substance dependence and is diagnosed by a rating system as follows:

- *Mild:* Person has three of the foregoing symptoms, but social functioning is only minimally affected.
- *Moderate:* Person's symptoms are between mild and severe categories.
- *Severe:* More than three of the foregoing symptoms exist, and social obligations are impaired.
- *Partial remission:* Over 6 months, some symptoms have occurred.
- *Full remission:* Over 6 months, no symptoms have occurred.

Not all patients who have a substance abuse disorder go through all stages, and not everyone goes through them in the same order. Nurses need to develop a particular interest in chemical dependency for several reasons. First of all, many medical/surgical patients are chemically dependent, which has an impact on their healing and the effect of their medications. Second, as part of the human experience, your chance of being in a close personal relationship with a person who is chemically dependent is great. Third, and maybe most important, nurses are part of a profession that has statistically high use and abuse of drugs and alcohol. It is estimated that 10 to 20 percent of all nurses are chemically dependent at some point in their lifetimes (Skinner, 1993).

Substance abuse is not a one-person illness; it affects the personal and professional relationships of the people associated with the user. The term **dysfunctional** is often used to refer to the relationships within an alcoholic family. While learning the symptoms of abuse and dependence, nurses will see that dishonesty and an inability to discuss the situation are strong components. Many times, the people who live in the dysfunctional family group begin to cover up for the user's behaviors and lack of responsibility. Family members or significant others take sides, begin to be dishonest with each other, and erode the bond that once was cohesive within that family.

Eventually, this leads to a condition called **codependency,** which is as serious as the use and abuse of the substance. In codependency, the significant others in the family group begin to lose their own sense of identity and purpose and exist solely for the abuser. Their actions take away the opportunity for the user to become responsible for his or her own actions. This is counterproductive for someone who already has a challenge to his or her self-esteem; the person who is addicted sinks deeper into the addiction and the codependent person becomes more codependent. It is a downward spiral. Melody Beattie is an author who has lived the life of codependency. She is well known in the area of recovery and continues to write books about recovery from a codependent lifestyle.

Another question that plagues the minds of professionals and researchers is "Why do some people become addicted or dependent and others do not? Can it be the chemical, or is it the person?" Some theorists are using a new term *addictive personality,* which includes all kinds of addictive behaviors. This term may begin to explain addictions to food, sex, and gambling as well as alcohol, chemicals, and any other dependency that people develop. Let's explore some possibilities as to why people might become chemically dependent.

■ ETIOLOGIC THEORIES

Psychoanalytic theories state that people who develop addictions to alcohol or other substances are those who failed to successfully pass through the oral stage of development. They therefore need constant oral satisfaction. It is not clear at this time whether the person who is chemically dependent is that way because of low self-esteem and a passive personality or whether the substance abuse causes those behaviors. Theorists disagree.

Biologic theories include numerous studies implying a familial connection—some sort of metabolic genetic disorder. Many of these studies were of twins born of at least one alcoholic parent and separated from those parents. The number of twins who were born of alcoholic parents but raised by nonalcoholic parents and yet developed alcoholism is consistently high. It can also be a behavioral or cognitive learning experience. The cognitive-behavioral theorists suggest that a person's perception of being high may influence the actual act of becoming high. It can be a very innocent beginning. For example, obtaining pain relief from medications from the physician or dentist can, according to cognitive theory, leave a patient perceiving that the use of these drugs is a "miracle cure." It becomes very easy to want that kind of relief again, and very soon a pattern is formed and other substances may be involved. For this reason, some theorists believe that chemical dependency is a learned behavior.

■ DIFFERENTIAL DIAGNOSIS

Frequently, the alcoholic patient is admitted to the unit with primary medical diagnoses including dehydration, hyperemesis, or respiratory infections.

■ TYPES

ALCOHOL ABUSE AND DEPENDENCE

Use and abuse of alcohol are present in all walks of life, on all economic levels, and in both men and women (Fig. 17-1). There is sometimes a very fine line between the person who is a "social" drinker and the person who has an alcohol abuse condition. One factor used to make that differentiation is the degree of need or compulsion to drink. Approximately 10 to 15 million people in the United States are classified as alcoholics. Teenagers and younger children are using alcohol in greater numbers. There

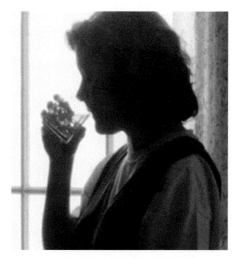

FIGURE 17-1. The use—and abuse—of alcohol occurs in persons of all ages, races, and cultural backgrounds, and in women as well as men. (Courtesy of National Institute on Alcohol Abuse and Alcoholism, National Institutes of Health, Bethesda, MD.)

is a high incidence of alcohol use and abuse among older adults as well. Alcoholism either directly or indirectly decreases a person's life expectancy by an average of 10 to 12 years. Box 17-1 presents a ranking of alcohol use and abuse among the main minority groups within the U.S. population.

The main defense mechanism used by people who are substance abusers is denial. The alcohol-dependent person will often

---

BOX 17-1	*A Ranking of Alcohol Use and Abuse among the Main Minority Groups in the United States*

ADULT RANKING HIGHEST TO LOWEST:
American Indians/Alaska Natives (nearly equal)
African Americans/Hispanics (nearly equal)
Asian Americans and Pacific Islanders

ADOLESCENT RANKING HIGHEST TO LOWEST:
Hispanic
White
African American
Data also indicate that alcohol consumption and abuse is growing most rapidly in the Asian American population and that across all demographic groups, men are more likely than women to be heavy drinkers.

use statements such as "I can quit anytime I want to" or "I just need a little bump to loosen me up."

Alcohol dependence includes improper use of alcohol and impaired social or occupational functioning, ultimately leading to signs of tolerance or withdrawal. **Alcohol abuse** is a pattern of compulsive use of alcohol. Alcohol dependence usually includes several main symptoms:

- Inability to cut down or stop using; daily use is common
- Binges that last 2 days or more
- Blackouts (amnesia while intoxicated)
- Social function impaired
- Last 1 month or longer

E. M. Jellinek, a pioneer in the field of alcohol use and abuse, has developed another classification system for alcoholism. His stages are as follows:

1. *Prealcoholic:* This involves occasional use, constant use/relief drinking, increase in alcohol tolerance.
2. *Prodromal*
   - Onset of and increases in number of blackouts
   - Drinking in secret
   - Preoccupation with alcohol
   - Gulping first drink
   - Inability to discuss problem
3. *Crucial*
   - Loss of control
   - Rationalizing drinking
   - Failure in efforts to control drinking
   - Grandiose and aggressive behavior
   - Trouble with family, employer
   - Self-pity
   - Loss of outside interests
   - Unreasonable resentment
   - Neglecting food
   - Tremors (hands)
   - Morning drinking
4. *Chronic*
   - Prolonged intoxication
   - Physical and moral deterioration
   - Impaired thinking
   - Anxiety that cannot be identified

- Obsession with drinking
- Constant use of alibis

5. *Other signs and symptoms*
   - Vomiting
   - Dehydration
   - Temper tantrums
   - Disorientation
   - Increased vulnerability to infections
   - Increased vulnerability to accidents and other forms of injury

■ TREATMENT MODALITIES OF ALCOHOL ABUSE AND DEPENDENCY

Perhaps the single most effective treatment for alcoholism is Alcoholics Anonymous (AA). AA is a nationwide organization, begun in 1935 by two alcoholic men who bonded and vowed to support each other through recovery. AA has groups in most communities. It is run by alcoholics, but there is no leader in the group.

One of the main tenets of AA is anonymity. People identify themselves by first names only. Someone usually starts the topic or introductions or asks an opening question, but the group runs itself. It is based on 12 steps, and frequently one step is discussed each week or on a designated week per month. AA meetings are closed—that is, nobody except the alcoholics themselves are allowed to attend. There is usually a group that has an open meeting monthly or quarterly. If the meeting is listed as open, any interested person may attend.

There are corresponding groups for families of the alcoholic (Al-Anon) and a special group for teenagers (Alateen). Adult Children of Alcoholics is a branch of AA formed for people who are now adults but grew up in an alcoholic home and were not able to get help at the time.

Table 17-3 lists the 12 steps of AA (Alcoholics Anonymous, 1981). Other 12-step groups serving other dependency needs

TABLE 17-3 ■ *The Twelve Steps and Twelve Traditions of Alcoholics Anonymous*	
The Twelve Steps of Alcoholics Anonymous	The Twelve Traditions of Alcoholics Anonymous
1. We admitted we were powerless over alcohol—that our lives had become unmanageable.	1. Our common welfare should come first; personal recovery depends upon A.A. unity.
2. Came to believe that a Power greater than ourselves could restore us to sanity.	2. For our group purpose, there is but one ultimate authority—a loving God as He may express Himself in our group conscience. Our leaders are but trusted servants; they do not govern.
3. Made a decision to turn our will and our lives over to the care of God *as we understood Him*.	3. The only requirement for A.A. membership is a desire to stop drinking.
4. Made a searching and fearless moral inventory of ourselves.	4. Each group should be autonomous except in matters affecting other groups of A.A. as a whole.
5. Admitted to God, to ourselves and to another human being the exact nature of our wrongs.	5. Each group has but one primary purpose—to carry its message to the alcoholic who still suffers.
6. Were entirely ready to have God remove all these defects of character.	6. An A.A. group ought never endorse, finance, or lend the A.A. name to any related facility or outside enterprise, lest problems of money, property, and prestige divert us from our primary purpose.
7. Humbly asked Him to remove our shortcomings.	7. Every A.A. group ought to be fully self-supporting, declining outside contributions.
8. Made a list of all persons we had harmed and became willing to make amends to them all.	8. Alcoholics Anonymous should remain forever non-professional, but our service centers may employ special workers.
9. Made direct amends to such people wherever possible, except when to do so would injure them or others.	9. A.A., as such, ought never be organized; but we may create service boards or committees directly responsible to those they serve.
10. Continued to take personal inventory and when we were wrong promptly admitted it.	10. Alcoholics Anonymous has no opinion on outside issues; hence the A.A. name ought never be drawn into public controversy.
11. Sought through prayer and meditation to improve our conscious contact with God, *as we understood Him,* praying only for knowledge of His will for us and the power to carry that out.	11. Our public relations policy is based on attraction rather than promotion; we need always maintain personal anonymity at the level of press, radio, and films.
12. Having had a spiritual awakening as the result of these steps, we tried to carry this message to alcoholics and to practice these principles in all our affairs.	12. Anonymity is the spiritual foundation of all our traditions, ever reminding us to place principles before personalities.

The Twelve Steps and Twelve Traditions are reprinted with permission of Alcoholics Anonymous World Services, Inc. ("A.A.W.S."). Permission to reprint the Twelve Steps and Twelve Traditions does not mean that A.A.W.S has reviewed or approved the contents of this publication, nor that A.A. agrees with the views expressed herein. A.A. is a program of recovery from alcoholism only—use of the Twelve Steps and Twelve Traditions in connection with programs and activites which are patterned after A.A. but which address other problems, or in any other non-A.A. context, does not imply otherwise.

have modeled themselves after the AA model.

Treatment for alcohol dependency and abuse is slow. One of the slogans of AA is "One Day at a Time." Members of AA believe that they are always in a state of *recovery,* not that they have *recovered.* Recovery from alcoholism is a process. With very few exceptions, an alcoholic who is recovering cannot ever have another drink, or he or she risks returning to the abusive patterns.

Rational emotive therapy (RET) is being used as well. This therapy is based on the idea that the way a person perceives being high makes the difference between normal use and abuse of the substance. RET uses the concept that, with homework and practice, a person can learn to think differently about the ABCs: (1) *A*ctivating event that led to the drinking. When the person changes the (2) *B*elief system about the activating event and the drinking, the (3) *C*onsequences of drinking will be less powerful. The person learns that he or she does not have to drink to handle the activating event but that, if the individual does drink, it will not be awful or terrible and there is the opportunity to do better the next time.

Psychoanalysis may also be used. This is a very costly method of treatment compared with AA, which is free. Psychoanalysis provides one-on-one therapy, whereas AA and RET are group activities.

Family therapy is important in reinstating honesty in communication. It is a safe place to intervene and explore the underlying feelings that have been ignored within that family unit.

Medications are used cautiously. It is not always wise to substitute the alcohol with another chemical. The chance for just transferring the substance of choice from the alcohol to the prescription drug is high in some instances. If, however, the anxiety level prohibits participation in therapy or if a depressive disorder accompanies the abuse, medications may be prescribed. Antidepressant or antianxiety classifications are prescribed in these cases.

Disulfiram (Antabuse), a drug that is sometimes prescribed for the person who abuses alcohol, is designed to be an aversive therapy. It falls in and out of the mental health community's graces. It is only effective if the person needing it is committed to not drinking. A person who takes Antabuse and then takes a drink of alcohol becomes violently ill. Patients soon learn that if they choose to drink, they simply will not take the Antabuse. Nurses must be aware that the person receiving Antabuse can also be adversely affected by using products that contain alcohol, such as colognes, mouthwash, and aftershaves.

The side effects of Antabuse include slurred speech, disorientation, personality changes, delirium, and impotence—many of the same symptoms as the person who is under the influence of alcohol. The obvious drawback to a medication such as this is that the person who chooses to drink quickly learns not to take the medication. For patients who are motivated to stop drinking, however, it can be very helpful. Sometimes patients who are actively using drugs when brought to the unit or who are cut off from their alcohol abruptly experience a condition called "delirium tremens" (DTs). In DTs, the individual's sensory activity becomes hyperexcitable. Visual hallucinations (e.g., "pink elephants" and "snakes all over"), tremors, and possibly tonic-clonic seizures are typical.

Researchers are seeking new treatments for alcohol abuse. One such treatment is a drug called acampresate, which acts on neurotransmitters and alters the function of certain chemicals in the brain. Naltrexone (Revia) is used to decrease cravings for alcohol and increase a person's chance to abstain from using alcohol.

Because people often experience dual diagnoses, depression commonly accompanies alcoholism. For these people, antidepressants either alone or in combination with other drugs may be helpful. To date, however, total abstinence is the only solution.

Milieu can be varied as well. Therapy ranges from in-house hospitalizations of 2 weeks or more (Fig. 17-2) to independent attempts to help oneself by attending AA. The method of treatment depends on the patient's circumstances and the insurance available to that patient. It is not uncommon to see patients come to treatment more than once. Some people are in treatment for reasons other than their own desire to be there or because they are not convinced that they cannot use the alcohol or the drug again without reverting to abusive patterns. This is not to be interpreted as a weakness in the individual or the treatment program. It is only a sign that the person is learning more about the ramifications of this disorder.

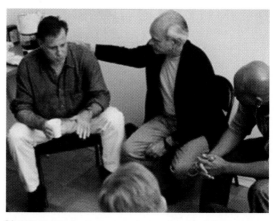

FIGURE 17-2. Treatment for alcohol problems can occur in a variety of settings. Here patients in a rehabilitation hospital engage in a group therapy session. (Courtesy of Cedar House Rehabilitation Center, Bloomington, CA. Used with permission.)

◾ NURSING CARE FOR TREATING PATIENTS WITH ALCOHOL DEPENDENCY OR ABUSE

1. *Honesty:* Effective therapeutic communication is essential. Nurses need to be in touch with their own thoughts and feelings about addictions in general. Any unresolved conflicts you may have involving personal experiences with addiction must be worked out to make it possible to confront and help your patients.

2. *Group:* If you are working on a chemical dependency unit, you may become part of the patient's treatment group. You need some knowledge of the type of therapy that is being used with the patient so that you can maintain that kind of communication in your other interactions with the patient.

3. *Awareness of use of defense mechanisms:* Alcohol and drug abusers are usually deeply rooted in the defense mechanism of denial. You need to confront this mechanism with your patient when you identify denial

behaviors. Rationalization is also frequently used by people with addictions.

4. *Support:* Positive reinforcement for successes is important when helping a person with an addiction. Every step is a big one in this field; every step taken is a new one.

5. *Safety:* Patients who are chemically addicted may become suicidal or display other bizarre behavior (e.g., during DTs). Maintaining a safe milieu and calm demeanor will help the patient through this time of panic. Also, the fact that a patient is hospitalized does not guarantee that he or she does not have access to the chemical and may not use it right in front of you! Do not let your guard down. Observe *always!* Confront all your suspicions honestly and nonjudgmentally with the patient and document all findings and behaviors that are suspect. Thorough patient teaching relating to medications and treatments is crucial.

6. *"Tough love":* This concept encourages the patient to be responsible for his or her own healing. "Doing for" the patient may be tempting, but it is not in the patient's best interest most of

the time. Nurses must toughen up the caretaking side of their personalities when working with patients who are alcohol or drug dependent.

■ DRUG ABUSE AND DEPENDENCE

Many substances can be addictive to humans: caffeine and nicotine are two that are very readily available. Coffee, tea, soda, and cigarettes are everywhere in our society and yet are very addicting. It has been said that the single most difficult addiction to overcome is the addiction to nicotine (Fig. 17-3). Anyone who is or was a smoker can probably attest to that.

Illegal substances such as marijuana, cocaine, crack, PCP (phenylcyclohexyl piperidine), and prescription medications for pain and mental health treatment are also potentially addictive substances (Box

17-2). In addition, **methamphetamine** (Fig. 17-4) is becoming more and more common, with directions for cooking on the Internet and supplies able to fit into a common briefcase. Some of the supplies used to make methamphetamine (also called speed, chalk, meth, ice, crank, and other terms) include pseudoephedrine (Sudafed), Coleman-style camping lantern fuel, freon, lye, batteries, coffee pots and filters, styrofoam coolers, etc.—common household materials.

It is becoming more and more popular among the youth in the United States to use inhalants such as lighter fluid, paint, paint thinners, and gasoline to get high. These are highly toxic, potentially lethal, and usually available in the house or garage. They are legal to buy and possess.

In addition, studies are showing that tobacco use among adolescents in the United States is again on the rise. Not necessarily the traditional tobacco, but hand-

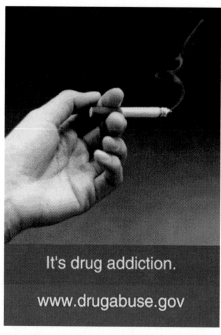

FIGURE 17-3. As this poster says, nicotine is an addiction, and it can be the most difficult one to overcome. (Courtesy of the National Institute on Drug Addiction, National Institutes of Health, Bethesda, MD.)

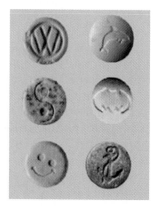

FIGURE 17-4. "Homemade" methamphetamine tablets. (Courtesy of Drug Enforcement Agency, U.S. Department of Justice, Washington, DC.)

rolled cigarettes called "bidi" or "rokok" are finding their way into the hands of adolescents and young adults (Fig. 17-5). These are flavored cigarettes that are coming primarily from India and other Southeast Asian countries. They may also be obtained on the Internet.

Bidis produce higher levels of carbon monoxide, tar, and nicotine than traditional cigarettes. Some estimates are that bidi users inhale three times the amounts of those toxins. Bidis are also less expensive than traditional tobacco cigarettes, making them easier for younger people to afford. Some are using them as "dessert" after meals. They have flavor and no calories!

Nurses need to be aware of these substances and incorporate data collection techniques that may help detect use of these substances that are becoming more widely used among all age groups.

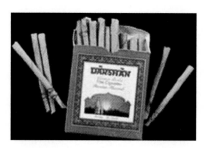

FIGURE 17-5. Bidis, flavored cigarettes from India and Southeast Asia, are less expensive than traditional cigarettes but may be even more toxic. (Courtesy of Campaign for Tobacco-Free Kids Store Alert; www.storealert.org. Used with permission.)

■ SIGNS AND SYMPTOMS OF DRUG ABUSE OR DEPENDENCE

The signs and symptoms of drug abuse and dependence can be very similar to those of alcohol abuse. Signs and symptoms that may also be seen in people who abuse drugs are

- Red, watery eyes
- Dilated pupils
- High blood pressure
- Runny nose
- Hostility
- Paranoia
- Needle tracks on arms or legs

■ TREATMENT MODALITIES FOR PATIENTS WITH DRUG ABUSE OR DEPENDENCE

1. *Narcotics Anonymous*
2. *Group therapy*
3. *Psychotherapy*
4. *Methadone programs:* Methadone acts as a sort of "step-down" for drug addicts. It, too, is potentially addicting, and its critics say it is only a substitute. Methadone is typically given once a day. It has the ability to help patients return to a more normal lifestyle, and, as treatment progresses and the need for chemicals decreases, it is easier to wean people from methadone than from the drug they were addicted to. Psychotherapy is also provided for patients in methadone programs.
5. *Office-based therapy for opiate addiction*: In 2003, The National Institute on Drug Abuse, part of the National Institutes of Health approved a treatment that can be administered in an office setting by physicians who have completed a special 8-hour training and certification by the Department of Health and Human Services. The medication is called Suboxone (buprenorphine and naloxone). It is not meant to replace any of the current treatments such as methadone programs, but rather to fill an existing gap in treatment for a large number of patients who were not able to be treated previously. Suboxone does not tend to produce the same high dependency as methadone and does not have the same level of "pleasure response."

■ ALTERNATIVE TREATMENTS FOR PATIENTS WITH A SUBSTANCE ABUSE DISORDER

Alternative modalities for this group of disorders are geared toward self-help. Some success has been achieved with the following modalities.

BIOFEEDBACK AND HYPNOSIS

Biofeedback has been used for quite a while in addiction treatment and is believed to have many calming effects as well as assisting in managing the strong desire for nicotine, frequently present with alcohol and other addictive illnesses.

NUTRITIONAL SUPPLEMENTS

Thiamine (vitamin B1) is known to be deficient in alcoholics. Replacement may help decrease alcohol-related psychosis. It can be taken as an oral pill or may be supplemented in the diet with foods such as liver, peanut butter, and whole grains.

Herbs such as valerian are believed to assist in decreasing anxiety during withdrawal. Milk thistle is said to have a positive effect on liver detoxification.

NEUROLINGUISTIC PROGRAMMING

Communicating in a method to which the patient can truly relate may help the person identify the underlying problems and place them in a different framework that may allow more effective self-help.

■ NURSING CARE FOR PATIENTS WITH DRUG ABUSE OR DEPENDENCE

Nursing care for those who are drug dependent is essentially the same as for those who are alcohol dependent. It is very important to remember that nurses and physicians do not "fix" the patient who is chemically dependent. With this type of disorder, as with many others, the desire to be chemical-free must come from the patient. The motivation to participate in the treatment program must come from within the patient. Nurses and health-care workers are tools for the patient to use to learn the new life skills that will be needed to be successful.

Table 17-4 summarizes the symptoms and nursing interventions for the alcohol and drug abuse disorders discussed previously.

TABLE 17-4	*Alcohol and Drug Abuse Disorders*	
TYPES	**SYMPTOMS**	**NURSING INTERVENTIONS**
ALCOHOL ABUSE	■ Inability to cut down or stop using ■ Daily use common ■ Binges that last 2 days or more ■ Blackouts, which increase ■ Impaired social function ■ Symptoms that last 1 month or longer ■ Increase in alcohol tolerance ■ Drinking in "secret" ■ Preoccupation with alcohol ■ Gulping first drink ■ Inability to discuss problem	■ Communicate honestly. ■ Assist patient in identifying thoughts and feelings. ■ Encourage participation in group and maintain consistency with new behaviors learned in group. ■ Confront use of maladaptive defense mechanism. ■ Support and give positive reinforcement of progress. ■ Exhibit "tough love."

(continued)

TYPES	SYMPTOMS	NURSING INTERVENTIONS
ALCOHOL ABUSE	■ Loss of control ■ Rationalization of drinking ■ Failure in efforts to control drinking ■ Grandiose and aggressive behavior ■ Trouble with family, employer ■ Self-pity ■ Loss of outside interests ■ Unreasonable resentment ■ Neglecting food ■ Tremors (hands) ■ Morning drinking ■ Prolonged intoxication ■ Physical and moral deterioration ■ Impaired thinking ■ Free-floating anxiety ■ Obsession with drinking ■ Constant use of alibis	
DRUG ABUSE AND DEPENDENCE	■ Similar to alcohol abuse ■ Red, watery eyes ■ Runny nose ■ Hostility ■ Paranoia ■ Needle tracks on arms or legs	■ See "Alcohol Abuse." ■ Encourage patient to be tested for HIV if drug use included use of needles.
CODEPENDENCE	■ Significant others beginning to lose their own sense of identity and purpose, existing solely for the abuser. ■ Actions of significant others taking away opportunity for user to take responsibility for his or her own actions ■ Lowered self-esteem	■ See "Alcohol Abuse." ■ Encourage participation in assertiveness classes.

Key Concepts ■ ■ ■

1. Abuse of and dependence on alcohol and other substances is a growing disorder in the United States. Much time and money are spent on treating the disorders and the illnesses associated with them.
2. Signs and symptoms of alcohol and chemical abuse can be masked as other symptoms. Good observations and careful documentation by the nurse can help attain the information needed for accurate diagnosis.

3. Medical care and nursing care are similar for both alcohol and drug disorders. It is important to remember that physicians and nurses do not "cure" the person with an addiction. The person must *want* to be chemically free; healing must come from within. Physicians and nurses are tools to help the patient learn to do that.

4. Alcoholics Anonymous and Narcotics Anonymous are groups of people who are chemically dependent. AA has a very high success rate. There are corresponding 12-step groups for family members who also need help for the illness.

5. Codependency is also an illness. Codependent people are generally closely linked with the chemically dependent person. People who are codependent need some kind of therapy to help regain their identity and allow the chemically dependent person to again become responsible for his or her own actions.

6. Tobacco use in several forms is on the rise among adolescents and young adults in the United States.

7. Dangerous, addictive, and lethal chemicals such as methamphetamine can be made from common household items.

COMMONLY USED MEDICATIONS ■ *Substance-Related Disorders*

ALCOHOL WITHDRAWAL
- **Chlordiazepoxide** (Librium)
- **Diazepam** (Valium)
- **Oxazepam** (Serax)
- **Nutritional supplements** (vitamins, magnesium)
- **Disulfiram** (Antabuse)

COCAINE WITHDRAWAL
- **Amantadine** (Symmetrel)
- **Bromocriptine** (Parlodel)
- **Desipramine** (Norpramine)

NARCOTIC AND ALCOHOL WITHDRAWAL
- **Naltrexone** (Revia)

HEROIN WITHDRAWAL
- **Methadone hydrochloride** (Dolophine)

REFERENCES

Alcoholics Anonymous. (1981). *12 Steps and 12 Traditions*. General Service Office of Alcoholics Anonymous, New York.

Beattie, M. (1987, 1992). *Codependent No More*. Hazelden Foundation, Center City, MN.

Beattie, M. (1990). *Codependents' Guide to the Twelve Steps*. Fireside-Parkside, New York, NY.

Bidi-use among urban youth—Massachusetts March–April 1999. (1999). *Morbidity & Mortality Weekly Report, 48*(36), 796–799. http://www.cdc.gov/epo/mmmr/preview/mmwr.html/mm4836a2.htm.

Foreman, J. (1999). Finding the keys to alcohol abuse. *Boston Globe and Minneapolis Star Tribune*, April 11.

Griffin, K. (2000). *Milwaukee Journal Sentinel* Drug appears to safely reduce craving for alcohol, study says. *Minneapolis Star Tribune*, February 6.

Peterson, D. (1992). Hennepin's alcoholic treatment questioned. *Minneapolis Star Tribune*, July 19.

Rasmussen, E. (2001). Clean and sober—treatment programs help nurses addicted to drugs save their licenses. *Nurseweek*, March 19.

Skinner, K. (1993). The hazards of chemical dependency among nurses, JPN, pg. 8.

Tobacco Use among Middle and High School Students—United States, 1999. (2000). *Morbidity & Mortality Weekly Report*, 49(3), 49–53. http://www.cdc.gov/epo/mmwr/preview/mmwr.html/mm4903a1.htm.

Special Mention

Michael B. Koopmeiners, MD, Associate Professor, University of St. Augustine for Health Sciences; Diplomate of the American Board of Family Practice; Diplomate of the American Society of Addiction Medicine; Minneapolis, MN

WEBSITES

www.alcoholics-anonymous.org
www.allaboutcounseling.com/codependency.htm
www.solutions4recovery.com
www.nurseweek.com/
www.heroin-drug-rehab.com/buprenorphine
www.nida.nih.gov
http://www.medicalcareersource.com/articles/ChemDepNurse.html
http://www.nurseweek.com/news/features/01–03/sober.asp

CRITICAL THINKING EXERCISES ■ ■ ■

1. Trent and Shawna are your neighbors. Shawna babysits for your two young children several times a week so that you are able to work your day-evening rotation at the hospital. You know that Shawna is a recovering alcoholic. Recently, at a neighborhood block party, you saw Shawna drinking a beer. Trent was drinking a soda. Shawna was laughing and behaving in a flirtatious manner. You comment to both Trent and Shawna about your surprise at her behavior. Trent responds, "She has one or two every now and again. It helps her to relax. It's no big deal." Shawna tells you very bluntly that it's none of your business and that if you are uncomfortable with her drinking a beer, maybe you should find a new babysitter.

   You recall that, on several occasions over the past two months, your 7-year-old has told you that Shawna "didn't make us supper tonight. She was real tired and said she wasn't hungry. She gave us some soda and potato chips and she slept a lot. Trent was gone, too." You are concerned with the welfare of your children and the health of your neighbors.

   What do you feel when Shawna responds to you this way? What are your thoughts about what is happening with Trent and Shawna? How will you alter your communication techniques to speak with them effectively right now?

2. Using the suggested nursing diagnoses listed here (or others you can think of), complete a nursing process for Shawna.

   SUGGESTED NURSING DIAGNOSES

   1. Denial, Ineffective
   2. Powerlessness
   3. Nutrition, Altered: Less than Body Requirements
   4. Individual Coping, Ineffective

ASSESSMENT/ DATA COLLECTION	NURSING DIAGNOSIS	PLAN/ GOAL	INTERVENTIONS/ NURSING ACTIONS	EVALUATION CRITERIA

3. Using the suggested nursing diagnoses listed here (or others you can think of), complete a nursing process for Trent.

SUGGESTED NURSING DIAGNOSES

1. *Self-Esteem Disturbance*
2. *Role Performance, Altered*
3. *Verbal Communication, Impaired*
4. *Social Interaction, Impaired*

ASSESSMENT/ DATA COLLECTION	NURSING DIAGNOSIS	PLAN/ GOAL	INTERVENTIONS/ NURSING ACTIONS	EVALUATION CRITERIA

ACTIVITY

1. Find an open Alcoholics Anonymous meeting. Explain that you are a student and ask permission to take notes. Listen and participate as invited to do so. Write a short paper on your impressions about the meeting.

TEST QUESTIONS ■ ■ ■

MULTIPLE CHOICE QUESTIONS

1. The *desired* effects of Antabuse include:
   A. Nausea, vomiting, palpitations
   B. Delirium, impotence, personality changes
   C. Euphoria, delusions of grandeur, mania
   D. Hepatitis, gastritis, esophagitis

2. The defense mechanism most frequently demonstrated by the chemically dependent person is:
   A. Undoing
   B. Rationalization
   C. Denial
   D. Reaction formation

3. The best nursing action for people who are in active withdrawal is to:
   A. Tell the patient how destructive the behavior is.
   B. Assess the patient.
   C. Explore hallucinations with the patient.
   D. Maintain safety for the patient.

4. Nurses know that alcohol functions as a:
   A. CNS depressant
   B. CNS stimulant
   C. Major tranquilizer
   D. Minor tranquilizer

5. The patient who is experiencing delirium tremens is most likely to exhibit which of the following types of hallucinations?
   A. Auditory
   B. Visual
   C. Tactile
   D. Olfactory

6. Sally and Susie are twins. They are 20 years old. Susie has a habit of drinking too much when they go out. They were out celebrating their birthday last night, and this morning Susie is vomiting. Sally calls her sister's teacher. "Susie is really ill. I think she has the flu; anyway, she can't come to school today. She said she has a test today and an assignment that she was supposed to pick up. I can come in and get the assignment for her. When can she make up the test?" Sally's behavior might indicate:
   A. Collaboration
   B. Compensation
   C. Lying
   D. Codependency

7. You are Sally and Susie's friend. A therapeutic response to them might be:
   A. "Sally and Susie, you are really going to get in trouble if you keep partying like that. It's bad for you."

B. "Sally and Susie, I care for you both, but Susie, you misuse alcohol. You both need help. Sally, you are not helping Susie by 'taking care' of her; she needs to do it herself."

C. "Sally, why do you keep lying for Susie? Just because she's in trouble doesn't mean you have to cover up for her."

D. "Susie, this is just a stage you're going through. Everybody does it; it's not a big deal. You're young! Have fun!"

8. Sally and Susie seek treatment. Susie is treated as an inpatient and Sally as an outpatient. The nurse planning discharge teaching will encourage them to:

   A. Attend weekly AA and Al-Anon meetings.
   B. Check back into the hospital unit weekly.
   C. Attend weekly sessions with the psychologist.
   D. Attend weekly Adult Children of Alcoholics meetings.

9. Your patient admits to using an illegal substance daily, thinking about it when not actually using it, and spending a lot of time figuring out where to get it. This patient could have:

   A. A delusion
   B. DTs
   C. A dependency
   D. Dementia

10. One of the major skills a chemically dependent person/family can learn during treatment is:

    A. Honest communication
    B. Codependency
    C. Denial
    D. Scapegoating

11. Your spouse has been an alcoholic for many years. S/he has been sober for the last 2 years but has begun drinking again. S/he drives drunk. You fear for his/her life, so you begin buying the alcohol for him/her. You are displaying what kind of behavior?

    A. Dry drunk
    B. Codependent
    C. Compassionate
    D. Tough love

12. Your 12- and 13-year-old children and the neighbor children next door have been acting differently the past few weeks. They have had runny noses and have had poor appetites. They have been asking you for batteries, camping gear, and cold medication. You think:

    A. They are planning a camping trip for scouts.
    B. They are getting the flu.
    C. They could be making methamphetamine.
    D. All of the above.

MATCHING QUESTIONS
Directions

Match the best definition or symptom in Column B with the condition in Column A. Each answer will only be used once. There is one extra definition or symptom.

COLUMN A

1. Acampresate, naltrexone (Revia)
2. Withdrawal
3. Addiction
4. Bidis
5. Methamphetamine
6. Dysfunctional relationship
7. Alcohol dependence
8. Codependency
9. Tolerance
10. Alcohol abuse

COLUMN B

A. Becoming drug of choice; made from common household items
B. Pattern of compulsive use of alcohol
C. Ability to endure the effects of a drug or the need for higher amounts of the drug to produce the desired effect
D. Unpleasant physical, psychological, or cognitive effects that result from decreasing or stopping the use of the chemical
E. Physical dependence on a substance
F. New generation of medications for alcohol-related diagnoses
G. Dishonesty and inability to discuss the situation are strong components
H. Produce three times the amount of carbon monoxide, tar, and nicotine of traditional cigarettes
I. Single most effective treatment for alcoholism
J. Condition arising when well-meaning significant others' actions take away the opportunity for the user to become responsible for his or her own actions
K. Improper use of alcohol and impaired social or occupational functioning, ultimately leading to signs of tolerance or withdrawal

Learning Objectives ■ ■ ■

1. Define anorexia.
2. Define bulimia.
3. Define morbid obesity.
4. Discuss bariatric or "weight loss" surgery
5. Identify populations at risk for eating disorders.
6. Identify possible causes of eating disorders.
7. Identify symptoms of eating disorders.
8. List nursing care for patients with eating disorders.

Key Terms ■ ■ ■

- Anorexia
- Body image
- Bulimia
- Morbid obesity

One has only to turn on the television, go to a movie, or look at a fashion magazine to become aware of the American ideal for what bodies should look like. Women of the "baby-boomer" years grew up with the Barbie doll. Collectors love Barbie; professionals who work with disorders of **body image** are more critical of her. People, especially teenage girls in the United States, are bombarded with the messages that "you can never be too thin," "thinner is better," and "thinner is healthier." Teenagers see their thin, shapely peers as the "popular" girls. Although women are afflicted with eating disorders approximately 20 times more frequently than men, teenage boys are not exempt. The modeling industry is promot-

ing more and more male models who are serving as role models for teenage boys.

It is believed that approximately eight million people in the United States have an eating disorder. Approximately 7 million of those are women. Other studies postulate that approximately 56 percent of women between the ages of 25 and 35 and 80 percent of girls in the fourth grade are dieting to lose weight.

As with all other threats to emotional health, eating disorders know no boundaries. Karen Carpenter, a well-known pop music singer of the 1970s and 1980s, died tragically in 1983 from the effects of anorexia. She was 33 years old. Celebrities such as television talk show host Oprah

Winfrey and singer Carnie Wilson have pub-
licly shared stories of their struggles with
eating and dieting and being overweight.

■ ETIOLOGIC THEORIES

Psychologically, when we feel good, it is easier to take better care of our bodies; therefore, looks are improved. When looks are
improved, we tend to get positive reinforcement from the fit of our clothes and the
reflection in the mirror. This positive
response leads to self-confidence; others
may pay us compliments, as well. The mind
and body connection is strong enough to be
entwined in all areas of mental health.

Some psychoanalytic theorists would say
that, at some point in the development of a
person with an eating disorder, he or she had
negative experiences with parents or close
caregivers, which sent the message that the
individual was unworthy of love and care
from those parents or caregivers. When they
reached their teenage and adult years, the
unconscious message remained: "Nobody
cares about me; therefore I do not care about
myself and will take on destructive behaviors
of overeating or starvation." Sigmund Freud

would say that anorectic women are afraid
of womanhood and heterosexuality, as eating is considered an expression of sexual
drive (Brumberg, 1988).

Women or girls who are anorectic frequently state that their mothers were overbearing and dominant. The feelings of these
teenage daughters may be in response to
their mothers' concerns over their eating
habits. Regardless, the young women who
develop anorexia seem to have negative feelings toward their mothers. Regression as a
defense mechanism is believed to be activated, resulting in ineffective emotional
development.

Biologically, this idea is being refuted on
several accounts. First of all, there is the
gender difference. Men and women are built
differently. Women are given more body fat
in different areas for the purpose of supporting pregnancies. Second, studies point
toward a genetic link for body build, size,
and amount of body fat. Researchers are
attempting to develop "antifat pills" for people who are trying to fight chemically what
they were given genetically.

Another idea posed by biologic theorists
is that there is a disturbance in the functioning of the hypothalamus (which regu-
lates eating and sexual activities) or that

Age-Adjusted Prevalence of Overweight and Obesity in Racial/Ethnic Groups in the United States		
	MALES **% OBESITY**	**FEMALES** **% OBESITY**
Non-Hispanic Black	60.7	77.3
Mexican American	74.7	71.9
Non-Hispanic White	67.4	57.3

Numbers are based on statistics from the Centers for Disease Control/National Center for Health
Statistics for the year 2000 and "Statistics Related to Overweight and Obesity," Weight-Control
Information Network, National Institute of Diabetes and Kidney Diseases, National Institutes of
Health, Bethesda, MD; win.niddk.nih.gov. Body mass index (BMI) of greater than or equal to 25
is the standard measurement used to define overweight. Only three racial/ethnic groups were studied.

there is a disturbance in the neurochemical dopamine.

In their book *Black Health Library Guide to Obesity,* Mavis Thompson and Kirk Johnson indicate that there may be special concerns about obesity among the African American population. The authors state that "over 30 percent of African-Americans are obese," which compares with the national average of 25 percent. Blacks and whites alike tend to put on weight with age. This statistic concerns the African American community, which also shows disproportionately high percentages of poverty and illnesses such as diabetes and hypertension (Thompson and Johnson, 1993).

Behaviorists say that food is a mainstay of social and cultural activities. The holidays that people celebrate, parties, theater outings, and even business functions revolve around food. Because food is associated with many pleasant activities throughout life, it is a powerful reinforcer. When things are good, people celebrate with food; when things are not so good, food serves as a reminder of pleasant things. It temporarily nurtures and satiates people when they are feeling unhappy. All this eating, if not metabolized and used, can lead to obesity.

■ TYPES

ANOREXIA NERVOSA

Anorexia nervosa is an "aversion to food." *Aversion* means desire to avoid something—in this case, food. A condition that can cause death from malnutrition, anorexia is usually manifested initially in adolescence but can be seen in some patients as young as 8 years old. Patients refuse to eat.

Some of the behaviors, signs, and symptoms associated with anorexia nervosa are

- Excessive weight loss, usually more than 25 percent of body weight prior to dieting

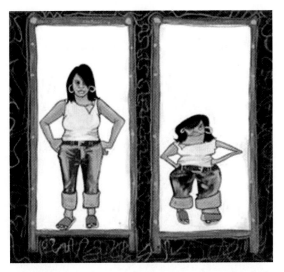

FIGURE 18-1. In anorexia nervosa, patients view their bodies in a distorted way. They may see themselves as being fat, when they really are not. (Courtesy of Ontario Women's Directorate, Toronto, Ontario, Canada.)

- Refusal to maintain normal weight
- Intense fear of being fat; consumption of only 200 to 400 calories daily
- Obsessive thoughts
- Excessive exercising
- Shy, introverted personality
- Perfectionism
- Lack of trust in one's own emotions
- Feeling inadequate and seeing self as fat, no matter what the weight
- Absence of menstrual periods
- Sleeping very little (2 or 3 hours per night)
- Distorted body image (Fig. 18-1)

BULIMIA NERVOSA

Bulimia is binge eating. Those with bulimia consume huge amounts of food—as much as 8,000 calories in a 2-hour period several times daily. A person who is bulimic can consume up to 50,000 calories per day. The binge eating is followed by forced vomiting. Bulimia also tends to be manifested during adolescence. Exercise expert Jane Fonda has been very open about discussing her binge-purge episodes while in college and at the beginning of her acting career.

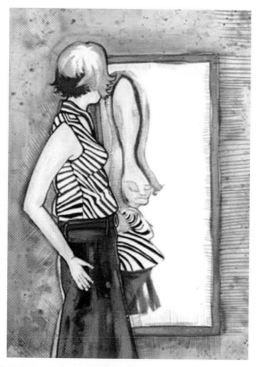

FIGURE 18-2. Like anorexia, bulimia nervosa involves a patient's having a distorted sense of body image. Bulimia also involves some form of purging to get rid of unwanted food and calories. (Courtesy of Ontario Women's Directorate, Toronto, Ontario, Canada.)

Some of the behaviors, signs, and symptoms associated with bulimia nervosa are

- Extreme dieting
- Use and abuse of laxatives or syrup of ipecac (induces vomiting)
- Use and abuse of diuretics
- Obsession with food and eating
- Extreme sensitivity to body shape and weight (Fig. 18-2)
- Poor self-concept
- Thoughts of harming self, possibly suicide
- Impulsiveness
- Feeling depressed, guilty, worthless
- Erosion of teeth enamel or hoarseness as a result of the hydrochloric acid from vomiting

The *American Journal of Nursing* (1993) quotes a study by the Boston University Medical Center. These researchers studied 91 women: 30 who were bulimic and 61 who were healthy (the control group). The study was retested with 63 in the second control group. The results averaged 77 percent who tested positive for bulimia by asking these two questions:

1. Do you eat in secret?
2. Are you satisfied with your eating patterns?

These are still valid, effective questions today.

The nursing interventions for the person with bulimia are essentially the same as for the person with other eating disorders. In addition, the nurse will monitor electrolytes from lab reports and notify the supervisor and physician of any abnormality.

MORBID OBESITY

Obesity is defined as body weight greater than 15 percent of the established ideal height-weight charts. **Morbid obesity,** or hyperobesity, is the condition of being more than 100 pounds above ideal body weight. It is associated with the number of fat cells in the body. Biologically, it is believed that the number of fat cells does not change with dieting. The number of fat cells present during childhood stays the same in adulthood.

Among the biologic reasons for obesity are hypothyroidism and diabetes. Among the negative concepts of obesity is the fact that much of society may blame the overweight people and assume that they are weak or lazy individuals.

The psychoanalytic view of obesity indicates that the oral stage of development is the highest level achieved by these individuals. The person is said to be fixated, or stuck, at that need for oral gratification. Obese people satisfy that oral need with food, according to the psychoanalytic theorists.

Costs Related to Obesity in the United States

CONDITION	APPROXIMATE COST (in billions of dollars unless otherwise specified)
TYPE 2 DIABETES	98.0
OSTEOARTHRITIS	21.2
HEART DISEASE	8.8
CANCERS (TOTAL):	7.0
*COLON CANCER	3.5
*BREAST CANCER	2.9
*ENDOMETRIAL CANCER	933 (million)
HYPERTENSION	4.1
GALLBLADDER DISEASE	3.9
PRODUCTIVITY (LOST WORK DAYS, RESTRICTED WORK DAYS, BED DAYS, AND VISITS TO DOCTORS' OFFICES)	3.4

Data from "Statistics Related to Overweight and Obesity," Weight-Control Information Network, National Institute of Diabetes and Digestive and Kidney Diseases, National Institutes of Health, Bethesda, MD; http://win.niddk.nih.gov.

■ MEDICAL COMPLICATIONS OF EATING DISORDERS

- Electrolyte imbalances
- Cardiac irregularities
- Edema and dehydration
- Gastrointestinal problems

■ BARIATRIC SURGERY

Many people who are chronically one hundred pounds overweight or more are choosing to have "stomach stapling," or bariatric, surgery. Carnie Wilson of WilsonPhilips fame, opted to have hers performed live on the Internet in 1999. It is not uncommon for candidates to wait upward of a year to be placed on a surgery schedule. Your nursing clinicals may include pre- or postoperative care for a patient with this type of surgery. How is caring for this patient any different from other postoperative patients? How is this any more stressful than, for instance, a patient who has just had surgery for cancer? In many ways, there are no differences. Both require high degrees of compassionate nursing care from nurses with excellent data collecting and communicating skills. What is different is that bariatric patients often have had an entire lifetime of fighting with weight issues. In just a very short time, their lifestyle will change forever. There are issues of learning new relationships with food, as seen with people who have anorexia and bulimia. There are potential unpleasant gastrointestinal side effects, such as dumping syndrome, that patients must accept. Potential postoperative complications are numerous. The surgery does not always work. For those feeling surgery is a last resort to feeling more healthy and looking more "normal," an unsuccessful surgery and less than optimal weight loss can be emotionally devastating. Nurses caring for patients who have undergone weight loss surgery must be very broadscoped in their approach to care and care planning for these patients.

Most bariatric surgery programs employ nurses to work with patients in clinic before and after surgery. The programs include components of education before and after surgery. Nurses frequently facilitate these sessions in partnership with the surgeon. It is common for patients to be followed for at least one year after surgery. As the nurse in the clinic, you will take the usual vital sign measurements and will be educating on diet, exercise, and medication, which, for some patients, includes taking vitamin B12 injections for the remainder of their lives.

Visit http://www.nursing.ecu.edu/bariatric for further physical and emotional nursing care for this group of patients.

■ ALTERNATIVE CARE FOR PATIENTS WITH EATING DISORDERS

Alternative care tends to center around the individual symptoms. Nutrition is stressed in the treatment program. In addition, underlying conditions, such as depression or other negative emotional states, may be addressed. The following alternative treatments may be helpful.

BIOFEEDBACK, HYPNOSIS, AND NEUROLINGUISTIC PROGRAMMING

See Chapter 9 to review these techniques. Learning to reframe one's relationship with and messages about food and messages about reinforcing a new lifestyle are two areas that could be worked on by using these techniques.

NUTRITIONAL SUPPLEMENTS

Nutritional supplements are discussed and prescribed from within the program. Eating real, "normal" food is stressed, but vitamins, such as B12 injections and oral multivitamins, are generally prescribed to supplement for what will be a mechanical decrease of nutrients via food.

■ NURSING CARE FOR PATIENTS WITH EATING DISORDERS

1. *Promote positive self-concept:* Gaining trust and giving positive reinforcement for the progress the patient makes will help the patient learn to change his or her lifestyle.
2. *Promote healthy coping skills:* Nurses who understand that developing healthy coping skills is time consuming and difficult for an anorectic person are able to demonstrate confidence that the patient can change. Empathy for the depth of this disorder will help gain the patient's trust and cooperation. The nurse must be careful not to be manipulated into negative behaviors by the patient with anorexia. Setting limits on behavior is part of the plan of care. Having the patient consistently stay within those limits is part of teaching new lifestyle behaviors. The American Anorexia and Bulimia Association is an advocacy group for people with eating disorders. The local phone book can be checked for a nearby chapter, or the social worker may have information.
3. *Promote adequate nutrition:* The physician and dietitian or nutritionist will meet with the patient to discuss calorie and nutrient requirements.

Nurses are responsible for monitoring the patient's ability and willingness to consume the specified amount of food. Usually, smaller and more frequent meals are tolerated better than the traditional three larger meals. For a person with an aversion to food, presenting a large tray of food can be overwhelming and discouraging. Positive reinforcement for increasing the caloric intake can be helpful. *Note:*

When implementing this type of behavior modification, the nurse would be better served to praise the caloric intake, *not* the weight gain. How nurses word the reinforcement can be crucial to the patient's willingness to continue the plan of care.

Table 18-1 summarizes symptoms and nursing interventions for the eating disorders discussed earlier.

TABLE 18-1 ■ *Eating Disorders*		
TYPE	**SYMPTOMS**	**NURSING INTERVENTIONS**
ANOREXIA NERVOSA	■ Weight loss of more than 25% of body weight prior to dieting ■ Refusal to maintain normal weight ■ Intense fear of being fat ■ Consumption of only 200–400 calories daily ■ Obsessive thoughts ■ Excessive exercising ■ Shyness and tendency to be introverted ■ Perfectionism ■ Lack of trust in own emotions ■ Feeling of inadequacy; seeing self as fat, regardless of weight ■ Absence of menstrual periods ■ Sleeping very little (2 or 3 hours per night)	■ Promote positive self-concept. ■ Promote healthy coping skills. ■ Promote adequate nutrition.
BULIMIA NERVOSA	■ Extreme dieting ■ Use and abuse of laxatives or syrup of ipecac ■ Use and abuse of diuretics ■ Obsession with food and eating ■ Extreme sensitivity to body shape and weight ■ Poor self-concept ■ Thoughts of harming self—possibly suicide ■ Impulsivity ■ Feelings of depression, guilt, worthlessness ■ Possible erosion of tooth enamel or hoarseness	■ See "Anorexia Nervosa." ■ Approach with positive, realistic expectations of food intake. ■ Allow patient some control in decision making.

(continued)

TABLE 18-1	*Eating Disorders (Continued)*	
TYPE	**SYMPTOMS**	**NURSING INTERVENTIONS**
MORBID OBESITY	■ More than 100 pounds above ideal body weight ■ Associated with the number of fat cells in the body ■ May have hypothyroidism and diabetes	■ Work with patient, family, physician, and dietitian to formulate healthy meal plans. ■ Encourage patient to participate in groups to promote acceptance of self and development of self-esteem.

Key Concepts ■ ■ ■

1. Eating disorders of one type or another affect large numbers of people in the United States. Statistics reflect primarily women with these disorders. Men are also becoming more affected with eating disorders as a result of the increase in popularity of male models.
2. Bariatric surgery is becoming far more common than in years past. There are many physical and emotional considerations required when caring for patients undergoing this surgery.
3. Eating disorders are serious and can be fatal as a result of malnutrition and electrolyte disturbances.
4. Eating disorders may be related to emotional or physical causes. Obesity per se may have genetic and emotional causes.

COMMONLY USED MEDICATIONS ■ *Eating Disorders*	
Alprazolam (Xanax)	**Hydroxyzine** (Atarax, Vistaril)
Buspirone (BuSpar)	**Lithium** (Eskalith, Lithotabs)
Chlordiazepoxide (Librium)	**Oxazepam** (Serax)
Fluoxetine (Prozac)	**Phenytoin** (Dilantin)

REFERENCES

Bailey, D. and Bailey, D. (1997). *Therapeutic Approaches in Mental Health/Psychiatric Nursing*, 4th ed. FA Davis, Philadelphia.

Brumberg, J.J. (1988). *Fasting Girls—The Emergence of Anorexia Nervosa as a Modern Disease.* Harvard University Press, Cambridge, MA.

Carson, R.C., Butcher, J.N., and Coleman, J.C. (1988). *Abnormal Psychology and Modern Life*, 8th ed. HarperCollins, New York.

Fast screen for bulimia. *American Journal of Nursing*, July, 1993.

Thompson, M. and Johnson, K.A. (1993). *Black Health Library Guide to Obesity.* Holt, San Mateo, CA.

Williams, S. (2004). Lean times—patients with eating disorders encounter difficulties obtaining treatment under managed care coverage limits. *NurseWeek,* August 23. Pages 10–13.

WEBSITES

http://www.nimh.nih.gov
www.edreferral.com/males_eating_disorders.htm

http://www.nursingcenter.com
http://www.nursing.ecu.edu/bariatric
http://www.scrippshealth.org
http://www.mentalhealth.com
http://www.nami.org
http://win.niddk.nih.gov

CRITICAL THINKING EXERCISES ■ ■ ■

1. Interview an overweight classmate, family member, or coworker. Ask about this person's attempts at weight loss. What was the success rate? What was the attitude of the physicians who were helping this person? What is this person's perception of the social view of obesity? What is your attitude about people who are overweight? If possible, plan a diet and exercise regimen with the person you interviewed. Be sure the individual has the permission of his or her physician before starting the program. Follow and document the individual's progress for this school term.

2. Watch television with a new eye. Which are the popular shows? Which commercials appeal to you? What do the characters look like? What roles do thin people play on the shows and commercials? What is selling the product on the commercial? How many fat people do you see on these same shows and commercials? What roles do they play? What messages are being sent?

3. Using the suggested nursing diagnoses listed here (or others you can think of), complete a nursing process for the subject you chose in exercise 1.

SUGGESTED NURSING DIAGNOSES

1. *Body Image Disturbance*
2. *Knowledge Deficit (Nutritional Requirements)*
3. *Self-Esteem Disturbance*

ASSESSMENT/ DATA COLLECTION	NURSING DIAGNOSIS	PLAN/ GOAL	INTERVENTIONS/ NURSING ACTIONS	EVALUATION CRITERIA

4. Using the suggested nursing diagnoses listed here (or others you can think of), complete a nursing process for a patient with anorexia nervosa.

SUGGESTED NURSING DIAGNOSES

1. *Body Image Disturbance*
2. *Knowledge Deficit (Dietary Needs)*
3. *Self-Esteem, Chronic Low*
4. *Fluid Volume Deficit, Risk for*

ASSESSMENT/ DATA COLLECTION	NURSING DIAGNOSIS	PLAN/ GOAL	INTERVENTIONS/ NURSING ACTIONS	EVALUATION CRITERIA

TEST QUESTIONS ■ ■ ■

MULTIPLE CHOICE QUESTIONS

1. The eating disorder that is characterized as an aversion to food is called:
   A. Morbid obesity
   B. Bulimia nervosa
   C. Anorexia nervosa
   D. Pica

2. The group of Americans that appears to have the highest percentage of obesity is:
   A. White Americans
   B. Hispanic Americans
   C. Asian Americans
   D. African Americans

3. Your 19-year-old patient has a diagnosis of anorexia nervosa. You notice that she seems to spend more time playing with her food than eating it. You know that patients with anorexia:

    A. Will eat normally if ignored
    B. Fear being fat
    C. Have an accurate body image
    D. Will binge and purge

4. An appropriate nursing diagnosis for a patient with anorexia might be:
    A. Altered nutrition; less than required amount, as evidenced by disinterest in eating
    B. Altered nutrition; more than required amount, as evidenced by eating meals of 2000 calories or more six to seven times per day
    C. Altered body image as evidenced by stating the wish that others look as good as the patient
    D. Fluid excess related to increased weight gain

5. A key nursing intervention to help patients with eating disorders is:
    A. Let the patient know he or she will be watched closely at mealtimes.
    B. Have the patient chart his or her own intake and output.
    C. Insist that the patient stay with a staff person for 2 hours after each meal.
    D. Encourage the patient to express underlying feelings about food, body image, and self-worth.

6. Bulimia nervosa is characterized by all the following *except:*
    A. Binging on food
    B. Purging the food after eating it
    C. Being able to control eating pattern
    D. Obsession with body shape and size

7. Donald has just been admitted to your surgical unit. He has had stomach stapling surgery. You prepare your list of postoperative cares and you include therapeutic communication statements such as:
    A. "You must be so relieved to be on your way to being thin."
    B. "What is the first meal you plan to eat?"
    C. "I'm interested to know if the rest of your family is also heavy?"
    D. "I'm here to help you any way I can."

8. It is Donald's second postoperative day. He is scheduled to have his first oral liquids. As you check on his progress at lunch, you note he hasn't touched his food. "I'm afraid to eat," he tells you. Your response might be:
    A. "It's OK for you to eat now. You won't choke."
    B. "Afraid to eat, meaning...?"
    C. "It's important that you eat, or the doctor may need to order the IV feedings again."
    D. "Why are you afraid to eat?"

9. Your new admission, a14-year-old female, presents with multiple symptoms including recent extreme dieting, use of laxatives and diuretics, thoughts of suicide, impulsive behavior, and erosion of the enamel on her teeth. The patient's medical diagnosis is _____

CHAPTER 19

Suicide

Learning Objectives ■ ■ ■

1. Identify main populations at risk for suicide.
2. Consider religious and cultural views of suicide.
3. Identify myths and truths about suicide.
4. Identify warning signs of suicide.
5. Identify nursing care for people who are suicidal.

Key Terms ■ ■ ■

- Suicide
- Suicide contract
- Suicide pact

Suicide is "the act or an instance of taking one's own life voluntarily and intentionally especially by a person of years of discretion and of sound mind" (Webster Online, 2004). Suicide is occurring more frequently in our society today. Estimates vary according to the various agencies that publish those numbers. It is a safe estimate that approximately 39 percent of people over age 65 try to commit suicide. Suicide is the third leading cause of death among adolescent and young adult Americans. It is estimated that 500,000 suicide attempts occur in this country annually and that approximately 30,000 of those attempts are successful (Shives and Isaacs, 2002).

This topic, once one that people preferred to ignore, is now a civil rights issue. People are demanding the right to choose to end their life when the quality of that life is unac-

ceptable. Legal cases are cited that make physicians liable for successful suicides, especially when the patient has attempted suicide previously. These cases were the beginning of the duty to warn of potential suicide. Today, physician-assisted suicide is happening and is being tested again in the legal system. A popular television show of the 1970s and 1980s, *M*A*S*H*, used the theme song "Suicide Is Painless." Suicide is also permanent and is becoming an option for certain populations in the United States.

People elect to make this choice for many reasons. Depression is a major cause. People with a terminal illness often consider suicide as the only way to carry out the remainder of their life and their death with dignity. The elderly, especially elderly white men, have difficulty dealing with loss, loneliness, and depression and sometimes look

U.S. Suicide Statistics (2001): Breakdown by Gender, Ethnicity, and Age

	NUMBER	PER DAY	RATE PER 100,000	PERCENTAGE OF DEATHS
Total	30,622	83.9	10.8	1.3
Males	24,672	67.6	17.6	2.1
Females	5,950	16.3	4.1	0.5
Whites	27,710	75.9	11.9	1.3
Nonwhites	2,912	8.0	5.6	0.9
Blacks	1,957	5.4	5.3	0.7
Elderly (65+ yrs)	5,393	14.8	15.3	0.3
Young (15–24 yrs)	3,971	10.9	9.9	12.3

for a means to terminate their life (Fig. 19-1). People who are unemployed and people who belong to minority groups are also at risk.

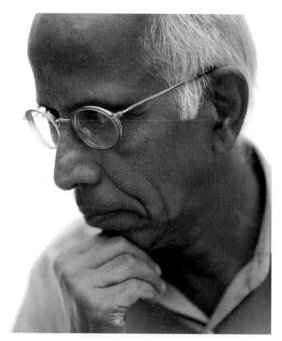

FIGURE 19-1. Older adults often have difficulty coping with loss, loneliness, and depression, and they have very high rates of suicide.

Teenagers are taking their own lives in growing numbers and overwhelmingly state feelings of anger and frustration about not being listened to or not being taken seriously as the reason for their actions (Fig. 19-2). **Suicide pacts** or "copycat suicides" among some adolescent groups and some religious groups may be a reason for the increase in these suicides (Came, 1994). Statistics from one study compared the rates of suicide in teenagers ages 15 to 19 in seven countries during the years 1962 to 1992. Canadian numbers have increased at a rate of 13.5 percent. That is just slightly higher than the rate for teens in the United States, which increased 11.1 percent over those same years (Came, 1994). Throughout all these groups runs the possibility for alcohol and chemical abuse in addition to other problems that seem insurmountable to the person considering taking his or her own life.

Religion and culture may influence one's outlook on suicide, just as it may affect the chance of our patient's attempting it. For example, it may be more honorable to orchestrate one's own death than to bring dishonor to the homeland. A religion may refuse to bury someone in the church or with the full blessing of the particular religion if that person died as a result of suicide. Terrorist acts by some radical groups, seemingly on the rise in recent years, demonstrate this kind of suicide. These groups profess an extreme hatred toward other groups of people and claim that it is a holy war they are fighting, as demanded by their religion. The tragedy, of course, is the large numbers of innocent people victimized by those who believe they are doing their religious duty. Understanding any group's or individual's motives for taking his or her life along with the lives of many others is often confusing at best and seems to foster more anger and mistrust of people assumed to be associated with those groups. Reactions to these "suicide bombings" are highly emotional and often prejudicial. The chance of a nurse being assigned to care for someone involved in such attacks is today very probable. Nurses will be asked once again to take stock of their beliefs and limits and to remember we are caring for the human being, not the "terrorist." Nurses are not exempt from the post-traumatic effects of tragedy. We are highly trained, true, but we are still parents, friends, siblings, and

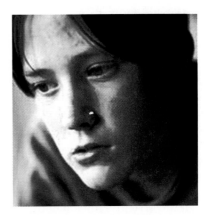

FIGURE 19-2. Suicides among teenagers are growing alarmingly. Many of the teens who attempt suicide state feelings of anger and frustration about not being listened to or not being taken seriously as the reason for their action. (Courtesy of Centers for Disease Control and Prevention, National Center for Injury Prevention and Control, Atlanta, GA.)

humans who experience the same pain and fear as everyone else. Some facilities provide grief counseling for employees. Please be sure to seek assistance if necessary.

In nonhospitalized people, the most common methods of suicide are shooting oneself with a gun, overdosing with medications,

U.S. Suicide Statistics (2001): Suicide Methods

	NUMBER	RATE PER 100,000	PERCENTAGE OF TOTAL
Firearms	16,869	5.9	55.1
All Other Methods	13,753	4.8	49.9
Hanging or Suffocation	6,198	2.2	20.2
Poisoning	5,191	1.8	17.0
Falls	651	0.2	2.1
Cutting/Piercing	458	0.2	1.5
Drowning	339	0.1	1.1
Fire	147	0.1	0.5

frequently taking prescription drugs, and hanging. Men tend to choose the more violent types of ending their lives; women tend to choose the overdose method. This may be one reason for the statistics showing that men kill themselves more frequently than do women. People who have overdosed have a better chance of being found alive, which makes intervention possible.

Some truths and myths about suicide are shown in Table 19-1.

What are some of the signs and symptoms? How do you know whether or not your patient is suicidal? Some of the signs and symptoms are

1. *Noticeable improvement in mood occurs:* When this happens, it is often a sign that the person has made the decision that has been causing personal conflict. The pain that is being experienced will soon be over for that person. The feelings of those who will be left behind may or may not be a consideration. It has been said that

suicide is the ultimate controller. For some people, this may be the only situation they have felt they could control in their lives. Some people are not concerned about the survivors because their own pain overrides that of others. Some people, especially young people, don't truly understand that death is final. Television, movies, and computer games that show death often do so in a way that is glamorous or humorous, and young people do not make the connection between the fantasy of the media and the reality of life.

2. *Person starts giving away personal items:* When someone has made the decision to terminate his or her own life, it becomes no longer necessary to keep certain things. Some people will even attempt to give away a beloved pet. However, these individuals do want those items cared for. In an attempt to "tie up loose ends," they decide who will get certain items. The items will be given away for reasons

TABLE 19-1	*Myths and Truths about Suicide*
MYTHS	**TRUTHS**
1. Most people who are suicidal do not leave suicide notes.	1. Approximately 80% do leave a note.
2. Children are not at risk for attempting suicide.	2. Children *do* attempt suicide. They often do not have the means to be successful, however. They will use aspirin or similar substances to attempt an overdose.
3. Once a person has attempted suicide and has been stopped, the person will not attempt suicide again.	3. If someone is convinced that suicide is the only option, chances are good that he or she will attempt several times and may be successful if intervention is not successful.
4. Suicide happens when the person is in the depths of depression.	4. It is more likely that the patient will appear happier just before suicide. When people are deeply depressed, they may lack the energy and motivation to end their lives.
5. People who slit their wrists or use pills are just asking for attention. They are not really serious about suicide.	5. It is true that these are slower methods of death; however, *all suicide attempts should be taken seriously.* Chances are that these people are asking for help and can be helped if we take them seriously at this point.

other than "because I am going to kill myself," although people sometimes use that honest approach and are not taken seriously. Usually, these persons will simply say that it's time to clean out a certain room or that they no longer need a certain item and they would like it to go to a special friend. Individuals may also write or change a will when contemplating suicide.

3. *Person starts talking about death and suicide or becomes preoccupied with learning about these things:* Curiosity about death is not unusual. People tend to be curious about what they don't know (even nursing students who are learning about mental health and mental illness!). When this curiosity becomes a preoccupation and a single thought for the patient, it signals that the person has ideas of attempting suicide. Reporting this to the charge nurse and documenting the concerns are required.

4. *Person has difficulty sleeping or awakens frequently very early in the morning:* This symptom is especially true for adolescent and adult patients. Older adults generally require less sleep or take frequent naps to meet their sleep needs. Young children may have problems sleeping, especially in unfamiliar environments. Episodes of sleep difficulty should never be ignored; be especially cautious if difficulty occurs in those in age groups who normally sleep for a 6- to 8-hour period every night.

■ ALTERNATIVE TREATMENT FOR PATIENTS WHO ARE SUICIDAL

This is a very serious condition. Immediate intervention is crucial. Once the patient is past the crisis stage, therapy that addresses the underlying emotion would be appropriate. Treatments that teach the patient how to help him- or herself are the best choices. Therapy could include the following.

NEUROLINGUISTIC PROGRAMMING (NLP) AND BIOFEEDBACK

See Chapter 9 for specific information on these techniques. Helping the patient learn to put his or her problems into a different context may keep the patient from reaching the unpleasant place that leads to suicide attempts. It should be noted that the person must be committed to helping him- or herself and must work hard at resolving the problems leading up to the suicide attempt in the first place. Biofeedback and NLP should be used in conjunction with other modalities, such as medication, as directed by the physician.

■ NURSING CARE FOR PATIENTS WHO ARE SUICIDAL

Nursing responsibilities for patients who are suicidal are many. The goal, of course, is always to prevent the suicide. Because the nurse may not know when suicide potential exists, especially for a first attempt, using excellent observational skills and communication skills is mandatory. Nurses are bound (under the *Meier v. Ross General Hospital* case) to report any reasons they have to suspect the patient may be suicidal. You must enter your observations and actions in your documentation for this patient.

1. *Monitoring frequently:* Every 10 to 15 minutes is the usual interval for monitoring suicidal patients. Note any changes in the person's grooming and dietary habits. Loss of interest in self-care may be a sign that someone is slipping deeper into depression or schizophrenia and may be at higher risk for suicide attempt.

2. *Safety:* Keep any potentially harmful items from the patient, such as knives, scissors, glass, razor blades, belts, nail files, electrical cords, and linens. It is common for patients who are considered suicidal to wear paper gowns and to have paper bedding. Some patients find a way to become wet over their entire body and then attempt to electrocute themselves by holding onto a metal object and sticking it in an electrical outlet.

3. *Medications:* Always be sure your patient has swallowed all medications. Patients find ways to "pocket" medications in their cheeks, roof of their mouth, or under their tongue and then save them until they think they have enough to successfully end their lives.

4. *Communication:* Listen to the physical concerns of the patient. The physical manifestations may be the method of communicating the desire to commit suicide. Ask outright if the person is considering suicide and, if so, how and when. Ask about any specific plan the individual may have. Also ask if this patient has attempted suicide in the past.

5. *Contract:* Develop a **suicide contract** with your patient. Sometimes this is enough to allow the patient to feel responsible and respected. In a suicide contract, the nurse and patient work out a system by which the patient will seek out a staff person (or a significant other) when he or she feels suicidal.

6. *Crisis intervention:* Review the information on crisis. Suicide is certainly a crisis situation. Nurses must be ready to think on their feet, perform professionally, and remain calm through it all.

Medical and therapeutic management of patients who have attempted suicide depends on the individual and the extenuating circumstances. The person may be taking an antidepressant medication. The type of therapy might include individual, group, or family therapy, and possibly all three types. Self-esteem and alternative methods for dealing with emotional pain should be discussed and practiced by the patient. Family and significant others may need to learn to reshape their relationship and change their methods of communication. Honesty is emphasized as an important basis for healing.

Table 19-2 summarizes symptoms or warning signs of suicide and nursing interventions for people who are suicidal.

TABLE 19-2 ■ *Suicide*	
SYMPTOMS OR WARNING SIGNS	**NURSING INTERVENTIONS**
■ Noticeable improvement in mood	■ Monitor frequently (every 15 minutes).
■ Giving away personal items	■ Provide safe milieu.
■ Preoccupation with talking or learning about suicide	■ Be certain that medications are swallowed.
■ Difficulty sleeping	■ Use effective, therapeutic communication.
■ Frequent very early morning awakening	■ Initiate a suicide contract.
	■ Implement crisis intervention when necessary.

Key Concepts ■ ■ ■

1. Suicide is listed as a leading cause of death among different risk groups in the United States. It crosses cultural, age, gender, and socioeconomic boundaries.
2. Many myths and diverse belief systems are related to suicide. Nurses must be aware of the facts and understand the warning signs that may signal suicide.
3. Safety, communication, and excellent nursing skills may be the tools to prevent a suicide. Using care with medications when working with people at risk for suicide is crucial.

REFERENCES

Came, B. (1994). The last trip. Three teens die in a shocking suicide. *Macleans'* (Canada), October 31, p. 14.

Montross, L., et al. (2003, August) Preventing late life suicide: 6 steps to detect the warning signs. *Current Psychiatry Online, 2*(8).

Shives, L.R. and Isaacs, A. (2002). *Basic Concepts of Psychiatric-Mental Health Nursing*, 3rd ed. JB Lippincott, Philadelphia.

WEBSITES

www.mentalhealth.org/suicideprevention
www.cdc.gov/ncipc/factsheets/suifacts.htm
www.currentpsychiatry.com
http://preventsuicidenow.com/suicide-statistics.html

CRITICAL THINKING EXERCISES ■ ■ ■

1. You are at home alone and the telephone rings. It is your best friend, "just calling to say goodbye. I just took a whole bottle of pills and I want to go to sleep. Talk to me until I go to sleep, please. You've always been there for me; help me to sleep now." What will you do? What will you say to this friend? Whom will you get to intervene? What are your feelings about your friend?

2. A patient in your facility is found unconscious. Heart rate is 50, pulse is 8 and thready, blood pressure is 90/40. The paramedics transport the patient to the local emergency department. The patient is revived. Results of the workup show large quantities of an antidepressant medication that is given to several patients on that wing. You remember seeing the patient near the medication cart on several occasions recently. Your supervisor has been making the med passes on that wing to help out while the other regular staff nurse is on vacation. What actions will you pursue?

3. Your family practice clinic is located within a larger hospital in a mid-sized town. It is a beautiful Tuesday morning. You are rooming patients as usual. It is a very busy day and the waiting room is full. Your daycare is also in this facility and your 3 year old is there today. He has the sniffles. You are con-

cerned he may be coming down with something. While you are thinking about your child, you assist Patient X to his room, take his vital signs, and offer him his gown to prepare for the doctor to come in for the physical evaluation of Patient X's respiratory symptoms. Patient X takes off his shirt, reveals a device of some sort attached to his chest and instructs you not to leave the room or he will set off the bomb immediately. What are you feeling right now? What actions can you take? What communication skills, especially those pertaining to suicide, will you use with Patient X?

4. Using the suggested nursing diagnoses listed here (or others you can think of), complete a nursing process for your friend in exercise 1.

SUGGESTED NURSING DIAGNOSES

1. *Self-Esteem, Chronic Low*
2. *Hopelessness*
3. *Violence, Risk for: Self-Directed or directed at others*
4. *Fear*
5. *Anxiety*

ASSESSMENT/ DATA COLLECTION	NURSING DIAGNOSIS	PLAN/ GOAL	INTERVENTIONS/ NURSING ACTIONS	EVALUATION CRITERIA

5. Using the suggested nursing diagnoses listed here (or others you can think of), complete a nursing process for the patient in exercise 2.

SUGGESTED NURSING DIAGNOSES

1. *Individual Coping, Ineffective*
2. *Thought Processes, Altered*
3. *Poisoning, Risk for*

ASSESSMENT/ DATA COLLECTION	NURSING DIAGNOSIS	PLAN/ GOAL	INTERVENTIONS/ NURSING ACTIONS	EVALUATION CRITERIA

TEST QUESTIONS ■ ■ ■

MULTIPLE CHOICE QUESTIONS

1. A nursing intervention that is appropriate for a patient who is suicidal is:
   A. Report the patient to the police.
   B. Ignore the patient's suicidal comments, considering them "attention getting."
   C. Tell the patient that he or she "has so much to live for!"
   D. Teach healthier problem-solving skills.

2. A person is more likely to commit suicide when he or she:
   A. Is in deepest depression
   B. Is apparently feeling "better"
   C. Is confused
   D. Is feeling loved and appreciated

3. Your patient tells you, "I am just a burden. Everyone would be better off if I was dead." Nurses are aware that:
   A. Suicide talk is just an attention-getting device.
   B. Suicide is an impulsive act; it is not thought out.
   C. Suicidal talk or ideation can lead to suicidal behavior.
   D. Suicidal people seldom really attempt suicide.

4. Mr. P is brought to the hospital by his wife. She states that he has been treated for depression recently but that tonight he is saying that "you and the kids don't need me messing up your lives." Mr. P tells you he has been thinking about suicide for some time now. A nursing diagnosis for Mr. P would be:
   A. Knowledge deficit related to family needs
   B. Ineffective individual coping as evidenced by manipulation of wife's feelings

    C. Anxiety related to hospitalization

    D. Potential for violence, self-directed, as evidenced by stating suicidal thoughts

5. Your charge nurse tells you that Mr. P must be placed on suicide precautions. The first intervention you begin is:

    A. Place Mr. P in a locked unit.

    B. Begin one-on-one observation at least every 15 minutes.

    C. Call the security code over the public address system.

    D. Allow Mr. P to shave and carry out his bedtime cares.

6. Further discussion with Mr. P reveals he is of a religious sect that believes there is honor in dying for one's religion. He does not understand why everyone is so afraid to die in this country. As his nurse, you:

    A. Document the discussion and remove the suicide precautions, citing religious freedom

    B. Encourage him to present his beliefs at group tomorrow.

    C. Document the discussion but tell him that the suicide precautions remain in effect.

    D. Thank him for his explanation and bring him his next dose of medication.

7. All of your good techniques fail. At 2 AM, the RN doing rounds found Mr. P dead in his room. The unit plans a debriefing for the other patients and a separate one for staff. It is believed another resident "smuggled" the items to Mr. P to make it possible for him to end his life. In the debriefing you learn:

    A. A person with a strong suicide plan will usually be successful.

    B. Not every suicide will provide a note.

    C. Religious and cultural beliefs are very strong predictors of behavior in certain individuals.

    D. All of the above.

8. You are working second shift in a small, rural hospital. It is about 10 PM. There has been an industrial accident. Details are sketchy, but your hospital is preparing to admit about 30 people. As they arrive and are triaged, you note a diverse group of injured people; many of them seem to be of Mid-Eastern or African descent. You are assigned to admit a 21-year-old man who claims to be from Iraq. He answers no other questions, but repeats a religious phrase over and over. You assume he has been severely injured, but your supervisor directs you to stay at his side and place him on suicide precautions. You are confused, but follow directions. What data will you be watching for with this particular patient as it may relate to a suicide threat? What is the rationale for that piece of data? There is no specific number of "correct" possibilities.

Data Rationale:

1.

2.

3.

20

Dissociative Disorders

Learning Objectives ■ ■ ■

1. Define dissociative disorders.
2. List four dissociative disorders.
3. Define multiple personality disorder (MPD)/dissociative identity disorder (DID).
4. List possible causes of MPD/DID.
5. State possible medical treatment for people with MPD/DID.
6. State nursing care for people with MPD/DID.

Key Term ■ ■ ■

■ Dissociate

Dissociative disorders are very rare. Perhaps because of the media play they have been receiving lately, they are beginning to be more frequently diagnosed. Movies such as *Dr. Jekyll and Mr. Hyde, The Three Faces of Eve,* and *Sybil,* books such as *When Rabbit Howls,* and even some TV soap operas have focused on the multiple personality disorder in their main character.

In persons with dissociative disorders, it is believed that ideas split off from the personality and become buried in the unconscious. It is the result of severe overuse of the defense mechanism of dissociation. People with dissociative disorders are not aware that they have a disorder until it is brought to their attention—usually quite abruptly.

This text does not go into depth describing this group of illnesses but mentions them very briefly.

■ ETIOLOGIC THEORIES

Psychogenic means from a psychological or emotional rather than an organic cause. It is believed that anxiety or severe psychological trauma is the underlying cause of the dissociative disorders. Individuals who develop the ability to **dissociate** are thought to have created the other personalities or conditions in an effort to separate from their severe emotional pain.

Some theories suggest possible biologic influences, but these are inconclusive at present. Ross, Anderson, Heber, and Norton

(1990) found a significant number of cases of multiple personality disorder in prostitutes and exotic dancers. Kluft (1987) began studying jailed male sex offenders and also found a proportionately large number of cases in that population. Today, there is continuing debate on the very existence of this disorder. Because *DSM-IV-TR* and other nursing texts continue to discuss the topic, and because the behaviors certainly do exist within the population, we will continue a discussion on dissociative disorders here.

■ TYPES

Four types of dissociative disorders exist: psychogenic amnesia, psychogenic fugue, depersonalization disorder, and multiple personality disorder. Each has its own set of symptoms, yet the medical and nursing care of people with these disorders is very similar.

PSYCHOGENIC AMNESIA

Psychogenic amnesia is the sudden inability to recall personal information as a result of some physical or psychological trauma. It is not organic. It goes beyond ordinary forgetfulness and is not the kind of memory dysfunction found in dementia. It is seen more frequently in adolescents and young women. Symptoms of psychogenic amnesia are wandering, confusion, and disorientation. The condition is usually temporary.

PSYCHOGENIC FUGUE

Psychogenic fugue is even more dramatic in its symptoms than psychogenic amnesia. People who have psychogenic fugue often suddenly leave town and take on a new identity, which fools people for a short time. The person does not appear to be confused or disoriented. It takes time before the stories get mixed up or do not flow well together.

This usually tips off someone that the person is not quite "right."

Psychogenic fugue is also usually short lived. It lasts a few hours to a few days. Psychogenic fugue usually follows some sort of severe stress and is often triggered by alcohol use. It reverses quickly with therapy most of the time, and once the patient has recovered, it is rare for this condition to recur.

DEPERSONALIZATION DISORDER

This disorder usually affects people under age 40. In depersonalization disorder, the person remains oriented to person, place, and time, but the perception of reality has changed. The patient with this disorder can talk about it somewhat, often describing the feeling that he or she is "floating" or "out of my body." The perceptual change may relate to the person's identity or to parts of the body. The patient may express the fear of "going crazy." It is quite possible that the person will attempt suicide.

Depersonalization disorder can coincide with other disorders such as schizophrenia, personality disorders, and seizure disorders.

MULTIPLE PERSONALITY DISORDER OR DISSOCIATIVE IDENTITY DISORDER

We must begin this section with yet another caveat: depending on the professional offering information, these two disorders may or may not be the same disorder! For purposes of this text and the population of nurses to whom it is directed, multiple personality disorder and dissociative identity disorder will be considered one and the same.

In multiple personality disorder (MPD), or dissociative identity disorder (DID), two or more completely separate personalities exist within one body. These personalities are usually quite opposite from the dominant or primary personality—so different that they can be different sexes, can have different medical diagnoses, and even manifest with different eye color. The mechanisms that allow differences of eye color or of one personality to be diabetic while another (in the same body) is *not* diabetic are unknown. This type of phenomenon, however, has been documented.

No matter how many personalities are living within one body, the main, or primary, personality is the one that is "forward" most of the time. The primary personality has no knowledge of the other parts, or "alters," as they are called. The other personalities all know each other, as well as the primary personality, however.

Confused? Imagine that your best friend, Pat, is a kind, gentle, loving person. That is the personality that is "forward" most of the time and the person you work with and share with. All of a sudden, you and Pat are at the mall and Pat's personality changes. Pat has a different voice and a different walking gait. You say, "Pat, are you all right?" and, to your amazement, Pat says, "I'm not Pat! Pat's a bore. I'm Chris and I'm a lot more fun! Let's blow this place!" You, of course, are stunned and probably at a loss over what to do. Now, imagine that "Chris" is also the opposite gender of "Pat." As time passes, you meet several other "parts" of Pat. When Pat is "forward," he or she has no idea that "Chris" or anyone else was there. Pat may well think that you are the one who needs help!

The "alters" all are their own identities and they have all split from Pat. Current thinking is that the real Pat probably had some horrible trauma early in life that caused the other parts to develop. Frequently, this trauma is related to physical or sexual abuse and the split developed as a mechanism to escape the pain and guilt of what happened.

The goal of treatment for people with MPD/DID is ideally to integrate the personalities into one personality or into as few personalities as possible. This can take years of work. If the cause can be found, then appropriate psychotherapy can help the person in an effort to prevent recurrence of the "alters."

■ MEDICAL TREATMENT FOR PATIENTS WITH DISSOCIATIVE DISORDERS

Medications, usually of the antianxiety classification, are ordered for many people with dissociative disorders. Sedatives, mood elevators, and antidepressants are also effective for some patients.

Psychotherapy is used individually and possibly in groups. Hypnotherapy is also quite effective in treating individuals with dissociative disorders. A hypnotherapist in many instances can help the patient explore those other sides of the self that are painful and repressed.

ALTERNATIVE TREATMENT FOR PATIENTS WITH DISSOCIATIVE DISORDERS

Depending on the person's emotional state, methods that stabilize into reality are most appropriate. Care under a trained professional would be appropriate, especially soon after the episode. Independent alternative treatment could include biofeedback and aromatherapy.

■ NURSING INTERVENTIONS FOR PATIENTS WITH DISSOCIATIVE DISORDERS

1. *Focus on short-term goals:* It is believed that several small successes will help to integrate the personality into a better, overall healthier state.
2. *Maintain a calm milieu:* Reducing anxiety is a major goal in treating these types of illnesses.
3. *Keep communication open:* Encourage the patient to verbalize thoughts, feelings, and concerns. If you are working with a patient who has MPD, address the "alter" by his or her name, not by the name of the primary personality,

unless advised to do so by the physician. Document very carefully the interaction with the "alter" and the activities that directly preceded and followed the presence of that personality.

4. *Observe for signs of suicidal thought:* This will be especially appropriate for patients with depersonalization disorder and MPD. The feeling of being "crazy" or the personality of any of the "alters" can result in suicidal thoughts. The nurse's responsibility is to observe and be alert for any signs of suicidal thoughts and to take the appropriate precautions.

5. *Document any changes in behavior:* Never assume that what you observe in a patient is insignificant. Document any and all changes that you perceive in the patient's behaviors and attitudes.

Table 20-1 summarizes the symptoms and nursing interventions for the dissociative disorders discussed here.

TABLE 20-1 ■ *Dissociative Disorders*		
TYPE	**SYMPTOMS**	**NURSING INTERVENTIONS**
PSYCHOGENIC AMNESIA	■ Sudden inability to recall personal information ■ Not organic ■ Goes beyond ordinary forgetfulness ■ Not dementia ■ Seen more frequently in adolescents and young women ■ Wandering ■ Confusion; disorientation ■ Usually temporary	■ Maintain calm milieu. ■ Maintain open communication; speak to the personality who is "forward." ■ Focus on short-term goals and small successes. ■ Observe for suicidal ideation. ■ Document all changes in condition.
PSYCHOGENIC FUGUE	■ Taking on "new identity," apparently not confused or disoriented ■ Lasts a few hours to a few days ■ Usually follows some sort of severe stress; often triggered by alcohol use	■ Same as for "Psychogenic Amnesia."
DEPERSONALIZATION DISORDER	■ Usually affects people under age 40 ■ Remains oriented to person, place, and time, but perception of reality has changed ■ Able to talk about condition somewhat; describes the feeling as one of "floating" or "out of my body" ■ May relate to their identity or to parts of their body	■ Same as for "Psychogenic Amnesia."

(continued)

TYPE	SYMPTOMS	NURSING INTERVENTIONS
	■ Expresses the fear of "going crazy" ■ May attempt suicide	
MULTIPLE PERSONALITY DISORDER/ DISSOCIATIVE IDENTITY DISORDER	■ Two or more completely separate personalities within one body ■ Primary personality having no knowledge of the other "parts" or "alters"	■ Same as for "Psychogenic Amnesia."

Key Concepts ▪ ▪ ▪

1. Dissociative disorders occur very rarely.
2. Theories relating to the underlying causes of dissociative disorders revolve around psychological or emotional issues rather than physical or biologic issues at the present time. Biologic etiologies are being considered, however.
3. Careful nursing assessment and communication skills are important tools in nursing care for people with dissociative disorders.
4. Medical treatment for dissociative disorders includes medications, psychotherapy, and hypnotherapy.

REFERENCES

4Women.gov. (2004). Women with disabilities—dissociatve disorders. http://www.4woman.gov/wwd/wwd.cfm?page=45.

Kluft, R.P. (1987). First rank symptoms as a diagnostic clue to multiple personality disorder. *American Journal of Psychiatry, 144,* 293–298.

Ross, C.A., Anderson, G., Heber, S., and Norton, G.R. (1990). Dissociation and abuse among multiple personality patients, prostitutes, and exotic dancers. *Hospital Community Psychiatry, 41,* 328.

WEBSITES

www.sidran.org/didbr.html
www.4woman.gov/wwd

CRITICAL THINKING EXERCISES ▪ ▪ ▪

1. Read the case study of Shirley, which follows. As the nurse caring for her when she returns, what questions might you consider including in your assessment? What communication skills will you want to use with her? Using the suggested nursing diagnoses listed here (or others you can think of), complete a nursing process for Shirley.

CASE STUDY 1

Shirley is a 32-year-old mother of three children. She has been married and divorced four times. Shirley suddenly disappeared and was found 3 days later in a town several states away from where she lived with her current husband and children.

Shirley was "discovered" when she began working at a local fast-food chain restaurant. The stories she told to different coworkers were inconsistent. The coworkers began asking her specific questions about her background, which she was either unwilling or unable to answer. Shirley's husband has reported her as a missing person, and, through the flyers and the media, it was soon decided that Shirley was that missing person. Her husband and the local authorities joined the medical team that was dispatched to return Shirley to her husband and family.

SUGGESTED NURSING DIAGNOSES

1. *Denial, Ineffective*
2. *Post-Trauma Syndrome*
3. *Individual Coping, Ineffective*

ASSESSMENT/ DATA COLLECTION	NURSING DIAGNOSIS	PLAN/ GOAL	INTERVENTIONS/ NURSING ACTIONS	EVALUATION CRITERIA

2. Read the case study of Peter, which follows. Using the suggested nursing diagnoses listed here (or others you can think of), complete a nursing process for Peter.

CASE STUDY 2

Peter is a 40-year-old business professional. He is the owner of his own business, which has been very successful for him. Peter has very few close friends, largely because his behavior has always been erratic. Recently, Peter was arrested for disorderly conduct in a local bar. Much to his embarrassment, Peter was dressed in women's clothing and identified himself as "Marti" when questioned by the police.

After a physical examination and psychological workup, Peter received a temporary diagnosis of dissociative identity disorder (also known as multiple personality disorder). More psychologic testing will be done with "Peter."

SUGGESTED NURSING DIAGNOSES

1. *Personal Identity Disturbance*
2. *Social Interaction, Impaired*
3. *Individual Coping, Ineffective*

ASSESSMENT/ DATA COLLECTION	NURSING DIAGNOSIS	PLAN/ GOAL	INTERVENTIONS/ NURSING ACTIONS	EVALUATION CRITERIA

TEST QUESTIONS ■ ■ ■

MULTIPLE CHOICE QUESTIONS

1. Peter is admitted to your unit in severe diabetic crisis. You note in his chart that he also has multiple personality disorder. You understand that MPD:

   A. Is consciously created to avoid stress
   B. Is an unconscious maladaptive response
   C. Is done to manipulate the feelings of significant others
   D. Is fairly easy to treat

2. When you go in to check on Peter one-half hour later, he is calm. His skin is of normal temperature and color. You call him by name, but "Marti" answers. You perform his glucometer check, and his glucose level has gone from 600 to 112 within that half hour. "Marti" informs you that *she* is not diabetic. You document:

   A. "Patient confused and disoriented. Refers to self as 'Marti.'"
   B. "Glucometer reading is 112. 'Marti' is responding. Skin is normal temperature and color—no flushing noted."

C. "Hallucination related to drastic drop in blood sugar as evidenced by referring to self by incorrect name."

D. "Denial related to situation as evidenced by stating: I don't have diabetes."

3. You know that the goal of treatment for this patient is:

A. Integration of personalities

B. Hopeless; nothing can be done

C. Easy, with antianxiety medications and psychotherapy

D. Accomplished only when the primary personality is "forward"

4. Which of the following is not a *dissociative* disorder?

A. Psychogenic fugue

B. Psychogenic amnesia

C. Obsessive-compulsive disorder

D. Multiple personality disorder

5. The main symptom of psychogenic amnesia is:

A. Sudden inability to recall personal information

B. Development of one or more distinctive personalities

C. Selective forgetfulness

D. Altered perception of reality

3

Special Populations

CHAPTER

21

Childhood and Adolescent Issues in Mental Health

Learning Objectives ■ ■ ■

1. Identify child and adolescent populations at risk for mental health disorders.
2. Define selected mental health conditions of childhood/adolescent age groups.
3. Identify treatment modalities used in childhood/adolescent age groups.
4. Identify age-appropriate nursing care for selected mental health issues.

Key Terms ■ ■ ■

- ■ ADHD
- ■ Adolescence
- ■ Autism
- ■ Childhood
- ■ Encopresis
- ■ Enuresis
- ■ Mental Retardation
- ■ Schizophrenia

In the world of neurology, professionals are beginning to ponder and study the possibility that today's young people are actually growing up with differently wired brains than those of their parents. The seemingly endless hours spent on computers and with computerized games seems to support a theory that brains are being stimulated differently and may, in fact, be chemically rewriting the brain's "schematic." If that proves true, then in the not-so-distant future, behaviors that today are termed "disorders" of childhood or adolescence may, in reality, become "norms." Once again, stay tuned! This text, however, is

about psychology and what is considered normal or not in real time!

Whether a sign of the social times, or whether part of human evolvement in the world, children and adolescents are growing up faster and with harsher realities of life than even their parents experienced. Times change quickly. Children are growing up sooner. Physically, they are maturing sooner and although they want to behave, dress, and experience things as their peers, older siblings, and parents do, it seems that younger people are still not mentally and emotionally prepared for life as it happens today. Who could have predicted Columbine? Who could have predicted the terror of September 11, 2001, and who could successfully avoid the continuous bombardment of the terror presented by the worldwide media? Violence is portrayed in television shows and videos targeted for younger populations. In the younger mind, it is not always easy to distinguish reality from fantasy or "make-believe."

Parents are also under additional stress. Jobs come and go at breakneck speed. Money and budgets are stretched beyond maximum. Children are no longer satisfied with anything but the best, and parents, for the most part, try very hard to provide that for their family. Sometimes the stress is out of control and people begin hurting those they love. Child abuse, abductions, and kidnappings are becoming all too common in the news today. Children hurting children by bullying or worse is becoming more frequent.

Tragically, mental health issues are not reserved for adults. Children are affected each and every day by the same stressors as adults, but in differing degrees and often with different manifestations. Children, depending on their age and ability, may not know how to verbalize a fear or concern and may repress the emotion rather than try to express it. Mental illness in children is a contributor to children not succeeding in school or in social interactions.

■ DEMOGRAPHICS: GROUPS OF CHILDREN AT HIGH RISK FOR DEVELOPING MENTAL HEALTH DISORDERS

What groups of children seem to be at highest risk for developing mental health disorders?

Today, children are displaying behaviors and being diagnosed with mental illnesses that two or three generations ago were nonexistent or at least not so readily observed in society. Popular estimates of people ages 9–17 who develop a mental health disorder is approximately 21% in the United States. It is important for nurses to remember that age is defined not only in chronological years, but also in developmental years. This chapter provides nurses with basic information on some of those illnesses. It also provides some tips for assisting parents of those children.

Children and adolescents who are at risk for developing a mental health disorder fall into the same demographic categories as adults with mental health disorders. Children with chronic illness or who have one or more disabilities, children born into poverty or certain minority/ethnic groups, children born of parents with addictive/abusive tendencies, children born to teenage parents, and children born to parents with certain genetic or biological disorders are those groups considered at highest risk for developing a threat to their mental health. Special age-appropriate testing tools, or inventories, have been developed for children and adolescents with threats to their mental health. Depending on the tool and the condition being tested, parents and school personnel (teachers) may also be asked to complete an inventory.

It is important to note that "mental retardation" is related to intellectual functioning and is not in and of itself a "mental illness." *DSM-IV-TR* defines "mental retardation" as "significantly subaverage general intellectual functioning that is accompanied by significant limitations in adaptive functioning," which must be in at least two of the following areas: communication, self-care, home living, social or interpersonal skills, use of community resources, self-direction, functional academic skills, work, leisure, health, and safety, with onset before age 18. Intelligence parameter is measured at IQ (intelligence quotient) of 70 or below and is measured by one of several standardized tests. Societal terms for "mental retardation" are "mentally challenged" and "developmentally challenged/delayed." Because impairments in adaptive functioning are frequently observed before IQ is determined, some professionals find it difficult to discuss "mental health/illness" without also including "mental retardation." For purposes of this book and the LPN/LVN scope of practice, discussions involving "mental retardation" will be kept to a minimum.

Before we address some childhood and adolescent mental health disorders, remember that cultural considerations must always be considered when working with people of any age who have mental health threats. *DSM-IV-TR* allows for cultural differences. Intelligence and behavior scales are adjusted to account for differences among cultures. One common example of a cultural and even gender-specific difference is the act of communicating. Some cultures will not or cannot speak a language comfortably. Individuals of that group may opt not to speak at all rather than risk being embarrassed personally or risk insulting the nurse or teacher or other figure they may actually respect. For example, a behavior being assessed in a child perhaps of Southeast Asian descent, may be "lack of verbal communication skills." The child may be of a developmental age at which speech would be expected, say 4 or 5 years of age. In this case, however, it may be a condition of culture rather than a symptom of a mental or developmental disorder.

■ CHILD ABUSE/NEGLECT

Abuse of children may take the form of sexual abuse, physical abuse, and/or emotional abuse. It is an act of *commission*, meaning an act of doing. Children are often terrified of reporting an act of abuse. The abuser is frequently a beloved relative, parent, or sibling. The child is afraid that it is his or her fault. Children are confused about what is happening and why. The abuser is often physically larger and therefore intimidating to a child.

"Shaken baby syndrome," which has been in the news far too frequently in recent years and months, is the condition of a baby being shaken so violently that severe head trauma, including subdural hematoma, cerebral edema, and retinal hemorrhage occur (Fig. 21-1). Frequently, death is the

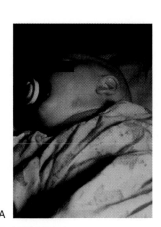
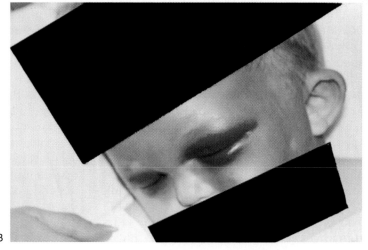

A   B

FIGURE 21-1. A, Bruise on the mandible of a victim of shaken baby syndrome (SBS). Any bruise on a nonambulatory infant is concerning and should warrant further search for other injuries. (Courtesy of Children's Hospital Boston Child Protection Team, Boston, MA.) B, Retinal hemorrhages and subdural hematomas are the hallmarks of SBS. What might appear to be only an orbital injury may be Battle's sign, indicating a potentially life-threatening basal skull fracture. (From Olson, Richard J., Child abuse primer for ophthalmologists, *Review of Ophthalmology*, www.revophth.com. Copyright Jobson Publishing, LLC. Reprinted with permission.)

outcome. Also frequently, it is the parent, relative, or primary caregiver who is the perpetrator of the abuse. The story is usually "I found the baby on the floor, not breathing," or "I moved the baby a little, but I certainly didn't shake the baby." In most states, nurses are mandatory reporters for suspected abuse.

Neglect is an act of *omission,* or of not doing something that should be done. Neglect may be manifested in children's not being fed or bathed, not being dressed appropriately, not being housed properly, or not being supervised and schooled if they are of school age. Any area in which a child's basic needs are not being met adequately and safely is an area of neglect.

Sexual abuse and exploitation of children is a discussion that could go on for a very long chapter. The Internet has many good qualities but it is a "safe" place for perpetrators to post child pornography. Adults and even other children and adolescents visit those Web sites. Many times, behavior then escalates from an act of voyeurism to actual need to commit the act. The young victim is usually a family member or has been entrusted to the care of the perpetrator. It may be an aunt, uncle, grandparent, neighbor, or teacher, but is most frequently someone known to the child and trusted by the child. The child or adolescent is, as in spousal abuse discussed in Chapter 23, usually physically weaker than the adult and is dependent on that individual. "This will be just our secret! Don't tell anyone, or the fun will have to stop." The perpetrator will spend time and money, and there is usually a pleasant time had by all, until the sexual abuse begins. The child is confused and unsure if it is right but believes the adult would not do anything wrong or hurtful. The cycle begins. It will continue for years sometimes, until the child becomes physically or financially secure enough to be able to confront the person committing the acts.

Children do not always have the words they need to express what is happening to them. They may be so fearful of the perpetrator that they say nothing. Or they try, but the person to whom they are talking is not understanding what the child is trying to say. Often, children will act out the abuse in their own play behaviors. Parents and nurses should watch children at play with a fresh set of eyes.

Also, sometimes the abuse is detected by accident on the part of the parent or caregiver. Blood in underwear, torn clothing, bruises or finger marks in unusual places, may be indicators of force, rough touch, or penetration and should be investigated. Nurses, as mentioned earlier, are considered mandatory reporters in most states. If this child is in your clinic and you have reason to suspect that the child is being abused, it is your duty to report your concern per your facility's policy for abuse reporting.

Children need to be taught "good touch" versus "bad touch" and to tell an adult when something is bothering them. Adults must then take the information seriously and attempt to help find the reason for the child's statements.

MEDICAL TREATMENT FOR CHILD AND ADOLESCENT SURVIVORS OF SEXUAL ABUSE

Medical treatment will depend on the type of abuse and the age of the child. Surgery, wound care, and medication are all probable treatments. The young abuse survivor may need to undergo testing for HIV and hepatitis B. If the child is a young woman who has entered or is near puberty, rape and pregnancy testing may be appropriate. It is possible that some perpetrators may have used drugs on these children. Blood testing may be done if that is a possibility, so that the child can be observed for signs of toxicity or addiction. Treatment would also include detoxification if necessary.

Medications could include antidepressants, antianxiety medications, antibiotics, and perhaps drugs to combat HIV/AIDS and hepatitis.

Counseling for mental trauma associated with physical or sexual abuse is also appropriate. Counseling may be done in conjunction with medication and may be one-on-one counseling, group counseling, or a combination of types of counseling. In very young children, therapists may use playing or drawing to help define the feelings of the patient. Playing and drawing may also be part of the treatment for very young patients (Fig. 21-2).

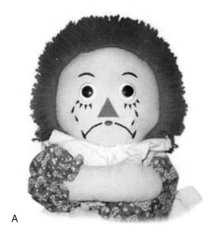

A

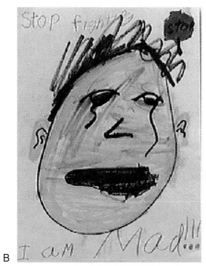

B

FIGURE 21-2. A, This "sad doll" is used to help very young children identify their feelings about abuse experiences. (Courtesy of T.A.L.K. Theatre, Seattle, WA.) B, Drawing may also be an important part of the treatment of young abuse victims. (From English, Susan, and Wohlmut, Thomas, Child Abuse in Stepfamilies: Is It Worse? www.stepfamily.net. Courtesy of Professor Stephen George.)

NURSING CARE FOR CHILD AND ADOLESCENT SURVIVORS OF SEXUAL ABUSE

Nurses may fill a variety of roles in treating young children who have been sexually abused. Nurses tend to have the trust of the child, who may then divulge information she or he is not comfortable divulging to other adults. Nurses may work actively with a care plan developed with mental health professionals and may be asked to observe for specific behaviors that would tell the mental health team if the child is progressing or not.

Some general nursing actions for working with children who have been sexually abused are

1. Communicate honestly and effectively and at an age-appropriate level.
2. Identify limits and boundaries. Some children may exhibit sexual acting-out types of behavior. Explain what is appropriate behavior and what is not acceptable.
3. Support the individual; encourage verbalization of feelings and thoughts.
4. Reinforce that the child is not to blame for the abuse inflicted on him or her.
5. Provide a safe environment for the child while in the nurse's care.

■ DEPRESSION IN CHILDREN AND ADOLESCENTS

DSM-IV-TR indicates that while it may be less common in these age groups, children and adolescents do exhibit symptoms of depression—particularly major depressive disorder, bipolar disorder, and dysthymic disorder. The symptoms are the same as in adult illness. There is some indication that adolescents who exhibit bipolar disorder may have been children with certain conduct disorders in earlier years. Estimates are that approximately 5% of children and up to 20% of adolescents in American society exhibit symptoms of depression. The numbers are essentially equal between males and females. Significant is that suicide, which may be a result of depression, is the third leading cause of death in teenagers.

In children, it is believed that depression is caused by factors such as family influence. If parents are depressed, the children are three times more likely to be depressed than their age-mates. Environment and biochemical imbalances in the brain are also possible causes.

In addition to the classic general symptoms of depression, children may exhibit a change in their school routines. They may become inattentive, experience a drop in grades, or become anxious about being at school.

Adolescents who become depressed may show all of the classic symptoms of depression and those connected with childhood, but may also be trying to deal with changes happening in their bodies, hormones adjusting, and social role and peer group changing.

Adolescent symptoms of depression may include rebellion, intense ambivalence, anger, rage, pessimism, and low self-esteem (Fig. 21-3). Diagnosis is done carefully, as some of these behaviors occur in this age group as part of the developmental stage. Always remember to look for a *change* in the patient's behavior and the degree to which the behavior is exhibited.

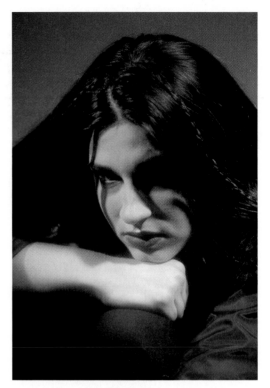

FIGURE 21-3. Adolescent symptoms of depression may include rebellion, intense ambivalence, anger, rage, pessimism, and low self-esteem.

MEDICAL TREATMENT OF CHILDREN AND ADOLESCENTS WITH DEPRESSION

Treatment of depression in these age groups is often difficult. Medications are not always helpful and can be dangerous. In September 2004, the Food and Drug Administration (FDA) of the United States recommended that a strong caution be placed on antidepressant medications for children and teenagers. The caution that suicide can be a side effect of antidepressants is suggested to be placed in a black box on the label, to draw attention to families and caregivers of children and adolescents taking antidepressants.

Monoamine oxidase inhibitors (MAOI's) are not often used, because of the food contraindications associated with them. Some tricyclic antidepressants can cause cardiac arrest and death in children and adolescents. Still, medications may be needed and should be used cautiously and monitored carefully.

Group therapy, family therapy, and partial or day-hospital programs have been shown to be helpful for many in this age group who are dealing with depression.

NURSING CARE FOR CHILDREN AND ADOLESCENTS WITH DEPRESSION

1. Communicate honestly and effectively and at an age-appropriate level.
2. Identify limits and boundaries. Explain what is appropriate behavior

and what is not acceptable. Be clear and concise. Place the limit in the "positive." For example, to an angry individual a nurse might say, "You may hit the punching bag in the gym, but not another person."

3. Care plans should focus on the child/adolescent's strengths. They should be structured, but able to flex frequently with the child/adolescent's needs.

4. Support the individual; encourage verbalization of feelings and thoughts.

■ ENURESIS AND ENCOPRESIS

Enuresis and encopresis are called "elimination disorders." The behaviors occur after the child would normally be expected to be toilet trained. Depending on the child that means generally between the ages of 2 and 5. Sometimes, the child has actually been "potty trained" for a period of time and reverts to the wetting or soiling behavior for some reason. Sometimes, reverting to elimination disorders is related to physical or emotional trauma such as sexual abuse.

Enuresis is the act of urinating in the bed or into clothing, either on purpose or accidentally (Fig. 21-4). The age at which this becomes labeled a "disorder" is approximately age 5—chronological age or developmental age. It is more common in males than females.

Encopresis is the accidental or purposeful passing of feces inappropriately. With encopresis, the chronological or developmental age of 4 is the cutoff point at which the behavior of incontinent stooling into clothing, the bed, or the floor is considered abnormal. Both of these definitions are consistently supported in the *DSM-IV-TR* as well as medical-surgical and mental health nursing textbooks.

A child with encopresis or enuresis is at risk for further psychological involvement. As a child ages and continues with the disorder, his or her peers and family become increasingly intolerant of the behavior. The family unit feels discouraged and frustrated. Peers begin teasing. Children can be ruthless and hurtful to each other. Name-calling and teasing begins. The child with the disorder feels even further separated from his or her social group and may fall deeper into the incontinence behaviors or may slip into further psychological trouble.

Physical causes must be ruled out. Enuresis can be related to diabetes mellitus or diabetes insipidus, congenital anomalies, and other internal disorders. Encopresis may be related to spinal cord lesions, anal fissure, Hirschprung's disease, cerebral palsy, hypothyroidism, and other medical disorders. If physical causes are ruled out, psychological causes such as anxiety, stress, adjustment reactions, and dysfunctional relationships with parents, particularly the mother figure, are evaluated. Occasional accidents should not be labeled as a disorder. Typically, a 3-month period demonstrating fairly consistent incontinence of urine or stool is the standard for diagnosis.

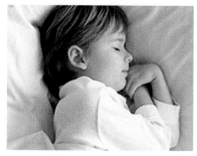

FIGURE 21-4. Sometimes a child who has already been potty trained will revert to wetting the bed for some reason. (Courtesy National Institutes of Health, Bethesda, MD.)

MEDICAL TREATMENT FOR CHILDREN WITH ELIMINATION DISORDERS

Medications are used sparingly and are related to the suspected underlying problem. Even mineral oil is cautioned in the very young child or infant. Aspiration is possible. Rather, education for parents and child is stressed. Age-appropriate activities such as watching very young children for signs they are ready to be toilet trained (such as pulling at wet diapers or trying to copy-cat parent's toileting behavior), scheduling routine times to sit on the toilet, and rewards for successful toileting attempts are strongly recommended.

NURSING CARE FOR CHILDREN WITH ELIMINATION DISORDERS

Nurses have excellent chances to impact this condition. Parents are usually perplexed as to what to do.

1. *Communicate effectively:* In this case, discussions about the family dynamic and interpersonal relationships may be helpful. Parental behavior may be partially causing the child's behavior. Helping the parents to identify possible negative behavior in the home and helping them to identify ways to change those behaviors may help the child to stop the incontinence. Be careful not to "blame" a parent; most parents have already tried everything they can think of to stop the problem before they bring their child in to the clinic. Remain positive in your interactions.

2. *Provide teaching materials:* Parents will be thankful for any assistance available that provides suggestions to solve the problem for the child and themselves. If the doctor has prescribed medications, ensure that the parents understand the dosing, side effects, and dietary information pertaining to the medication. Be certain they can identify when they need to contact the doctor.

3. *Work with the family and doctor to assist with dietary suggestions:* A diet high in roughage is frequently suggested for the child with encopresis. Children are not typically fond of the foods contained in this type of diet. It is important to work with parents on encouraging the child to eat the fruits, vegetables, and grains required, while not forcing or coercing.

4. *Sleeping arrangements:* Teach parents that allowing the child to sleep with them or scolding excessively may actually worsen the problem. The child who has soilage nocturnally should be assisted to clean up and then returned to his or her bed. The parents should remain outside the child's door until the child settles.

5. *Play therapy:* As with situations of child abuse, play therapy or allowing the child to see toileting behavior demonstrated by using a doll or stuffed animal may give the child a visual idea of toileting and may alleviate fear that could be associated with the toilet.

■ ATTENTION DEFICIT HYPERACTIVITY DISORDER

Attention deficit hyperactivity disorder **(ADHD)** is a disorder in and of itself. It is a combination of two disruptive behavior patterns but given one name. It is grouped with other "disruptive behavior disorders."

ADHD is a disorder that affects all, including adults. It is characterized by a variety of age-inappropriate behaviors. The two most obvious are inattentiveness and hyperactivity (Fig. 21-5). Other behaviors exhibited in people with ADHD include but again are not limited to inability to focus on task, underachievement (academic, social, etc.), hyperactivity, noncompliance (with rules, regulations, norms, etc.), and impulsive actions. Poor self-concept, leading both into the disorder and after exhibiting the inappropriate behavior, is also a characteristic of this disorder. According to *DSM-IV-TR*, some symptoms must be present before the child reaches his or her seventh birthday

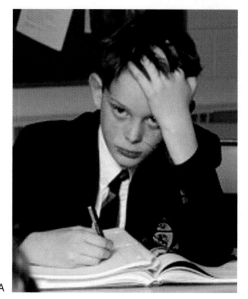

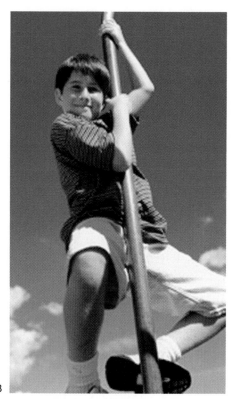

A

B

FIGURE 21-5. The two most obvious signs of ADHD are inattentiveness (A) and hyperactivity (B). (A, Courtesy of Aspen Education Group, Cerritos, CA. B, Courtesy of Blue Cross/Blue Shield of Georgia, Atlanta, GA.)

and must be exhibited in at least two locations. For example the child may display the impulsiveness at home and in church, school, or while in the shopping mall. *DSM-IV-TR* cautions that diagnosing ADHD in children younger than age seven is a bit more challenging, since the younger child is prone to shorter attention as a result of the child's developmental stage. ADHD is more common in males and does seem to have a pattern of running in families.

Children with this disorder are generally of average or above average intelligence, but do not always perform at their level of intelligence. ADD and ADHD disorders may carry over into adulthood.

Causes of ADHD are not yet confirmed. Genetics, certain brain disorders, and maternal drug use during pregnancy are being researched. Dual diagnosis of ADHD with learning disorders, drug use by the child, or depression and other mood disorders is not uncommon.

MEDICAL TREATMENT OF CHILDREN AND ADOLESCENTS WITH ATTENTION DEFICIT/ HYPERACTIVITY DISORDER

As with other illnesses affecting young people, use of medication is controversial. Physicians must consider the physical maturity of a child's brain, liver, and kidneys as well as the child's ability to handle other effects of medication before prescribing. Typical medications used are Ritalin (methylphenidate hydrochloride) and Cylert (pemoline). These are both stimulants. Occasionally, antidepressants such as Wellbutrin (bupropion) may be used, especially in older children and adolescents.

Forms of psychotherapy for the child and family are also indicated.

NURSING CARE FOR CHILDREN AND ADOLESCENTS WITH ATTENTION DEFICIT/HYPERACTIVITY DISORDER

1. *Effective communication*: Therapeutic communication with the child/adolescent and the involved family members is always indicated. Teaching/modeling skills to assist with interpersonal family communication is helpful.

2. *Assist with behavior modification tools:* Limit setting, reward systems, and positive reinforcement may be helpful. Facilitate agreement between the parents and child/adolescent regarding what will be used as the tool, what is fair, and what the consequence to inappropriate behavior will be. Consistency among all parties is crucial in this modality.

3. *Reinforce information about medications:* The physician should discuss the effects and side effects of any medications ordered. Family members may have further questions for nurses. Be prepared to assist with clarification about the medication(s).

■ CONDUCT DISORDER

Conduct disorder is a disorder of anger. The child/adolescent does not hide the anger outburst, which could be directed at humans or animals. What is hidden, however, is the underlying cause of the anger. This disorder seems to affect males two to three times more frequently than females and seems to occur around the time of puberty. Careful screening and medical testing is important, as much change is happening developmentally in this age group. Other mental health issues such as schizophrenia may also manifest during this developmental stage.

Conduct disorder manifests in many ways. Again, it is a pattern of behavior; a

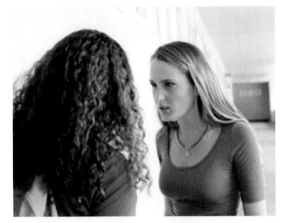

FIGURE 21-6. Recurrent bullying is a behavior that may indicate a conduct disorder, and it can be found among both boys and girls. (Courtesy of U.S. Department of Health and Human Services, Office of Women's Health, Fairfax, VA.)

one-time incident does not diagnose the condition. Some behaviors might be bullying, displaying or using a weapon, arson, lying, fighting, truancy from school, and running away from home (Fig. 21-6). *DSM-IV-TR* clarifies running away as either happening more than once or a one-time episode that lasts for an extended period of time.

Causes of conduct disorder may involve medical conditions such as lead poisoning, phenylketonuria, brain tumors, head trauma, or having been exposed to cocaine while in utero. Nonmedical factors that may contribute to development of conduct disorder are poor parental relationships or lack of father or father figure.

MEDICAL TREATMENT FOR CHILDREN AND ADOLESCENTS WITH CONDUCT DISORDER

Sometimes, there is an underlying medical condition, perhaps a closed head injury or a seizure disorder. The physician will need to assess and treat the underlying disorder as well as the behaviors associated with the conduct disorder. Medications are directed at symptom control and work most effectively with counseling.

Medical treatment may include counseling for the parents and family as well as the affected child. Parenting skills, consistency in limit setting, and progressing maturity of the child may, over time, lessen or eliminate the behaviors of conduct disorder.

NURSING CARE FOR CHILDREN AND ADOLESCENTS WITH CONDUCT DISORDER

Nursing interventions are similar as those stated above.

1. *Maintain safety:* Maintaining physical safety and psychological and emotional safety is the primary nursing intervention for children and adolescents who have conduct disorder.

2. *Communicate honestly and effectively:* Communicate at an age-appropriate level behaviors that are acceptable. Communicate what the effect of inappropriate behavior has on others around the child. Communicate the consequences of inappropriate behavior and most importantly be consistent with enforcing those consequences.

3. *Assist with behavior modification tools:* Limit setting, reward systems, and positive reinforcement may be helpful. Set realistic expectations according to the child's age and ability level. Consistency among all parties is crucial.

4. *Model and educate family with respect to appropriate role:* In other words, parents need to be parents. The child needs to be the child. The parent should be in "control" of the situation. The child has input; negotiation is healthy, depending on the age of the child, but the child does not always "win." When the child does not "win" and behavior limits are exceeded or violated, the consequences for the inappropriate behavior must be enacted. Parents may find this diffi-cult and exhausting. They will need support and positive reinforcement from the nurse and medical or counseling staff.

5. *Reinforce information about medications:* The physician should discuss the effects and side effects of any medications ordered. Family members may have further questions for nurses. Be prepared to assist with clarification about medication(s).

■ AUTISM

Autism is believed to be the most common of the "pervasive developmental disorders." As such, it is also considered to be the most difficult to treat and the least likely to be reversed. There are two main kinds of autism and several alternative terms and subgroups within those two main types of autism. They vary quite a bit in type and severity of symptoms. One type is related to bilateral brain damage incurred early in life. The other is not related to brain damage, but rather to low levels of serotonin in the part of the brain responsible for language, the left frontal lobe.

The incidence of autism is on the rise. It affects males three to four times more frequently than females. Sadly, at this point in time, it is not curable. Children with autism are considered disabled for life. Autism should not be confused with or misdiagnosed as schizophrenia, although some behaviors may be similar.

The single most common symptom or manifestation of autism is impaired social interaction. Learning disabilities, avoiding making eye contact, inability to make friends or respond to other people's emotions are other symptoms. Children with this disorder may rock back and forth, twirl their hair, and perform self-hurtful or self-mutilating behaviors, such as biting themselves or hitting their head on objects.

Diagnosis may also look at failure to meet certain developmental tasks, such as a baby not babbling or performing gestures (pointing, grasping, etc.) by age 12 months, or at any age, losing any language or social skills that had been acquired. There are several inventories that the physician, psychologist, or psychiatrist might administer to help with diagnosing.

Causes of autism are not confirmed. Genetics, viral infections, and chemicals found in the environment are suspected causes or contributors to development of autism. For a family with one autistic child, there is about a 5 percent chance of having a second child with autism. As mentioned earlier, serotonin levels have been shown to be diminished in the left frontal lobe of many with autism. Fragile X syndrome, congenital rubella, and tuberous sclerosis may be medical causes of the disorder. As children with autism pass through adolescence and into adulthood, they have a 20–30 percent chance of developing epilepsy. The reason for that is also unclear but is suspected to relate to an imbalance of neurochemicals or perhaps brain injury.

Other theories include a reaction to early childhood immunizations. At this time, there is no evidence-based research that supports that theory.

MEDICAL TREATMENT FOR CHILDREN AND ADOLESCENTS WITH AUTISM

Doctors will prescribe medication for the symptom or behavior. Usually it will be a medication that contains or stimulates serotonin or an antipsychotic medication such as haloperidol (Haldol).

NURSING CARE FOR CHILDREN AND ADOLESCENTS WITH AUTISM

1. *Maintain safety:* Again, environmental and psychosocial safety is required. Therapists may prescribe special equipment or even special clothing to help maintain safety. The goal of this intervention is to discourage and prevent self-destructive behavior. Assisting parents to identify situations that may trigger the unwanted behavior is also helpful in preventing or de-escalating the behavior.

2. *Reinforce medical and counselor teaching:* Work with the parents and child on social skills. Provide praise and positive reinforcement for both the parents and child. Technology is assisting with interventions for some patients. Virtual reality equipment is being used in some settings and with some success to help with teaching and behavioral training.

3. *Maintain effective communication with all parties:* Speak to the child or adolescent in simple, direct, age-appropriate language. Ensure that the family and others involved in the day-to-day care of the patient feel comfortable discussing concerns.

■ PERCEIVED THREATS TO SAFETY

Today's society is a frightening place globally. Children are growing up in poverty and fear. Their homeland's safety is questionable. Parents and loved ones die, sometimes in front of them. In the United States, we have witnessed tragedy of child on child violence, as with the situation at Columbine High School and similar situations in other schools around the country (Fig. 21-7). Child abuse, sexual and otherwise, is in the news almost daily. Children rape other children. Children are abducted all too often by estranged parents or other people known to the child. Child abduction happens frequently enough that a national program called the Amber Alert has been signed and endorsed by President George W. Bush to assist law enforcement, in conjunction with high-speed Internet providers, with the swift dissemination of information to locate abducted children. Gangs of many different

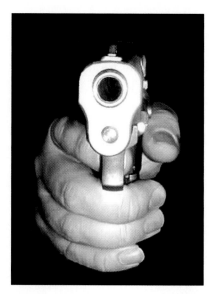

FIGURE 21-7. Today's society can be a frightening place for children. The fear of violence from adults or even other children is very real. (Courtesy of World Independent News Group, Sisyphus Press, State College, PA.)

MEDICAL TREATMENT FOR CHILDREN AND ADOLESCENTS WITH PERCEIVED THREATS TO SAFETY

Children and adolescents who have a real or perceived threat to their safety will react to that threat in different ways. As with other mental health conditions, physicians must do a comprehensive examination and evaluation of the individual and the threat. Medications or therapy will be ordered on an individual, as needed basis.

NURSING CARE FOR CHILDREN AND ADOLESCENTS WITH PERCEIVED THREATS TO SAFETY

ethnic and cultural groups, involving both genders, are a loud and dangerous presence in society. They are frequently drug-related and recruit other children and adolescents who may be in a vulnerable psychosocial state.

How can nurses help children and their families? Hilary Clinton coined a phrase and wrote a book on her belief, "it takes a village" to raise a child. Whether or not your personal belief system agrees with hers, there is some validity in communities—meaning full neighborhoods, cities, and municipalities, not a particular ethnic community—keeping their eyes and ears open for issues affecting the safety of their citizens. Watching for suspicious behavior, changes in the habits of the children and adolescents in your neighborhood, and reporting those observations to the parents and authorities can go a long way toward preventing abductions and gang activities. Adults acting on concerns brought to the attention of authorities such as police or school leaders is extremely important for the safety of children and the community at large.

1. *Provide safety:* Everyone, children and adolescents included, needs safety as identified by Maslow. Nurses provide safety in the examination area, the hospital room, and the school, for those who may become employed there.
2. *Communicate effectively:* Honest, age-appropriate communication is essential. Listen to the child's concerns and then *do something.* It may not be realistic to be able to "fix" the problem, but if the child or adolescent sees that someone took what they said seriously and made an attempt to address that concern, chances for continued meaningful communication are greatly improved.
3. *Maintain agency policies regarding apparel, items allowed onsite, etc.:* If the item of clothing is not allowed or the article in the backpack is not allowed in the clinic or the school, it simply is not allowed. This falls under enforcing boundaries and expected behavior. Parents and children must be expected to follow agency policy for the safety of all in the area. It may be necessary to provide a private area and summon supervisory or management staff in situations such as these.

■ ALTERNATIVE TREATMENT FOR CHILDREN AND ADOLESCENTS WITH MENTAL HEALTH DISORDERS

Children benefit from alternative therapies, as do adults. With herbal preparations and nutritional supplements, care must be taken that the child is getting adequate nutrition to support normal growth and development. Children do benefit from:

- Aromatherapy
- Play therapy
- Massage
- Neurolinguistic programming
- Biofeedback (when age-appropriate)

Key Concepts ■ ■ ■

1. Children and adolescents do experience threats to their mental health. They have the same illnesses as adults but may manifest them in different ways. Some illnesses continue into adulthood.
2. Medications and therapy are effective for a great many people in these age groups. Recently, black box warnings have been applied to certain antidepressants when used with children and adolescents: they may actually increase the chance for suicide.
3. Autism is thought to be the most serious of the pervasive-type disorders. Many professionals believe it has the least chance of being reversed.
4. Parents, family members, and other primary care givers need to be involved in treatment of children and adolescents. Consistency of care is crucial. Parents may need counseling as well, in order to become more effective in their role as parents.

CASE STUDY: ATTENTION DEFICIT DISORDER ■ ■ ■

AB is an attractive, intelligent 40-year-old man who has spent much of his life feeling miserable.

AB grew up in a military family, which, because of his father's job caused the family to move often enough so that he attended 12 grade/preparatory schools. As a child, AB was quiet, shy, and did not develop close friends easily. He did not socialize well or often. He was easily distracted and sometimes found himself in trouble for "misbehaving" in his classes.

As a teenager, he scored high on his standardized tests, yet despite constant studying, he "flunked" several of his classes. By the age of 20, he was attending more than one 12-step program. Much as he tried, he could not maintain interest in his classes. Even his "favorite" subjects became difficult to attend routinely. AB was often impulsive. He became obsessed with the paranormal and occasionally had suicidal fantasies. He survived and is today a successful nurse but admits he has difficulty organizing his thoughts and still feels dissatisfied with himself and his life at times.

AB now knows that the symptoms he suffered from as a child, such as inattention, misbehaving in the manner he did at school, and impulsivity, were more than just those of an unhappy child. He was diagnosed as a child with attention deficit disorder (ADD). About half of the children who are diagnosed with ADD develop skills that help them "outgrow" ADD; the other half do not. That half moves into adulthood with the same type of problems they had as children.

AB understands that the condition may be inherited and tends to run in the families. He has identified one aunt and one cousin who have been willing to talk with him and who experienced many of the same symptoms in childhood and into adulthood. The cousin has, in fact, been in trouble with the law and has a history of illegal drug use.

AB credits the military for his diagnosis. He had access to educators, physicians, and mental health professionals who were able to diagnose him at an early age. He was placed on Ritalin and later in life has had several other medications. Today, he remains on Clonidine. He remains in therapy and occasionally speaks to small church groups and nursing classes in his city.
He finds talking to others helps him as much as it helps them.

1. What questions would you like to ask AB? Those would very likely be the same questions a nurse would want to ask a patient on an intake interview to assist in diagnosing attention deficit disorder. List those questions.

2. What could you say to AB's parent(s) to help them as they begin the process of learning what AB is experiencing? Write those ideas, using therapeutic communication verbiage. Include information giving support and teaching techniques. If your class time allows, work in pairs, each taking turns as the "nurse" and the "patient/parent."

REFERENCES

American Psychiatric Association. (2000). *Diagnostic and Statistical Manual of Mental Disorders—Text Revision,* 4th ed. Author, Washington, DC.

Ballard, D. K. Office of Outreach and Graduate Studies, University of Wisconsin-River Falls, 410 S. Third Street, River Falls, WI 54022, ph: 715-425-3256, email: diane.ballard@uwrf.edu.

Hartman, T. (1998). *Healing ADD—Simple Exercises That Will Change Your Daily Life.* Underwood Books. Grass Valley, CA.

Prensky, M. (2001). Digital game-based learning. In Seroussi, K., *Unraveling the Mystery of Autism and Pervasive Development Disorder: A Mother's Story of Research and Recovery,* pp. 40–46. McGraw-Hill, New York. (Author has copyright. Published by Simon and Schuster, New York).

Ratey, J. and Miller, A. (no date). Foibles, Frailties and Frustration Seen Through the Lens of Attention. http://www.adhdnews.com/ratey.htm.

WEBSITES

http://www.adhdnews.com/ratey.htm
www.autism-society.org
http://www.cdipage.com/adhd.htm
www.childdevelopmentinfo.com
www.childabuse.com
www.codeamber.org
http://www.vinsight.org

CRITICAL THINKING EXERCISE ■ ■ ■

1. You go to your neighbor's house for a family party. You notice their 3-year-old son, Timmy, off by himself. You know he usually is eager to play with the other children, but this evening he seems particularly shy of your 7-year-old son. An hour later, you notice they are both gone. You find your son "playing doctor" with Timmy. Your son tells you that Timmy's daddy plays this with them all the time. What will you do?

TEST QUESTIONS ■ ■ ■

MULTIPLE CHOICE QUESTIONS

1. An 8-year-old child is in the waiting room. This child has a diagnosis of conduct disorder. You call another patient to the room but notice this child beginning to act out inappropriately. Your first concern and nursing action would be:
   A. Ask the parent to take the child outside until they are called for their appointment.
   B. Provide an environment of safety for the child and parent.
   C. Change the rooming order and take this parent and child ahead of the patient just called.
   D. Wait a few minutes; the child will probably calm down soon.

2. A young mother comes to your clinic with her 2-year-old daughter. The mother is crying and distraught. She explains that she is divorced from the child's father, but he has visitation rights. Tonight, when the little girl came back from her father's house, she noticed blood on the little girl's panties. She wants to know what to do. Your first action is:
   A. Get them a good lawyer.
   B. Show empathy and offer privacy.
   C. Call the police.
   D. Tell them you understand just how they feel.

3. The little girl is not talking to you or the social workers. You suggest giving her some toys and drawing materials. Your rationale for this is:
   A. It gives you one less person to work with at the moment.
   B. You know children can be bribed.
   C. You think she might talk if she were distracted.
   D. Children often communicate feelings through their play.

4. All of the following are factors that may lead to parental child abuse except:
   A. Stress and poor parenting skills
   B. Gender of parent
   C. Parent having been abused as a child
   D. Culture of the parents

5. Nurses involved with caring for a child who has been abused understand that the adult or other older child committing the abuse:
   A. Must be put in jail
   B. Is dangerous and must be supervised at all times
   C. Must understand the abused child will be placed in foster care away from the abuser
   D. Needs empathy and nonjudgmental attention

6. Martin is 7 years old and has a diagnosis of ADHD. He has broken his arm and requires surgery to have it set. You are the nurse doing the admission checklist with Martin and his family. You know that people with ADHD:
   A. Have normal or above average intelligence
   B. Are impulsive
   C. Are inattentive or easily distracted
   D. All of the above

7. The single most common symptom of autism is:
   A. Strong ability to make friends
   B. Impaired social functioning
   C. Appropriate emotional responses
   D. Achieving and maintaining age-appropriate developmental tasks

8. The parents of 6-year-old Anna say, "Nurse, why us? The doctors tell us Maria has the most difficult of all childhood developmental disorders to cure. What did we do wrong? What can we do for her?" Your best response might be:
   A. "The doctor is correct."
   B. "Her medications should help calm her somewhat."
   C. "We have specialists here who can help you. I will call someone."
   D. "Maybe she will outgrow the autism."

9. A 27-year-old man comes running into the clinic one afternoon. He is holding a 15-month-old child. The child is not breathing and has a cyanotic color around her lips. She wouldn't quit crying. I just tried to get her to stop crying. Then she went limp on me!" the man says. While the doctors work on the baby, you interview the man. He is her uncle. He was babysitting. You:
   A. Report your concern of child abuse to your direct supervisor
   B. Call the police to arrest this man
   C. Do nothing but express your sincere sympathy at this awful situation
   D. Attempt to determine how long he shook the baby

CHAPTER

22

Aging Population

Learning Objectives ■ ■ ■

1. Discuss concepts of aging.
2. Define ageism.
3. Discuss social trends in the aging population.
4. Identify five mental challenges of the older adult.
5. Identify medical treatment for the older adult.
6. Identify nursing actions for general care of older patients.

Key Terms ■ ■ ■

- Ageism
- Alzheimer's disease
- Aphasia
- Elder abuse
- Elderly
- Geriatrics
- Gerontology
- OBRA

Geriatrics, or **gerontology,** means the study of older adults. The study of older adults is a specialty in nursing. With more and more North Americans reaching age 65 within the next 10 to 15 years, learning the complications, abilities, and best ways to assist that population is a very timely study.

Aging begins at the moment of conception. Think about it. Aging happens to us and we have no control over it. It is a condition of time passing. It is also a condition that researchers are beginning to redefine: What *is* "old age"?

When we are 10, we can't wait to be 16 so we can drive a car. When we are 16, we want to be 18 so we can be out on our own. When we turn 30, the idea of time passing begins to take on a different tone for some people. In a society that promotes the image

of youth, we see youth vanishing. Perhaps we're not as fast or as thin or as healthy as we were in our 20s. Still, we see healthy, happy people over age 65 working, recreating, and socializing. Life expectancy in the United States is in the early 70s for men and the early 80s for women. So, what *is* this process of aging?

The majority of people over 65 are intellectually intact and are able to care for themselves (Fig. 22-1). Only about 0.4 percent of people over age 65 are institutionalized in long-term care centers or assisted-living facilities (Barry, 2002). These numbers are slowly on the rise as children of the 1950s and 1960s (often referred to as "baby boomers") enter advanced age. Older people are usually basically mentally healthy; that is, they are able to accept and

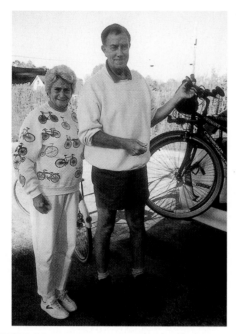

FIGURE 22-1. Most older adults are independent and fully able to care for themselves. (From Williams, L.S., and Hopper, P.D., *Understanding Medical Surgical Nursing,* 2nd ed. Philadelphia, FA Davis Company, 2003, p. 199. Reprinted with permission.)

deal with the changes and losses they are experiencing.

Of course, many challenges are involved with aging. People lose their visual and hearing acuity. Many of these individuals are living on fixed incomes that are not adequate to meet their needs for housing, food, and health care. Safety is also an issue. Criminals are finding older adults easy targets and are robbing and mugging them in higher numbers than in generations past. The need to face death becomes more of a reality.

Certain illnesses become more prevalent as we age. Alzheimer's disease (see Chapter 15) may become more prominently manifested in old age, rendering the individual incapable of caring for himself or herself and possibly requiring a major lifestyle change by necessitating the individual's move to a nursing home. Coronary disorders such as arteriosclerosis and respiratory disorders such as pneumonia occur more frequently in this age group, and patients are

less responsive to the treatments for them. People are sicker longer. Nutrition is challenged: Elderly people may not be able to afford to buy nutritious foods, and the food they do prepare does not taste as it once did because the taste buds are less sensitive.

A phenomenon called **ageism,** which is occurring in the United States, is discrimination against a group of people on the basis of their age. It assumes that most older people are incapable of functioning in and contributing to society. What thoughts cross your mind as you see that the car ahead of you is being driven by an older person who can barely see over the steering wheel?

Most people over age 65 have retired from their careers. Whereas people now may conceivably change careers at least five times during their working years, the **elderly** people of today most likely had one or two jobs over their lifetime and worked 20 to 30 years at each job. That job probably represented a large part of their identity, and retirement may lead to feelings of loss and depression when the person has to redefine who he or she is. Retirement also means a decrease in income, which can have a negative impact on a person's lifestyle.

The need for intimacy never leaves us. As human beings, the need to love and be loved is one of the primary needs for survival of the individual and the species (Fig. 22-2). As people age and spouses and friends die, who is there to love older people? Prospects for marriage are slim. Children and grandchildren may live on the opposite side of the country. In addition, older adults may be forced to live with their adult children, which is not always the ideal situation. Elderly individuals are at risk for **elder abuse** (physical and emotional abuse of older people) by their children or caregivers. Elder abuse is discussed further in Chapter 23.

Aging has many challenges, yet most individuals are able to cope with the changes brought about by aging and progress through this life stage with dignity. They are proud of their families and their personal accomplishments. They can see the contri-

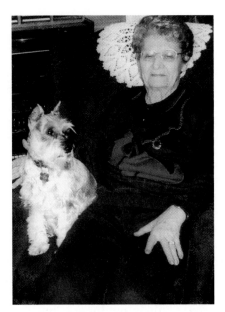

FIGURE 22-2. Pets can fulfill the need for companionship and intimacy in an older person's life. (From Townsend, M.C., *Essentials of Psychiatric Mental Health Nursing,* 3rd ed. Philadelphia, FA Davis Company, 2005, p. 194. Reprinted with permission.)

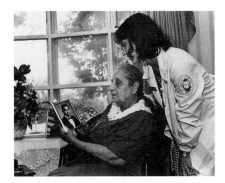

FIGURE 22-3. Increasingly, nurses are caring for older adults in their own homes. (From Sorrell, J.M., and Redmond, G.M., *Community-Based Nursing Practice: Learning Through Students' Stories.* Philadelphia, FA Davis Company, 2002, p. 421. Reprinted with permission.)

butions that they have passed on to others. People who have learned to adapt to change throughout life have the best chances of progressing through old age with the same kind of resilience. The Omnibus Budget Reconciliation Act (**OBRA**) is a federal act that provides standards of care for older adults. One of the provisions of OBRA is ensuring proper assessment of elderly people. It is for this reason that only registered nurses (RNs) may conduct or coordinate assessments of elderly individuals. Other health-care team members help with this assessment by providing input as to the patient's abilities and responses to the treatment plan.

Nurses are caring for the older individual not only in the health-care facility but also more and more in the privacy of the person's own home (Fig. 22-3). Because it is believed that people will stay healthier and maintain more control of their lives if they can stay in their own homes, the home health industry is growing. One of the primary concerns for nurses and others caring for older adults is to help them maintain a good quality of life. Nurses caring for clients in their homes need to be aware of some of the major mental and emotional disturbances they may encounter, as well as the physical diagnoses of the patient. Some of these mental disturbances follow.

■ ALZHEIMER'S DISEASE AND OTHER COGNITIVE ALTERATIONS

As stated in Chapter 15, when a person has been diagnosed with **Alzheimer's disease,** it has most likely been taking its toll on the individual for 20 years or more. It is now, in the later years, that the debilitating effects are most observable. This disease may necessitate the person's leaving the home he or she has lived in all of that person's adult life. It may mean living apart from a spouse who he or she may not appear to remember. Socializing will be curtailed because of the inability to relate to others easily. Alzheimer's disease has an impact not only on the patient but also on all the people in that person's life.

Further information on Alzheimer's disease and the care of patients with this disorder is included in Chapter 15.

■ CEREBROVASCULAR ACCIDENT (STROKE)

A cerebrovascular accident (CVA), or stroke, is a medical disorder that has implications for mental health workers. A CVA is a devastating and frightening experience for the patient and family. Depending on the location and size of the brain and blood vessel involvement, many physical and cognitive functions may be temporarily or permanently affected (Fig. 22-4). Some of the mental health issues associated with CVA follow.

DEPRESSION

Patients realize the losses associated with their stroke. They may not be able to express them verbally or physically, but they do realize that they cannot do things independently. Self-esteem decreases as they realize they may be incontinent, unable to eat independently, or unable to communicate with their families. Depression may develop.

Left-side infarct

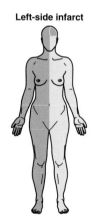

Right-side infarct

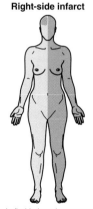

Right-sided weakness or paralysis
Aphasia (in left–brain-dominant clients)
Depression related to disability common

Left-sided weakness or paralysis
Impaired judgement/safety risk
Unilateral neglect more common
Indifferent to disability

FIGURE 22-4. The location of a stroke is a key factor in the physical and cognitive functions that may be affected. A stroke on the left side of the brain affects the right side of the body; a stroke on the right side of the brain affects the left side of the body. (From Williams, L.S., and Hopper, P.D., *Understanding Medical Surgical Nursing*, 2nd ed. Philadelphia, FA Davis Company, 2003, p. 834. Reprinted with permission.)

They worry about the effect of their stroke not only on themselves but also on their spouses and other family members. Will this be permanent or only temporary? Will it happen again? How long will I be this way?

As these worries become more pronounced, the patient may become more depressed. The physicians, nurses, and therapists will try to explain these concerns to the patient and family, but the patient still feels out of control of his or her destiny. You may see crying and refusal to perform tasks that the patient could do after the stroke. The patient may avoid eye contact with you or refuse to interact with family members. All these behaviors may indicate depression in the patient who has had a CVA. By recognizing and confronting these behaviors, you can help the patient understand that you really are there to help and that you are concerned with the patient's thoughts and feelings.

Being honest and generous with positive reinforcement for attempts to overcome the feelings of depression will also be helpful in building the patient's confidence and self-esteem.

APHASIA

Three classifications of **aphasia,** a speech disorder that may be found in patients who have had a CVA, are expressive, receptive, and global (see Chapter 2). A patient with aphasia needs to learn to talk all over again. Communication is such a basic need that any threat to this ability must be worked at very diligently by the nurse and the patient. The goal of communicating with a person who has aphasia is to stimulate the communication. Patience will be mandatory. Give the person time to speak, write, or show you what is needed. Praise him or her for all efforts to communicate. One communication technique that is effective, especially in expressive aphasia, is to associate the object with the word. The more senses a person can implement, the better the reinforcement for the learning.

The physician and speech therapist will determine the proper plan of speech therapy. Nurses need to pay close attention to following this plan and document the patient's progress and emotional responses to speech therapy.

■ DEPRESSION

It is not "normal" to feel depressed all the time when we are older. Major depression in the elderly population can show itself differently than in other age groups. In addition to the information discussed in Chapter 12, nurses observing and assisting elderly people should watch for constipation, headaches and other body aches, and difficulty breathing for which there is no diagnosis. Often patients will discuss these physical symptoms rather than admit to being depressed.

These symptoms are similar to other afflictions common in the elderly population such as drug reactions, electrolyte imbalances, and dementia. Nurses must get information accurately, document it, and be certain that appropriate medical care is obtained to rule out other ailments.

■ MEDICATION CONCERNS

The process of pharmacokinetics is slower and less complete in older people. Because circulatory and renal function is decreased, it is easier for these persons to become toxic. Nurses who work in facilities that care for older adults must be very alert to the effects of the medications they give their patients as well as to the possible signs of side effects and toxicity. You need to report any concerns to your charge nurse immediately and document your observations accurately. If your state allows you as a licensed practical nurse/licensed vocational nurse (LPN/LVN) to contact the physician by telephone, you will also take that responsibility.

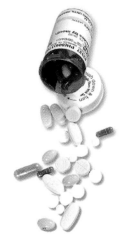

FIGURE 22-5. Older adults often take a large number of prescription and nonprescription medications, and they may lose track of their medication routine. (Courtesy of www.amarillo.net, Amarillo, TX.)

Patients who live at home may lose track of their medication routine (Fig. 22-5). They may forget to take medications or forget they have taken them and take another dose. Many pills look alike. When visual acuity is lessened and lighting inadequate, patients may mistake one pill for another—for example, they may take two lanoxin tablets instead of one lanoxin and one furosemide. These types of mistakes can be lethal.

To help with this situation, nurses have systems available for teaching patients and families. Containers are available for planning which medications are taken at what time, enabling the nurse and patient to set up the patient's medications for a week or longer and for different times of day. If the patient is reliable, this will serve as a reminder to take a particular dose. If the patient still needs some reassurance, the nurse can instruct the patient to immediately mark a calendar on the appropriate date each time a dose is taken. In this way, the patient can double-check that the medications are taken correctly and will be less anxious about it.

Nurses also must be aware of the patient's weight, nutrition, and activity levels. It is very easy for older people to become toxic from their medications, regardless of whether they are at home or in a facility. Patients with drug toxicity or overdose can present with symptoms similar to those of a mental illness or other physical illness. It is not uncommon for a proper dose of a medication for an older adult to be as little as 25 percent of the "usual" recommended adult dose. It is the nurse's responsibility to ask specific questions of the doctor regarding medication doses.

Similarly, side effects to medications can look like other symptoms. Nurses can teach patients and families about this possibility. Table 22-1 shows some of the common side effects of drugs on older people, disorders

that may have similar symptoms, and some nursing actions that can be taken and taught to the patient.

■ PARANOID THINKING

Paranoid thinking may be a result of fear about the social environment. As stated earlier, certain people see elderly persons as "easy marks." What was once a situation that was not threatening (such as a walk around the block) can become very frightening for the person who has slowed reaction time and diminished physical capacity for

TABLE 22-1	*Possible Drug Side Effects for Elderly Patients**
SIDE EFFECT	**OTHER POSSIBILITIES**	**NURSING ACTIONS**

SIDE EFFECT	OTHER POSSIBILITIES	NURSING ACTIONS
DRY MOUTH	■ Stress response; electrolyte imbalance ■ Vitamin B deficiency	1. Offer sips of water or ice chips. 2. Offer hard, sugar-free candy (such as lemon drops) if patient is able to suck on them without choking. 3. Provide oral care with light application of lubricant such as petroleum jelly. 4. Review lab work or call physician.
CONSTIPATION	■ Fluid and nutritional deficiency, hemorrhoids or rectal pain ■ Hypothyroidism	1. Assess diet for fiber and fluid intake. 2. Assess area for signs of hemorrhoids or other inflammation. 3. Assess need for laxatives as ordered by physician. 4. Discuss need for physical activity as condition warrants.
ORTHOSTATIC HYPOTENSION	■ Heart disorders	1. Assess vital signs. 2. Teach patient how to get out of bed or chair slowly. 3. Tell patient to stay sitting for a few minutes until dizziness goes away.
URINARY COMPLICATIONS	■ Prostate problems ■ Bladder problems ■ Uterus problems ■ Urinary tract infections ■ Cancers	1. Inform patient to: Take all medications by 1600 hours (4 PM). 2. Drink little or no fluids after 1600 hours (4 PM). 3. You must: Keep track of frequency, amount, color, and odor of urine and abdominal girth.

(continued)

SIDE EFFECT	OTHER POSSIBILITIES	NURSING ACTIONS
CONFUSION/ DISORIENTATION/ MENTAL SLUGGISHNESS	■ Hypoglycemia ■ Head injury [e.g., fall] ■ Infection/fever ■ Vitamin deficiency ■ Transient ischemic attack [TIA] ■ Brain tumor	1. Give sweetened drink. If patient is still confused after 10 minutes, call physician. 2. Check vital signs for signs of infection. 3. Attempt to validate whether patient has had recent head trauma.
FATIGUE	■ Infectious process ■ Anemia ■ Hypothyroidism ■ Stress ■ Narrowing of coronary arteries	1. Assess vital signs. 2. Assess stress level.
MOOD SWINGS/ IRRITABILITY	■ Psychological disorders ■ Electrolyte imbalances	1. Use verbal and nonverbal communication skills to assess cause. 2. Request lab work.

Always report these side effects to your charge nurse, document carefully, and notify the physician if that is allowed for LPN/LVN practice in your state.

self protection. Paranoid, fearful thinking can be a defense mechanism against these kinds of disabilities, making the fear the reason to avoid leaving the house. This self-imposed isolation can bloom into feelings of loneliness, which can lead to more serious illness.

■ INSOMNIA

Insomnia, or inability to sleep, is frequently seen in the older adult. It can be a result of many conditions, including depression, fear, pain, urinary incontinence, napping during the day, or sometimes a condition nick-named "sundowner syndrome," in which the person turns around daytime and night-time hours. These people sleep much of the day and are wide awake and active during the night. This syndrome is sometimes seen in patients who have Alzheimer's disease. Lack of rapid eye movement (REM) sleep can have negative effects on anyone, even contributing to psychotic behavior. To

someone with Alzheimer's disease or other cognitive problems, the effects of insomnia can intensify the symptoms of the cognitive disorder.

The nurse needs to concentrate on keeping communication open with these patients. You will need to be sure that you and your patient are using words in the same way. For instance, if the patient says, "I do not sleep at night because I am worried," the word *worried* should be explored. What is the patient worried about? What can be done to eliminate the worry? How severe is the worry? Using the 1 to 5 rating scale, the nurse can more objectively document the impact of the "worry" on the patient.

■ END-OF-LIFE ISSUES

Life can end at any age; however, death is more common among the older population. Nurses who work in areas such as long-term care, home care, or hospice have a great opportunity to learn about and assist people with end-of-life issues. In these days of managed care, it may not be economically feasible for professional counselors to meet the needs of older adults dealing with these profound issues. Many people in this population will prefer the services of their own spiritual leader, but since the duties of many such leaders are overwhelming, the appropriate clergy may not be available at the moment of immediate need. However, we nurses are there, and we have all the tools needed to be the helper. Nurses must take inventory of their beliefs surrounding the subjects of death and dying. It is also very important for nurses to talk about and understand their patients' religious and cultural beliefs about what the end of life means to them. It is the nurse's responsibility and privilege to be able to help someone through this stage of life according to that individual's needs and wants.

One issue a patient may experience is widowhood. The surviving spouse must learn to live independently or face an alternative form of housing. Finances and household chores may have been "gender-specific" in that relationship, and now the surviving person is forced to assume responsibilities formerly done by the deceased. The subjects of dating and working may become delicate issues for the person: Families may have strong opinions about what the newly widowed person "should" do. Nurses can play an advocacy role with widowed persons. Active listening skills, validating the person's thoughts and feelings, and offering information about various services available to widowed persons are skills that can be very helpful.

Nurses can be effective in helping people to die. Death of the body as we know it is inevitable. People need to know it is "OK" to die. Elizabeth Kübler-Ross and others who teach about death and dying tell us that helping people to resolve life issues can help them to die with peace and dignity. Again, nurses who choose to work in hospice, home care, and long term care settings have a special opportunity to be there for people at this very important stage of life.

Using humor and laughter appropriately, maintaining the hope they may still have, and reassuring them that they will not be forgotten after death are some truthful techniques nurses can learn to use to help people prepare to die.

We must not ignore the incidence of suicide among the aging populations. This chapter has alluded to many losses that people are likely to face as they age. Compound the sadness of losing jobs, friends, and other aspects of earlier life with physical illness and altered physical ability, and it may become more clear why some elders feel helpless or hopeless and opt for suicide. According to the National Institute of Mental Health, older Americans are more likely to die by suicide than other age groups. They account for approximately 13 percent of the U.S. population, yet persons age 65 and older accounted for 18 percent of all suicide deaths in the United States in the year 2000. The highest rates were found in white men age 85 and older. Follow the screening suggestions provided in Chapter 19 when considering the possibility that an older person may be at risk for suicide.

■ SOCIAL CONCERNS

Older adults, like younger adults, in today's world may find themselves in financial trouble. Medicare and Social Security benefits are decreasing. Retirement age has increased over the years, and politicians are discussing raising it yet again, potentially requiring people to continue working into their late 60s before they become eligible to receive the Medicare and/or social security benefits they have earned. Perhaps they have inadequate personal and supplemental insurance, so they will not seek medical help when they need it. They may find their heat and power cut off due to inability to pay utilities on their fixed income. Most municipalities are enacting laws and emergency funds to help avoid this life-threatening situation. Nurses can help provide the necessary information to help the elders who are opting to remain at home or in assisted living.

As baby-boomers age, nurses will see a significant increase in the patient demographic they are caring for. The average age of patients will be older, and the concerns nurses face will relate more frequently to issues pertaining to people in the ending stages of life.

It is worth mentioning again at this time that the family unit of the older population may have a different look as well. People are opting to have children later in life. Nurses may see much younger family members that we might anticipate. The upcoming older generation is very diverse. Those of varied ethnic and cultural backgrounds will be seeking assistance in long-term care facilities (Fig. 22-6). We need to be prepared to learn about those customs, ask the proper questions upon intake data collecting, and be ready to offer care according to customs that may be different from our own and different from those we were trained in.

One of the cultural demographics to consider is the group of elders who have lived a homosexual or bisexual lifestyle. We need to anticipate issues surrounding grooming, roommate, bathroom-sharing, family preferences, and even potentially a different definition of what will be "appropriate

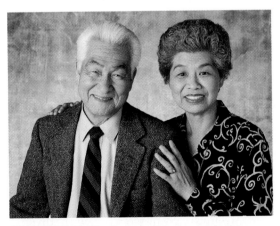

FIGURE 22-6. The demographic changes in the American population mean that a more ethnically and culturally diverse group will be seeking assistance in long-term care facilities. Nurses must be ready to offer culturally sensitive care.

behavior" for those of that lifestyle. Individuals may be reluctant to share this type of information unless we communicate acceptance. The nurse's role will need to become even more flexible. We will need to be very open with our communication and with the type of questions we must learn to ask in order to provide the best care to all entrusted to our care.

■ NURSING SKILLS FOR WORKING WITH OLDER ADULTS

The following are some general skills a nurse learns to use, which will make working with the elderly population more effective:

1. *Respect:* In the United States, a handshake is a sign of respect and cooperation. It is usually given at the beginning and ending of business meetings, and it is customary to shake hands at more formal social functions or when being introduced to someone new. Shaking the hand of your elderly patient will convey that respect and cooperation and is an effective way to begin your nurse-patient partnership.

   Using the proper name of the patient also shows respect for that person. "Mr. Washington" or "Mrs. Jones" is the best way to address the patient. If the patient prefers and asks you to, you may call him or her by the first name or the name that the person is called socially. Do not do this until invited to do so, however. Also, it is not acceptable to assign nicknames arbitrarily to patients. In home care and long term care, there is a danger of becoming too familiar. The facility becomes the patient's home, and they become friendly with each other. This informal atmosphere sometimes spreads among the staff. This is a time when you must remember your professional role. You can be pleasant and friendly while still being professional.

Under no circumstances should an older adult be treated as a child. As abilities leave and the older adult begins to become incontinent and loses the ability to feed and dress himself or herself, some people take on a parental role. It can be easy to deal with an elderly person as one would deal with a child. It is important to remember that this is a population of people who have been productive members of society. They have had careers and raised families. They are now adults who have special needs in order to help them maintain their adult dignity.

2. *Goal setting:* When preparing the plan of care with your older patient, remember to discuss goals that are attainable. Self-esteem and pride in one's accomplishments are as important when we are 80 as they were when we were 20. Success breeds success, and meeting small goals is an encouragement to the older person to attempt the bigger goals. The patient will see that the nurse was there to help reach that goal and, again, the relationship will strengthen.

3. *Patience and understanding:* Older patients who have some challenge to their physical or cognitive functioning may be slower to respond to verbal cues and may not be able to sprint down the halls at the pace that nurses generally travel. *Plan* for this. Attempt to convey the message that you have plenty of time (even though you may not). The patient who feels burdensome will be less likely to attempt activities or collaborate in the plan of care. He or she will be very sensitive to any nonverbal communication expressed by the nurses. It is therefore important to focus entirely on that person at that time.

4. *Humor:* Humor that is appropriate to the age and condition of the patient will help smooth over some of the harder times for you and your patient.

Caution: Not everyone appreciates humor and not everyone finds humor in the same things. Take your cues about humor from the patient. If the patient jokes about a situation, it is probably acceptable to go along with the humor. *Never* embarrass the person. Taking a situation in stride at the patient's suggestion, however, can be a very healthy mechanism for dealing with some of the hardships associated with aging.

5. *Safety:* Ensuring safety in the care facility and teaching safety to the patient who remains at home are very important. With vision, hearing, and other senses losing accuracy, it is easier for the older person to misjudge space, sound, and temperature. This could lead to falls, burns, and inability to hear the doorbell or the telephone ringing.

6. *Independence:* The older adult should be allowed to perform without assistance as much as possible. Do not assume that the older person is unable to do things independently. On the other hand, offer assistance as necessary. Let the person know that you would like to help in whatever way you can. Because of the loss in hearing and visual acuity that often accompanies aging, you may need to arrange for adaptive equipment that can help the patient to maintain as much independence as possible with daily activities.

7. *Acceptance:* In rapidly increasing numbers, people of diverse backgrounds and lifestyles are approaching the time of life that may require living in long-term care centers or assisted living communities. Those who will be caring for that population must be in touch with their own thoughts and feelings about working with diverse groups of people and must be prepared to flex care to meet their needs. Remember, however, that humans are much more alike than they are differ-

ent. Basic human needs as defined by Maslow and others are important for all groups of people.

Table 22-2 summarizes some of the concerns of aging adults and techniques nurses can use to more effectively help this population.

■ RESTORATIVE NURSING

Restorative nursing is part of rehabilitation and focuses on maintaining dignity and achieving maximum function for patients

and residents (Fig. 22-7). Some articles refer to restorative nursing as "good, old-fashioned nursing care"—arguably a subjective statement, and likely related to the professional age of the writer! Goals include independence, promoting self-esteem for the patient, and allowing the patient to maintain as much control over his or her life and daily living activities as possible.

Most skilled nursing facilities are required to provide at least one designated nursing assistant and nurse who are specially trained and part of the "restorative" team. They work in conjunction with physical therapy and rehabilitation departments to

TABLE 22-2	*Concerns of Aging Adults*	
CONCERN	**FACTORS ASSOCIATED WITH THIS CONCERN**	**HELPING TECHNIQUES**
ALZHEIMER'S DISEASE AND OTHER COGNITIVE IMPAIRMENTS	■ Debilitating effects are observable. ■ Patients need to leave the home they have lived in all of their adult lives; living apart from a spouse. ■ Socializing will be curtailed.	■ Respect for the individual ■ Realistic goal setting ■ Maintaining patience and understanding ■ Effective communication; allowing time for the patient to respond ■ Appropriate use of humor ■ Teaching and promoting safety ■ Promoting independence
CEREBROVASCULAR ACCIDENT (STROKE)	■ Physical and cognitive functions may be temporarily or permanently affected. ■ Depression is evident. ■ Aphasia may be present.	■ See "Alzheimer's Disease" ■ Allowing venting of emotions ■ Assisting with communication techniques ■ Allowing patient to verbalize; not automatically answering for patient
DEPRESSION	■ Symptoms may be different from those in other age groups. ■ Constipation; headaches and other body aches may be present. ■ Difficulty breathing for which there is no diagnosis may occur.	■ See "Alzheimer's Disease" ■ Allowing venting of thoughts and feelings ■ Teaching about patient's medications ■ Encouraging involvement in group activities as able

(continued)

TABLE 22-2 ■ *Concerns of Aging Adults* (Continued)		
CONCERN	**FACTORS ASSOCIATED WITH THIS CONCERN**	**HELPING TECHNIQUES**
MEDICATION CONCERNS	■ Pharmacokinetics is slower and less complete. ■ Circulatory and renal function is decreased. ■ It becomes easier for elderly people to experience side effects or become toxic. ■ Patients who live at home may forget to take medications or forget they have taken them and take another dose. ■ Visual acuity is lessened; patients may mistake one pill for another. ■ Nurse should advise patient to maintain weight, nutrition, and activity levels.	■ Providing patient with information about medication ■ Instructing patient to notify physician immediately if signs of side effects occur
PARANOID THINKING	■ Fear about the environment. ■ Slowed reaction time and diminished physical capacity. ■ Feelings of loneliness and isolation.	■ Allowing venting of feelings ■ Not reinforcing the paranoid thoughts ■ Speaking in terms of the "here and now"
INSOMNIA	■ Depression, fear, pain, urinary incontinence, napping during the day are common. ■ Decreased REM sleep can contribute to psychotic behavior; insomnia can intensify the symptoms of cognitive disorders.	■ Discussing underlying feelings ■ Teaching relaxation methods ■ Encouraging patient to seek medical evaluation

provide individualized restorative exercise and training to assist residents to achieve their maximum ability.

Restorative nursing is also part of a facility's documentation and reimbursement requirements. State and federal surveys grade the facility on its restorative program. OBRA long-term care laws require that residents either maintain or improve compared with their condition at the time of admis-

sion. Declines in residents' condition that cannot be proven to be medically unavoidable are not allowed. Including restorative nursing care in a person's care plan can prevent declines in condition that occur gradually, over time, such as loss of mobility, contractures, and loss of self-care ability. Restorative nursing is to be provided to any resident, regardless of his or her cognitive ability: The resident with dementia and the

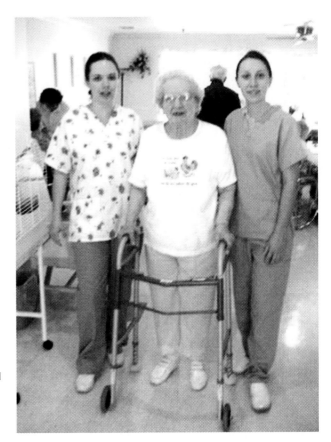

FIGURE 22-7. Restorative nursing is concerned with providing individualized restorative exercise to help patients achieve maximum function and maintain their dignity. (Courtesy of Little Brook Nursing Home, Califon, NJ.)

transitional care resident recuperating from knee surgery are equally in need of restorative nursing services.

■ PALLIATIVE CARE

Palliative care is end-of-life care. It is about keeping patients and families comfortable and promoting the best quality of life that one can provide to someone at the end of his or her life. In addition to working with grief and bereavement with the patient and significant persons in that patient's life, nurses choosing to work in a palliative setting will need to be comfortable with issues such as pain, symptom management, sedation and opioid medication at end of life, artificial nutrition and hydration, assisted suicide, and coordinating or providing complementary therapies. In addition, nurses will need to hone their communication skills and be very cognizant of religious, cultural, ethical, and legal issues, especially surrounding the heavy medications and assisted suicide issues.

It is widely documented that the preferred place of death of a patient is in his or her own home. Sometimes that is not possible. Because of that, many long-term care facilities are designing special units dedicated to palliative care (Fig. 22-8). Organizations such as The Center to Advance Palliative Care are attempting to show the need for hospital-based palliative care, as well.

Nurses are receiving special training and certification in this new specialty area. The good news is that LPN/LVN-prepared nurses

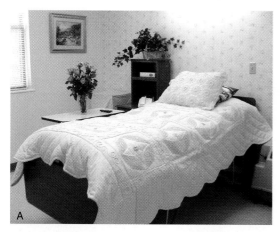 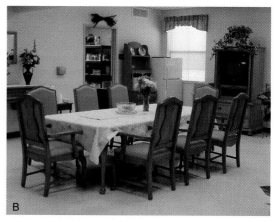

FIGURE 22-8. Many long-term-care facilities are designing special hospice units to give dying patients a more homelike environment. (Courtesy of Chandler Hospice, San Antonio, TX.)

are more than welcome into the fold. To encourage LPN- and LVN-prepared nurses to participate in palliative nursing, the Hospice and Palliative Nurses Association (HPNA) has developed a set of competencies that can be purchased from them online (Web site at end of chapter). The publication is called *Professional Competencies for the Hospice and Palliative Licensed Practical/ Vocational Nurse* (ISBN: 0-7575-0916-9).

Most nurses are familiar with the concepts mentioned above as components of palliative care. A bit nebulous yet for nurses is the idea of "complementary" and "alternative" treatment. This text provides information on alternative options in several chapters, but a basic definition is presented here. Complementary and alternative therapies are those that are not necessarily part of traditional nursing or medicine. As such, they may or may not be governed by a nurse's license. Each state has its own laws surrounding nurses engaging in alternative or complementary treatments. The terms refer more to the way in which they are delivered than any particular modality. To help define the terms *alternative* and *complementary,* let's use aromatherapy as an example. When used alone, aromatherapy would be considered an alternative therapy, but when used in conjunction with traditional medication and counseling, for example, it would be considered a complementary therapy.

Key Concepts ■ ■ ■

1. The concept of old age is changing. People are living longer and better after age 65. Older patients are being cared for in facilities and in their homes. Diversity among aging persons is on the rise. Nurses must be prepared to flex the care required to provide the best care possible to many different groups of elders. Nurses have an active part in helping the patient maintain a good quality of life.
2. Normal conditions of aging include diminishing hearing, vision, and other sensory acuity. Alzheimer's disease and other cognitive disorders are not considered a part of normal aging.

3. Afflictions affecting the older adult can be mental or physical or a combination of these. Medication side effects and drug toxicity can share the same symptoms as disorders that affect the elderly population. Accuracy of observation, documentation, and prompt reporting are crucial to a nurse's responsibility in caring for elderly people. Excellent communication skills are necessary.

4. Palliative care and other end of life treatments are becoming strong modalities in the treatment of patients with terminal diseases.

REFERENCES

Spotlight on Aging: A Newsletter for Seniors and Their Families. St. Paul: Minnesota Board on Aging. November 2002.

Barry, P.D. (2002). *Mental Health and Mental Illness,* 7th ed. JB Lippincott, Philadelphia.

Ferrell, B.R. and Coyle, N. (2001). *Textbook of Palliative Nursing,* Oxford University Press, New York.

Kaplan, B.J. (November 2002). Gay Elders Face Uncomfortable Realities in LTC. *Caring for the Ages* (American Medical Directors Association), Vol. 3, No. 11.

Koffman, J. and Higginson, I.J. (2004). Dying to be Home? Preferred location of death of first-generation Black Caribbean and native-born White patients in the United Kingdom. *Journal of Palliative Medicine,* 7/5, 628–636.

WEBSITES

www.capc.org
www.currentpsychiatry.com/2003
www.hospicecare.com
www.hpna.org
www.nimh.nih.gov
www.mnaging.org
www.palliativecarenursing.net
www.restorativenursing.com

CRITICAL THINKING EXERCISES ■ ■ ■

1. You are celebrating your retirement when the room goes dark. You wake up in a busy room with lights and noise and many people. You think you recognize some of them and you try to call out to them, but they just stand there and look at you. Someone you don't know is trying to say something to you and keeps shining a flashlight in your eye. Your life partner is crying. What happened to you? Why won't they answer you? What are you feeling now? What do you wish someone would do to help you?

2. Mr. Jacobs is admitted as a new resident in your nursing home. He is 76 years old and has a diagnosis of congestive heart failure (CHF). He has fallen at home several times recently and his adult children are concerned that he will become seriously injured. They have told him he needs to "go there for a while until you get stronger." They tell the staff, confidentially, they plan this to be a permanent placement and will be selling Mr. Jacobs' home to pay for his care. Mr. Jacobs will be started on digoxin, furosemide, and potassium for the CHF and has an order for acetaminophen with codeine for pain.

Five days later, Mr. Jacobs has had a change in mood. His family comes to visit and finds that he is combative and forgetful. One of his children is crying. She looks at you and says, "What have you done to him? He's never been like this before." What thoughts cross your mind? How do you respond to the personal attack? How will you attempt to resolve this situation? How would you like to be treated if you were the family member?

3. Using the suggested nursing diagnoses listed here (or others you can think of), complete a nursing process for a patient who has had a CVA.

SUGGESTED NURSING DIAGNOSES

1. *Verbal Communication, Impaired*
2. *Fear*
3. *Sensory/Perceptual Alterations (visual, auditory, verbal, tactile)*

ASSESSMENT/ DATA COLLECTION	NURSING DIAGNOSIS	PLAN/ GOAL	INTERVENTIONS/ NURSING ACTIONS	EVALUATION CRITERIA

4. Using the suggested nursing diagnoses listed here (or others you can think of), complete a nursing process for Mr. Jacobs in exercise 2.

SUGGESTED NURSING DIAGNOSES

1. *Anxiety*
2. *Injury, Risk for*
3. *Thought Processes, Altered*

ASSESSMENT/ DATA COLLECTION	NURSING DIAGNOSIS	PLAN/ GOAL	INTERVENTIONS/ NURSING ACTIONS	EVALUATION CRITERIA

TEST QUESTIONS ■ ■ ■

MULTIPLE CHOICE QUESTIONS

1. One effective communication technique for assisting a patient with aphasia is:

    A. Try to guess the word or finish the sentence.
    B. Associate the word with the object.
    C. Tell the patient to think about it while you make the bed.
    D. None of the above.

2. According to OBRA, who is responsible for completing the assessment of an older adult?

    A. All health staff
    B. Nursing assistants
    C. LPN/LVN
    D. RN

3. Mrs. Brown, who is usually alert and oriented, is showing signs of confusion. Her vital signs are all within normal limits. She has recently been started on furosemide for congestive heart failure. The nurse suspects:

    A. Just normal aging
    B. Stroke
    C. Medication side effect
    D. Depression

4. A 73-year-old patient in your long-term care center has become withdrawn and cranky. You try to find a method to initiate communication and activity with the person. Which of the following statements would be the best choice to try communicating with your patient?

    A. "Why are you staying over here by yourself?"
    B. "Your daughter wants you to make friends here."
    C. "I need a partner for the card game; I'd like to have you be my partner."
    D. "The doctor said the more you do, the better off you'll be."

5. "Losses" that are associated with the process of aging frequently cause:

    A. Presbycusis
    B. Depression
    C. Dementia
    D. CHF

6. When an older patient begins to show signs of dementia, physicians and nurses should assess all of the following *except:*

    A. Medication routines
    B. Nutritional intake
    C. Circulatory function
    D. Behaviors assumed to be part of "normal aging"

7. The speech impairment that affects many people who have had a stroke is called:

   A. Affect
   B. Aphasia
   C. Autism
   D. Ageism

8. Nurses understand that one of the reasons that older people become toxic from their prescription medications is:

   A. Drugs are metabolized faster in older people.
   B. Drugs are metabolized slower in older people.
   C. Drugs are ineffective in older people.
   D. Drugs need to be ordered in stronger doses for older people.

9. Your patient is admitted with bruises on his head and upper arms. His son is with him and jokes about the bruises, stating, "Dad is getting so clumsy. He falls out of his wheelchair a lot." You glance at the patient, who says nothing, is looking down, and is avoiding eye contact. You become alert for the possibility of:

   A. Blood dyscrasias
   B. Vitamin deficiency
   C. Elder abuse
   D. Self-inflicted wounds

10. The federal law that mandates special care and assessment skills for the older population is called:

    A. OBE
    B. OPRAH
    C. COBRA
    D. OBRA

11. When orienting new nursing assistants and other staff to your long-term care facility, you remind them:

    A. Memory loss is a normal part of aging.
    B. Memory loss is not a normal part of aging.
    C. Stress decreases as people age.
    D. All of the above.

12. In the orientation class mentioned above, you notice one of the housekeepers crying. She shares with the group that her grandmother has "old timer's or something and she doesn't remember me anymore." You respond to her:

    A. "It must be difficult for you to see your grandmother with Alzheimer's disease."
    B. "It's called Alzheimer's disease. Many of our residents have that illness."
    C. "How old is your grandmother?"
    D. "Who else has a relative with Alzheimer's?"

13. Treena is a 72-year-old woman who is in end stage cancer. She is taking regular doses of chemotherapy and pain medications. She is an artist by profession and professes that the color pink always makes her calm and happy. Her room has been painted pink, and her linens are all in shades of pink. How is color therapy being used for Treena? _____

14. If Treena were using only the color therapy and no traditional medication, what would the color therapy be identified as? _____

23

Victims of Abuse

Learning Objectives ■ ■ ■

1. Define abuse.
2. Define victim.
3. Differentiate among different kinds of abuse.
4. Identify characteristics of an abuser.
5. Identify nursing care to help survivors of abuse.

Key Terms ■ ■ ■

- Abuse
- Abuser
- Date rape
- Elder abuse
- Emotional abuse
- Incest
- Physical abuse
- Rape
- Respite care
- Safe house
- Sexual abuse
- Sexual harassment
- Spouse abuse
- Survivor
- Verbal abuse
- Victim

Abuse is defined as **1:** a corrupt practice or custom **2:** improper or excessive use or treatment **3:** *obsolete*: a deceitful act **4:** language that condemns or vilifies usually unjustly, intemperately, and angrily **5:** physical maltreatment (Webster Online, 2004).

Victim is defined by Webster Online as "one that is acted on and usually adversely affected by a force or agent."

Experts who work in the field of abuse are divided regarding the term *victim*. This word connotes a dependency that many believe serves to place the target of abuse in a more dependent position emotionally.

Many prefer to use the term **survivor.** It is more positive and forward-thinking than the somewhat defeatist *victim*. Both terms will be used interchangeably in this text.

Abuse is not an easy topic to assess. For one thing, strong cultural influences surround abuse issues. In some cultures, rough treatment of children and wives is not only accepted but expected. Flogging of citizens is the law in some countries; in the United States, flogging would be a travesty. Increasingly, people are reporting instances of abuse in the workplace. Examples of workplace violence range from verbal assaults to hostile environments caused by supervisors to physical assault and homicide. Nurses are employees as well as caregivers. We find ourselves on both sides of the issue of abuse in the workplace.

The combining of many people in this country can cause much controversy. Consider this all-too-typical scenario: You, the nurse, witness a man from another country verbally berating his wife and threatening her with physical harm while they are in their child's room. You report this to your supervisor, who investigates. Two days later, your station receives a telephone call from the minority counseling office, informing you that you have infringed on the civil rights of this couple to practice the customs of their culture. "But there are laws in this country!" you say. You are told that people have a right to continue their customs and that it is abuse only if the person or persons involved consider it to be so. In this situation, the wife accepted the behavior of her husband, and your reporting the situation was insulting to them. What about the responsibility of nurses to report all suspected cases of abuse? If you are confused right now, you are paying attention!

One of the reasons abuse is so hard to prosecute is that it is so individualized. People are generally abused by someone close to them: a parent, relative, child, spouse, babysitter, clergy, or some other trusted person. The **abuser** often apologizes profusely and promises the abuse will never happen again. The survivor wants desperately to believe the abuser and does nothing. Sooner or later, the abuse repeats. The cycle repeats. The victim (survivor) may begin to cover up the abuse to protect the abuser. The victim may begin to feel responsible—"maybe if I were thinner . . . prettier . . . richer . . . younger . . ."—and it takes a serious hospitalization or near-death episode to convince the survivor to report the abuser and get some help.

Abuse covers all ages, genders, races, walks of life, and economic classes.

Statistics are skewed somewhat in favor of female abuse, primarily because men have been reluctant to report abuse by women. This chapter presents some of the larger groups that experience abuse. You will learn some characteristics of abusers as well as characteristics of victims. The final part of the chapter gives some ideas for developing a helping relationship with both the abused and the abuser, because both, in all probability, need treatment.

■ CHARACTERISTICS OF ABUSERS

ABUSED HIMSELF/HERSELF

"Violence begets violence. People—especially children—tend to imitate what they see" (Rubin, Peplau, and Salovey, 1993). That statement remains the belief of researchers today. It is accepted that, except in rare situations with a genetic or biologic connection, violence, aggression, and abuse are learned behaviors. Children who grow up witnessing violence in the home and on television are sensitized to believe that this is right behavior and will very likely continue into adulthood, retreating to these childhood memories and resorting to abuse when they are stressed.

LOW SELF-ESTEEM/NEED FOR POWER

Abusers have not learned to accept themselves. They feel frustrated and minimized as persons. They have poor interpersonal relationships and may not have their ideas and accomplishments validated by people they want to notice them. Therefore, they resort to physical, verbal, or emotional abuse of others in an attempt to bring a sense of power and importance to themselves. Sexual abuse is almost always not about sex; it is about conquering and winning. It is about berating another human being in order to feel a sense of strength. It is a short-term "fix" for the abuser and a life-long scar for the abused.

ALCOHOLIC/CHEMICALLY DEPENDENT PERSONS

These afflictions, as discussed in Chapter 17, also have psychoanalytic components relating to ineffective emotional development. Certainly some experts believe there are also genetic and biologic causes for these dependencies. There may be permanent cognitive impairment if the chemical use was intense and long term. Regardless of the underlying causes, the outcome may still be the ability to abuse another person.

PARENTS WITH UNWANTED CHILDREN

Parents who for some reason do not want a family are at risk for abusing each other and the unwanted child. Mothers who are victims of rape or who have no spouse, men who feel "tricked" into a relationship because of the pregnancy, and parents who are drug or alcohol users are among those at highest risk for becoming child abusers.

■ CHARACTERISTICS OF THE VICTIM

1. *Dependent or codependent personality:* Low self-esteem may again play a part in someone's becoming abused. People who have not learned to be assertive and to say what they think and feel or to speak out for what they need and want may not be able to call up the strength they need to ward off an attack. They may be easily manipulated by the abuser into believing either that they deserved the attack or that the abuser is truly repentant and will not abuse again. They will begin to make up reasons to excuse the abuser's behavior and may accept the responsibility for the abuser's actions.

2. *Reliance on abuser:* People who are reliant on the abuser for financial support are vulnerable to attacks from the abuser. This holds true for all age groups of people who are abused.

■ CATEGORIES OF ABUSE

SEXUAL ABUSE

Sexual abuse is violent or nonviolent sexual contact or sexual activity that is not wanted by the receiver. Sexual abuse can be part of other classifications of abuse as well. **Sexual harassment,** which involves physical or verbal sexual innuendo, may take place in many situations but typically occurs on a job by someone in authority. It may or may not include actual sexual activity but serves to leave the recipient uncomfortable and the workplace unfriendly to that person or group of people. Both sexual abuse and sexual harassment are forms of power play being used by the abuser. There are laws to protect people from these activities. In recent years, headway has been made into finding in favor of those being harassed on the job; prosecuting domestic sexual abuse is not as successful.

As suggested earlier, sexual abuse is generally inflicted on someone the abuser considers less powerful physically or emotionally. The abuser is usually a close, significant figure in the abused person's life and knows how to manipulate the potential victim into submission. This is sometimes referred to as "button pushing." Button pushing means the abuser knows what to say or do to get a particular response from the intended victim. When that response is achieved, the abuser uses it as an excuse to sexually abuse the victim. This is an example of stimulus and response, Skinner's theory on "operant conditioning."

Incest is defined as "sexual intercourse between persons so closely related that they are forbidden by law to marry; *also* : the statutory crime of such a relationship" (Webster Online, 2004). It can include foreplay, touching, kissing, and mutual masturbation, as well as oral sex and intercourse. The most frequent occurrence of incest is in very young children (ages 5 through 8), although it applies to persons of any age group.

Rape is forcible, degrading, nonconsensual sexual intercourse accompanied by violence and intimidation. Most hospital emergency rooms and urgent care centers have rape kits to assist in proper collection of evidence such as sperm, hair, and other fibers that may be compared with others to identify a suspect. It is important that the person who was raped not clean up before going to the emergency department. Although evidence must be kept intact, one of the victim's first instincts is to "wash away" the incident both physically and psychologically by showering. Nurses should discourage that activity until evidence and DNA sources can be collected. **Date rape** or **acquaintance rape** is seen frequently among high school and college students and young adults within that age group. A belief surrounding date rape is that the person who pays for the date (typically the male figure) is entitled to sex from the other person (typically the female figure).

An alarming reality in the United States is that rape happens to elderly people, as well as to children and other adults. That population is being assaulted in their private residences and in long-term care and assisted living facilities.

PHYSICAL ABUSE

Physical abuse includes any action that causes physical harm to another person. Hitting; burning; withholding food, water, and other basic needs; and other activities that go beyond accidental contact—these are all considered physical abuse. For example, a parent spanks a child. Many people believe it is never acceptable to touch another person out of anger. Spanking is a very controversial activity at best, but some individuals believe that a spanking, when other forms of discipline have failed, is a proper thing. When that spanking goes from one slap on the buttocks to repeated slaps or when it escalates into a "belt beating," that is beyond accepted limits of physical harm to that child. What is already a borderline-acceptable behavior has crossed the line into probable abuse. A wife who uses extraordinary means to "punish" her husband for extramarital relationships has gone beyond acceptable behavior.

A rule of thumb for defining the line between an accident and physical abuse is when the recipient says, "Stop. You're hurting me," or something similar. If the activity stops and does not repeat itself, that behavior may well have been just an accident. If the behavior persists, if the request to stop is ignored or mocked by the perpetrator, or if the activity is repeated in future situations, there is a strong chance that the perpetrator is guilty of abuse.

EMOTIONAL ABUSE

Emotional abuse is the willful use of words or actions that attempt to undermine the other person's self-esteem. This includes the "silent treatment," which causes the other person to "guess" at the problem and "game playing," which involves activities such as developing a relationship (business or personal) and then suddenly changing the ground rules of that relationship in such a way as to confuse the other person about the relationship.

Emotional abuse overlaps physical and spousal abuse very often. **Verbal abuse,** name-calling, and using foul language aimed directly at the person are ways to begin to undermine that person's confidence, opening the door to other types of abuse.

SPOUSE/DOMESTIC ABUSE

In a 2001 study of women visiting a pediatric clinic, researchers found that more than 16%, or 553 mothers, had been physically abused at some point in their lifetime.

The researchers strongly encourage screening for domestic violence as part of the office intake protocol (Parkinson, Adams, Emerling, 2001).

Many authors refer to this as "wife abuse." As mentioned earlier, **spouse abuse** or **domestic abuse** may appear to be wife abuse only; however, this information may be skewed because men do not report abuse as often. Counseling centers are beginning to develop programs to encourage men who are abused by their spouses to come forward for help. Hopefully, the stigma will diminish, and the statistics will soon reflect more accurate numbers of male spouse abuse.

Spouse abuse takes many forms. There is an old saying and song that uses the words, "You always hurt the one you love." As dysfunctional as that sounds, there is a great deal of truth to those words. We learn very intimate things about our life partners, and we know how certain situations will affect them. Popular estimates of wife abuse in the United States are that a woman is beaten by her partner (or ex-partner) every 18 seconds.

Emotional spouse abuse often incorporates the children: "If you go out with your friends tonight, I'll see to it that your kids are taken away; you're unfit to be their mother (father) if you go out at night and leave them without their mother (father). You do not deserve them!" Or "Leave and when you get back the kids and I will be gone and you won't see them again!" Words such as these are used to intimidate and frighten a parent. Parents usually love their children, and the last thing they want is to lose them. Button pushing such as this is very effective at negatively controlling someone's behavior out of fear of the consequences.

Three phases of the spousal abuse cycle are very predictable (Fig. 23-1):

1. *Tension-building:* The recipient of the abuse is compliant, believing that in some way he or she is at fault and deserves the abuse. These individuals remain accepting and continue to be supportive even though they know the

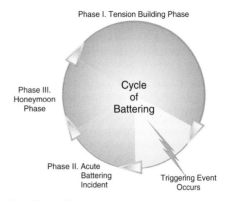

FIGURE 23-1. Phases of the spousal abuse cycle. (From Townsend, M.C., *Psychiatric/Mental Health Nursing: Concepts of Care,* 4th ed. Philadelphia, FA Davis Company, p. 776. Reprinted with permission.)

behavior is inappropriate. The victim is probably using denial as a defense mechanism. The perpetrator is using verbal abuse and minor beating and also is aware that the behavior is not appropriate.

2. *Acute battering:* The victim senses that the beating is coming and may even provoke it to get it over with. He or she may try to hide and will probably not seek help until the next day, if at all. The police may be called, but by the time they arrive, the victim may have already forgiven the perpetrator. This kind of physical abuse usually happens in private or when the perpetrator thinks they are alone.

3. *Honeymoon:* The perpetrator is contrite, loving, and very sad about the incident of abuse that has occurred. The abuser promises to get help but only after discussing how the abuse has taught the other a lesson, such as "Don't make me mad!" The victim wants desperately to believe this and will forgive the perpetrator and begin to think that the relationship will return to "normal." The victim is still very much in love with the perpetrator and believes this love will conquer all and the abusing will stop (Walker, 1979).

ELDER ABUSE

The National Elder Abuse Incidence Study suggests that more than 500,000 Americans aged 60 and over were victims of domestic abuse in 1996. While this is the currently quoted statistic, other agencies indicate that number rises somewhat annually.

Physical abuse of the elderly commonly includes slapping, hitting, and striking with objects, resulting in bruises, sprains, abrasions, skeletal fractures, burns, and other injuries (Fig. 23-2). **Elder abuse** takes place in private homes and established health-care facilities. Current estimates are that approximately 30 percent of older people who are abused are abused by their children.

Nurses who care for older adults either through home care or in a facility must be alert to signs that the older adult has been abused. Good physical and emotional observations on each home visit, after visits by friends and family, and when returning from passes from the facility are important.

Nurse and social workers can also serve as resource people for families or other caregivers who are caring for elderly people. Offering the names of such agencies as your state's agency on aging and Meals on Wheels and providing the phone numbers can be very helpful in enabling caregivers to get help from some services and to find some "respite care" so they can get away for

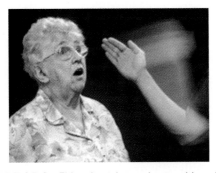

FIGURE 23-2. Elder abuse is a serious problem. It occurs in private homes and in health-care facilities. (Courtesy of Arkansas Adult Protective Services, Little Rock, AR.)

a while. **Respite care** is a service offered by various agencies throughout the community. It provides a relief caregiver to stay with the elderly person so that the primary caregiver can take a vacation or just have an afternoon away from the responsibility. Any period of time (up to approximately two weeks) can generally be arranged. The amount of time will depend on the availability and individual circumstances.

Neglect of the older person can include improper nourishment and improper use of the person's finances, as well as other situations that are not in the best interest of the older person.

■ GENERAL CRITERIA FOR SUSPECTING ABUSE

1. *Bruising:* Bruises in unexpected areas such as the head, rib cage, upper arms, wrists, or genitalia.
2. *Bleeding:* Bloody underwear; bloody emesis (may indicate internal abdominal injury).
3. *Absence from work or school:* Employees or children who have unexplained and/or frequent episodes of absence or truancy or who have patterns of absence.
4. *Depression:* Children and adults who are depressed may be attempting to deal with the abuse internally. Depression is often defined as "anger turned inward." People who for one reason or another cannot express their anger often show signs of depressed behavior.
5. *Withdrawal from friends and social activities:* People who are being abused may not only change their relationships but may also move from one location to another in an attempt to hide their shame and guilt. Any change in social pattern could be an indication of abuse.

6. *Frequent bladder infections:* Signs of infection in the urinary or reproductive tracts (itching, burning, pain, blood).
7. *Physical abnormalities:* Edema of the vulva, presence of semen, difficulty sitting or walking, or torn underwear.
8. *Frequent visits to the emergency room:* Parents or caregivers who are abusing children often make numerous trips to the emergency room or urgent care center with minor concerns, such as colds or excessive crying, or with a child who is "accident prone."

■ GENERAL NURSING ACTIONS TO HELP ABUSED PERSONS

1. *Ensure safety:* The survivor of abuse will be confused and fearful. The nurse needs to reassure the patient that everything possible is being done to ensure the patient's safety. Obtain a list of people who are considered "safe" by the patient. Ask if the patient would like those people to be called. If the patient wishes to press charges, offer assistance with making the appropriate phone calls. Call for assistance from a physician and counselor if none is in the immediate area. Alert security staff members according to your agency protocol. Maintain a calm milieu.
2. *Know your own thoughts and feelings about abuse:* The nurse is responsible for helping the patient through this initial horrifying experience. A nurse who has been abused or who has been an abuser may find it difficult to be therapeutic for the patient. Remember that you may be treating two people: the survivor as well as the abuser. You are responsible to help all patients. Abusers are in need of our help as much as the person who is abused. It is worthwhile to mention that nurses face stressful situations daily. In order to be healthy and helpful for our patients, we as nurses must be aware of our own mental health to avoid the possibility of becoming abusive of those in our care.
3. *Remain nonjudgmental/show empathy:* This is a crisis situation in many ways. Recalling your communication skills and helping the patient to verbalize any concerns, thoughts, and feelings are crucial. Remaining technically correct in performing any procedures or sample collections is imperative to avoid contamination. Maintaining professionalism and confidentiality for both the survivor and the abuser is mandatory. Calling for help from counselors, advocates, or people chosen by the patients will help maintain a calm milieu. *Note:* In their book, *Beginning to Heal,* Ellen Bass and Laura Davis (1993) state, "Don't sympathize with the abuser. The survivor needs your total loyalty" (p. 107). Nurses are not ethically allowed to make that kind of therapeutic decision. We attempt to help every patient to the best of our ability. You are not expected to condone or accept the action, but you are expected to respect and help the person, regardless of the situation.
4. *Know your agency policy:* Every clinic, emergency room, and urgent care center has its own policies and procedures for dealing with abused patients. Familiarity with these policies and procedures will help save time and convey confidence. The patient may be confused and embarrassed about the situation. It may well have taken every bit of courage the person had just to get to your facility. Your smooth handling of the situation may provide the extra bit of confidence the victim needs to actually go through with the examination. In most jurisdictions, with the exception

of persons legally classified as "vulnerable," notification of police, taking of pictures, etc. may only be done with the patient's consent.

Many hospitals and trauma centers have some sort of abuse-advocacy program. A representative should be contacted immediately to visit the victim. The abuse program representative will be able to offer support and provide information on safe houses and other services that may be available to the victim and his or her children.

Nurses who are caring for a survivor of abuse need to be aware of their state's law regarding children who may have witnessed the abuse. In some states, a child who sees or hears abuse is also considered to have been abused. Nurses and other health-care providers are most likely mandated reporters and, as such, find themselves in an ethical bind: They want to help and support the patient/survivor; however, they must tell that individual that if a child saw or heard the abuse, the nurse must, as a mandated reporter, report this fact to the child protection agency. The patient/survivor may be forced, in a sense, not to divulge the whole situation to the nurse.

The physician or counselor will discuss treatment options with the survivor and the abuser. The survivor may be referred to a **safe house,** that is, a shelter for temporary living for persons who have been battered. Legal counsel may be requested as well. A law enforcement agency may be present also. Nurses now can take a more advocacy-oriented role for the patient. Be supportive.

Table 23-1 summarizes the types of abuse discussed here and the general nursing interventions to care for people who are abused.

TABLE 23-1 *Abuse Disorders*		
TYPE OF ABUSE	**SIGNS/SYMPTOMS**	**NURSING INTERVENTIONS**
SEXUAL	■ Violent or nonviolent sexual contact or activity that is not wanted by the receiver ■ Foreplay, touching, kissing, and mutual masturbation, as well as oral sex and intercourse ■ Frequent bladder or vaginal infections ■ Bloody underwear Includes: ■ "Incest"—sexual intercourse between persons so closely related that marriage is illegal ■ Rape—forcible, degrading, non-consensual sexual intercourse accompanied by violence and intimidation ■ "Date rape"—seen frequently in high school and college students (belief surrounding date rape is that the person who pays for the date is entitled to sex from the other person)	■ Carefully use rape kit and preserve evidence. ■ Provide safety. ■ Be nonjudgmental. ■ Show empathy. ■ Be advocate for patient. ■ Maintain calm milieu. ■ Know own thoughts and feelings regarding abuse and abuser. ■ Know agency policies. ■ Assist with contacting outside agencies (e.g., lawyer, clergy), as requested by patient.

(continued)

TYPE OF ABUSE	SIGNS/SYMPTOMS	NURSING INTERVENTIONS
PHYSICAL	■ Any actions that cause physical harm to another ■ Hitting ■ Burning ■ Withholding food, water, and other basic needs ■ Other activities that go beyond accidental contact ■ Request to stop ignored or mocked by the perpetrator ■ Activity repeating itself in future situations ■ Frequent visits to emergency department (for all forms of abuse) ■ Excessive bruising or bruising on unusual areas of body ■ Withdrawal from friends and social groups	■ Provide safety. ■ Be nonjudgmental. ■ Show empathy. ■ Be advocate for patient. ■ Maintain calm milieu. ■ Know own thoughts and feelings regarding abuse and abuser. ■ Know agency policies. ■ Assist with contacting outside agencies (e.g., lawyer, clergy), as requested by patient.
EMOTIONAL	■ Willful use of words or actions that undermine self-esteem—includes the "silent treatment" (causes the other person to guess at the problem) and other types of game playing ■ Name-calling ■ Using foul language	■ Same as for "Physical Abuse."
CHILD ABUSE/ NEGLECT	■ Sexual, physical, and/or emotional abuse—act of commission (doing) or omission (not doing) ■ Fear that abuse is child's fault ■ Child confused about what is happening and why ■ Abuser often larger than the child, which is intimidating ■ Excessive absences from school	■ Same as for "Physical Abuse."
SPOUSE	■ Physical, emotional, and "button-pushing" kinds of abuse ■ Most typically reported by women ■ Seems to go through a cycle of abuse ■ Withdrawal from friends and social groups	■ Same as for "Physical Abuse."
ELDER	■ Slapping ■ Hitting ■ Striking with objects—bruises ■ Sprains ■ Abrasions ■ Burns ■ Occasionally skeletal fractures and other wounds	■ Same as for "Physical Abuse."

Key Concepts ▢ ▤ ▪

1. Abuse takes many forms and is being reported in higher numbers annually. Most of the abuse is being reported by women; however, estimates suggest that almost as many men are being abused. Men need to be encouraged to report abuse.
2. Symptoms of abuse are many but include commission of physical and emotional behaviors. Neglect is the omission of cares or nutrition for people who require these needs.
3. Abuse happens in all age and socioeconomic groups.
4. Nurses must be sensitive to the needs of the abused person as well as those of the abuser. Careful attention to physical assessment, communication, and emotional support are components of nursing care for people who are suffering the effects of abuse.
5. Screening for domestic abuse is strongly suggested as part of office intake protocol.

REFERENCES

Bass, E. and Davis, L. (1993). *Beginning to Heal— The First Book for Survivors of Child Sexual Abuse.* Harper Perennial/HarperCollins, New York.

Boyd, M. and Nihart, M. (1998). *Psychiatric Nursing—Contemporary Practice,* Lippincott, Philadelphia.

Davidson, M. (2001). The nurse practitioner's role in diagnosing and facilitating treatment in patients with post-traumatic stress disorder. *American Journal for Nurse Practitioners,* 5 (9), 10–17.

Parkinson, G., Adams, R., and Emerling, F. (2001). Maternal domestic violence screening in an office-based pediatric practice. *Pediatrics* September 1, 2001; 108(3 www.aappolicy. aappublications.org/cgi/content/full/pediatrics; 101/6/1091

House Select Committee on Aging. (1991). *Congressional Quarterly Almanac.* 102nd Congress, 1st Session, CQ, Inc., Washington, DC.

Webster Online. 2004. www.merriam-webster.com

Rubin, Z., Peplau, H., and Salovey, P. (1993). *Psychology.* Houghton-Mifflin, Boston.

WEBSITES

www.elderabusecenter.org/

CRITICAL THINKING EXERCISES ■ ■ ■

1. Contact an emergency room or clinic in your town. Request an appointment to interview the staff about their policies and procedures for treating abused persons.

2. Mrs. Jones leaves your long-term care facility for a weekend with her daughter and son-in-law. She seems apprehensive but tells you, "I just worry that

I'm a bother to them." You bathed her and helped her pack and now you document that she is gone until Sunday afternoon and that you were concerned about her apprehension. You noted no other physical or mental abnormalities. Sunday afternoon, she returns with skin tears on both arms and a bruise over her right eye and on her right cheek. She is crying. Her daughter says, "Doesn't that look awful? Gram took a tumble from the toilet." "Gram" says nothing until her daughter leaves, then says to you, "I worry about her. Her husband is a nice man, but he gets so mad at us sometimes. I really can't blame him; he has a lot on his mind, and I can't give them any more money." What are your responsibilities according to your facility? According to the state? According to your personal belief system?

3. Mrs. P is admitted to your surgical floor. She has multiple rib fractures and bruises, a broken jaw, and a broken right arm. Mrs. P is married to a popular public figure in your town. She was beginning to tell you about her 2- and 3-year-old children who saw the event. She stated to you that she "should have known better. I'm so uncoordinated. I should never have tried to climb that ladder myself." Mrs. P asks you to get something from the bathroom for her. As you are complying with her request, you hear Mr. P enter the room and say, "I told you to quit talking and just leave me alone. You know you make me mad when you nag at me." You hear Mrs. P say, "Ssh" as you emerge from the bathroom. Mr. P smiles broadly at you and says in a joking tone of voice, "I suppose she told you how clumsy she is. I told her not to do it, but she never listens. Too independent for her own good!" Mrs. P is no longer maintaining eye contact and you observe her looking toward the floor. What should your initial response be to Mrs. P? to Mr. P? What nursing actions would be appropriate in this situation? What confidentiality issues must you maintain? What reporting issues might you be required to address?

4. You are an LPN/LVN employed in your hospital's employee health service. Todd, who works in central supply, presents with lacerations on his arms and face, ranting about someone who attacked him: "He's crazy. That guy is crazy! I asked him to help me unload some boxes and he pulled a knife on me. Told me he'd heard I'd been with his girlfriend. I don't even know her. He just went crazy. What can I do?" What are your priorities for Todd? What are some options for Todd to resolve this situation? What are your reporting responsibilities?

5. Using the suggested nursing diagnoses listed here (or others you can think of), complete a nursing process for Mrs. Jones in exercise 2.

SUGGESTED NURSING DIAGNOSES

1. Injury, Risk for
2. Skin Integrity, Impaired
3. Anxiety
4. Ineffective Family Coping: Compromised

ASSESSMENT/ DATA COLLECTION	NURSING DIAGNOSIS	PLAN/ GOAL	INTERVENTIONS/ NURSING ACTIONS	EVALUATION CRITERIA

TEST QUESTIONS ■ ■ ■

MULTIPLE CHOICE QUESTIONS

1. When caring for someone who has been abused, the nurse can be therapeutic by:

    A. Showing empathy
    B. Ensuring safety
    C. Contacting counselors and advocates
    D. All of the above

2. Which of the following is a legal requirement for you (the nurse) to perform when caring for a rape victim?

    A. Ask why it happened.
    B. Document the information in the patient's own words.
    C. Offer to take the patient home after your shift.
    D. None of the above.

3. When a survivor of abuse and the abuser both present at your facility, your responsibility is to care for the:

    A. Survivor only
    B. Abuser only
    C. Both people
    D. Neither one; call the physician

4. Mrs. X has been caring for her mother at home. Mrs. X's mother has third-stage Alzheimer's disease and is requiring more of Mrs. X's time. She says to you, "I just don't know what to do. I can't stand it anymore. I love my mother, but I don't have any time for myself and I can't afford a nursing home." You say:

    A. "Mrs. X, hang in there. Things have a way of working out."
    B. "Why don't your sisters and brothers help out a little?"

    C. "There are agencies that provide respite care for people in your situation. If you like, I could tell the social worker that you would like some information on this service."

    D. "It's got to be hard to put up with this all day when you aren't trained for it."

5. A 38-year-old female presents to urgent care. She has a 3-year-old and a 4-year-old child with her. She is frightened and badly bruised. "He'll kill us all if he knows we came here," she screams. You:

    A. Ask her to please not scream—she is alarming the other patients.

    B. Ask, "Who will kill you?"

    C. Bring her and her children to a room immediately.

    D. Ask her to sit for a moment while you contact someone who can provide safety for her.

6. Mrs. Blackeye arrives for her appointment. She has had a positive home pregnancy test and suspects she is pregnant. She has a black eye and a lacerated upper lip and admits her husband hit her because "I did something stupid. I fell asleep and supper burned. It's my fault. He works hard. He deserves a decent meal. I'm OK." You tell her:

    A. "Nobody deserves to be hit. Here is the name of an organization that can help."

    B. "You need to leave him right away before he hurts your baby too."

    C. "Why do you stay and let him do that?"

    D. "Has he done this before?"

A Final Word to Students

You will soon be graduating, writing state boards, and beginning your first positions as licensed nurses. Some of you may be preparing to continue a mobility program into registered nursing or another professional direction.

Earlier in this textbook journey, we discussed the stress that may come with working with diverse groups of people with a myriad of conditions. We discussed the fact that nurses are humans. We have families and personal issues of our own. It is of paramount importance that nurses learn to "practice what we preach" when it comes to stress reduction techniques. You will be of no help to anyone if you do not first take care of yourself. How can we do that? How can you refuse an extra shift for the third time this week? Here are some things to try:

1. Learn to say "no" and mean "no." Respectfully. Politely. Firmly. Learn your facility scheduling policies. If you are a member of a union, learn those policies. Work within them. Do your part. Do more when you can. Sick people need someone to care for them. They deserve to be cared for safely by nurses who are well rested, who are in a stable state of mental health, and who are not distracted. Say "no" when you need to say "no." Say "yes" when it is possible and healthy for you to do so.

   On the lighter side, (humor is important as well), this author used to instruct nursing students in "the mechanics of saying no." Practice this together. Place the tip of your tongue against the roof of your mouth or against the back of your upper teeth. Begin a slight humming sound with the consonant "nnnnnnnnnn." When you have a good "nnnn" hum sound, allow your lower jaw to drop down loosely. The "nnnn" sound changes to something vaguely resembling an "o" sound. The "nnnn" and "o" done in quick succession will give you the word "no!" Mechanical help for a condition frequently found in nurses "no-o-phobia": fear of the word "no."

2. Many employers have an employee assistance program of some sort. These are usually free to employees and sometimes to their families. Some have fees for certain services after a designated number of free calls. Use this benefit. They are usually contracted by vendors other than your employer, and records are confidential and not available to your employer.

3. Recognize your limits. Not all of us can work full time. That's OK! Super-Nurse only exists in one's imagination. Those who must balance family, work, and single-parenthood may need to cut back a day or two per pay period. For those of us who are the majority of society today, it is frightening enough to live from pay check to pay check. We wonder how we can make it on 8 days per pay period when we can barely do it on full time hours. Again, consult your policy manual or your human resources department. Most employers offer some sort of financial planner or consultant. See how you can work smarter, not harder, financially.

4. Become involved in work groups or state groups that assist in policy-making. Make your voice and your professional concerns heard.

These are only a few simple suggestions, but they are ideas that can help relieve some stress of one's professional life and allow a bit of peace of mind. Be proactive, not reactive!

According to the United States Department of Labor Bureau of Labor Statistics, in the year 2000, LPN/LVN-prepared nurses held approximately 700,000 jobs. The breakdown was 29 percent in nursing homes, 28 percent in hospitals, and 14 percent in clinics and offices. The rest worked in schools, home health care, per diem agencies, or other industry and government agencies. Approximately 20 percent, or 1 in 5, worked part time. The rate of job growth is expected to increase rapidly into the year 2010.

The average or median age of working nurses is rising. It is now into middle age. That opens up a new set of challenges. Older nurses' working longer work days often leads to increases in work-related injuries. Nurses find themselves with restrictions on how much they can lift, push, pull. . . . Some can't squat, bend, or even climb steps. The Americans with Disabilities Act (ADA), a federal law, requires employers to make "reasonable accommodations" to allow disabled workers back to the workplace at whatever capacity they may be able to work. State workers compensation laws also provide for people to work with specific restrictions. Workers on "light duty" cause the workload to shift. Sometimes an extra and potentially uncomfortable burden is placed on the able-bodied nurses, causing them more wear and tear. Ultimately, that situation has the potential to create a safety issue for the patients who need to be lifted or transported by nurses picking up the extra work the restricted nurses cannot do. There are ethical, legal, and logistic challenges present in this situation. First of all, what is "safe" for the patient demographic in your agency? What legal responsibilities does the employer or staffer have to meet, again considering both the staffing needs for acuity of the patient group and the medical restrictions and accommodations needed by the injured worker? What is "fair" to both the disabled nurse and the able-bodied nurse? Research is currently being conducted and published looking for a correlation between the number of "older" nurses in the workforce, increased workload and patient acuity, and the amount of reports of nurses injured on the job.

Long term care facilities, clinics, and hospitals are still the primary employers for the LPN- and LVN-prepared nurse. Slowly, however, other opportunities are opening, perhaps due to the economy, perhaps because other industry sees the value of a nursing education as a base of knowledge and a strong skill set. Insurance companies, human resource agencies, job recruiters ("headhunters"), and human services (county, state, faith-based, etc.) are employing nurses in various positions for those interested in something other than traditional "floor" nursing. Nurses may become involved in facilitating groups or assisting with programs such as the "peer mentoring" program associated with Catholic Charities and the Mental Health Consumer Network, a group active in the central Minnesota area. Peer mentors are people who have been consumers of mental health services and who have positive attitudes about recovery. They assist those who currently need a one-on-one relationship with another recovering person.

The good news is that nurses will always be needed. Our roles may change. The environments in which we work may change. Our level of preparation for entry into nursing may change. Your nursing license is a wonderful springboard into a myriad of other professional opportunities.

What will remain constant is that people will continue to become physically and mentally ill. They will require health care professionals who are highly trained and highly skilled, yet who have managed to maintain that special something that makes us nurses: the art of caring.

Best of luck in your careers!

Kathy Neeb

REFERENCES

American Association of Occupational Health Nurses, Inc. (2003). *Shouldering the Burden of On-the-Job Injury, 23* (8), 1.

Hope Community Support Program, Catholic Charities. Peer Mentoring. 125 11th Avenue, North St. Cloud, MN 56303; Ph: (320) 259-0380.

USA Weekend (a division of Gannett Satellite Information Network, Inc.). (2003). Crisis in White, August 29–31, 6–7.

SPECIAL MENTION:
Lynn Keller, RN, BSN
Hope Community Support Program, Catholic Charities.

WEBSITES

www/bls.gov
www.usaweekend.com

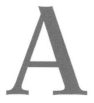

Answers and Rationales

■ CHAPTER 1

1. B. The main goal of deinstitutionalization was to allow as many people as possible to return to the community and lead as normal a life as they could. Not all mentally ill people would be able to do that because of the severity of their illness. On the other hand, not all mentally ill people had to be kept in locked units, nor do they today. Community hospitals were to be kept open, but many state hospitals closed because of the decline in census.

2. C. The development of psychotropic (psychoactive) medications in the 1950s was a keystone to allowing people to return to their homes. The Community Mental Health Centers Act came about 10 years later. The Nurse Practice Act dictates the scope of practice for nurses; and electroshock therapy, now called electroconvulsant therapy, took place in hospitals.

3. D. The Nurse Practice Act, which is written specifically for each state, is the set of regulations that dictates the scope of nursing practice. The NLN and the ANA are national nursing associations that set recommendations for the practice, education, and well-being of nurses. The Patient Bill of Rights is a document to protect the patient. Nurses must know the parameters of this document for ethical practice, but it does not dictate the scope of nursing practice.

4. D. Deinstitutionalization and changes in the health-care delivery system encourage people with mental health issues to be treated in a variety of health-care settings. Nurses will care for patients with mental illnesses in all of the settings listed.

■ CHAPTER 2

1. B. This option offers assistance in a way that encourages the patient to say what he or she needs. Option A used the word "why," which has negative connotations. C is closed-ended and allows a "yes" or "no" answer. D is also closed-ended. Adding the "please" does not make it a correctly formatted question.

2. C. Nurse-patient communication is purposeful and helpful. Option A would change the focus of the nurse-patient relationship and lower the chances for a successful therapeutic relationship. Sometimes nurses and patients do become friends, but this cannot get in the way of the professional relationship of the nurse to the patient. B suggests that the nurse is somehow "the boss." Patients sometimes have that perception, but the nurse is really a "partner" in collaboration with the patient. D suggests a distance that would place the nurse too far from the patient emotionally. It would be difficult to discuss some of the intimate details the patient needs to discuss if the relationship is too distant and formal.

3. C. This option combines an observation with a closed-ended question. In this instance, it can be effective. Even with the closed-ended question, it is the best of the four choices. Option A implies playing into a hallucination and assumes that the patient intends to be talking to someone else. B is intended to quiet the patient by using guilt. Asking the patient to be quiet will discourage the patient from wanting to confide in you. D uses the word "why" without prefacing it with an observation, thus opening up the possibility of the patient's feeling defensive.

4. D. This option honestly tells the patient that you cannot give that information. The physician must explain the results first. Option A oversteps the boundaries of the nurse. B uses the "why" word. C gives advice, by using the word "should."

5. C. This puts the conversation back to the patient and allows venting of concerns. Options A and B give advice; D gives false reassurance and also belittles the patient's concerns.

6. A. This is correct because it tells the patient the nurse is concerned yet leaves the patient responsible for stating what he or she needs at the moment. B uses the word "why," and C has a very authoritarian tone. D is a command that is very authoritarian and even threatening.

7. A. Here, the nurse tells the patient that he or she understands the special concerns of the religion and culture of Judaism but does not make a promise that the dietitian will come, which would build false hope. Option B is incorrect because it does make that promise. C does not give any indication that compromise is possible or that the nurse is "hearing" the true concern. D is agreeing and is a block to therapeutic communication.

8. D. This is stating an implied thought or feeling. The nurse is checking out the fact that the patient is feeling ignored. Option A makes light of the patient's concern to see the physician. B is not helpful for the patient and shows no sensitivity for the patient's desire to see the physician. C is a block because it shows disapproval for the patient's concern and sides with the physician rather than the patient.

9. A. This option is more correct than B because it offers an observation before using a closed-ended question. B and C are simply closed-ended questions. D is an observation, but it uses "why," which tends to leave people feeling defensive.

10. B. "I feel like" is not a "feeling" statement at all, but rather a thought statement. There is no emotion identified. Option B encourages the nurse and patient to explore what emotional response is being experienced by the patient in a safe environment. Options A and C are nontherapeutic techniques. Option D is nontherapeutic in many ways: changes the subject, does not reflect what the patient has said, and implies the nurse is not interested in pursuing the patient's feelings.

11. A. The nurse is trying to use an implied feeling. "That must feel very discouraging." Option B places a value or implies right/wrong actions or feelings. Option C uses "why," which tends to lead to feelings of defensiveness for the patient, and "D" diminishes the patient's concerns and again leans toward a "right/wrong" value.

12. It is a "thinking" statement. The speaker is expressing a thought. There is no emotion expressed after the word "feel." To turn this into a "feeling" statement, try, "I feel concerned that the patient's family does not understand the situation." To more correctly verbalize the thought, try, "I think/believe the patient's family does not understand the situation."

13. **A, B, E,** and **G** are therapeutic skills. Closed-ended questions, giving advice, and the word "why" are examples of nontherapeutic communication skills.

14. Matching

   1. D. General lead. Allows the patient to continue and gives the message that the nurse is willing to listen.
   2. K. Agreeing. A block.
   3. E. Sharing observations. Gives the patient an objective statement about a specific behavior, making it more difficult to deny a problem and encouraging better communication and better patient care.

4. C. Giving advice. A block: tells the patient what is valued by the nurse; may interfere with communication of the patient; does not have success with the nurse's idea of what "should" be done.

5. A. Reflecting. Parrots words said by the patient.

6. I. Giving information. A therapeutic technique (giving advice is a block).

7. G. Belittling feelings. A block: lessens the validity of the patient's concern.

8. H. Ensuring understanding. Makes certain that patient and nurse are using the words in the same way.

9. B. Reassuring clichés. A block: gives false reassurance to the patient.

10. F. Crying. Although crying has many functions and should be allowed, if nurse focuses on it, it may divert him or her from finding the real problem.

Conversational Practice

Therapeutic/Helping

1. "I need to talk to you about your attendance." Stating what one needs is an assertive, honest therapeutic communication technique.

2. "I see by your time card that you have been late for work four times this month." Stating a specific observation. This is honest and acceptable.

3. (Marie starts to cry.) Crying is a behavior that nurses allow from patients but that is not focused on. Crying can be helpful but can also be a manipulative technique.

4. Silence for a short time is a therapeutic technique that allows both the staff member and the employee time to collect their thoughts and decide whether to continue or terminate the conversation.

5. "I guess I'd like to improve my attendance." The therapeutic part of this statement is the assertive, "I'd like to improve my attendance." With these words, Marie is assertively making a choice for herself and taking responsibility for her actions.

Nontherapeutic/Blocks

6. "Why?" This word tends to leave people feeling frustrated and defensive and is best eliminated from helping communication.

7. "Is something wrong?" This is a closed-ended question.

8. "Can you tell me what the problem is?" This is a closed-ended question.

9. "Marie, you really should start exercising." The word "should" is nontherapeutic because it gives advice and places the staffer's value on the employee.

10. "You're wrong, Marie." This is disagreeing with the patient and again places the staffer's value system on the employee.

■ CHAPTER 3

1. B. Ethics is a code of professional expectations that does not have legal force behind it. The issues border on legal implications, but ethics comes more out of expectations that patients have of nurses than out of actual legal bounds.

2. C. Each state has a Nurse Practice Act that defines the scope of practice for RNs, LPNs, and LVNs in that state.

3. D. The Patient Bill of Rights is designed to define the rights of all patients in healthcare facilities. These will change somewhat from state to state. People who are institutionalized for some reason may be termed "vulnerable" because they may be unable to speak for themselves or provide for their own safety. All who care for people in these facilities must treat them in accordance with the Patient Bill of Rights.

4. B. This is an honest, assertive technique that shows one nurse voicing a concern to another nurse. Options A, C, and D are all forms of blocks to therapeutic communication.

5. D. Most Nurse Practice Acts require that LPNs follow the chain of command. In this situation, speaking with the nurse in charge is the best choice. Option A is a block to therapeutic communication because it is argumentative and voices disagreement with the patient. B is not safe: Even though it is always important to listen to patients, a nurse must never assume the patient is right. C is inappropriate at this time; it must first be determined that an error has occurred. Once this is established, the RN or the LPN, if allowed by state and/or agency policy, should inform the physician.

6. **C.** The Health Insurance Portability and Accountability Act allows patients to have a greater say in how their records are shared and with whom. It also has regulation relating to other areas of confidentiality and how files are shared among providers. It does not force anyone to treat in a particular facility, but it would raise questions about transporting records in personal vehicles, etc.

7. **B.** Offer another pain relief technique. Mr. Ouch does have the right to refuse medication. He also has the right to privacy, but the option provided borders on punitive and may be a threat to patient safety. It is also appropriate to discuss acceptable behavior and the effect he is having on the other residents...just not now. Wait for a time when he is reasonably comfortable and willing to negotiate treatment. Bringing in more staff and performing an invasive technique is not only threatening, but it violates many of the Patient Bill of Rights.

8. Matching

1. E	**5.** G
2. B	**6.** D
3. H	**7.** C
4. I	**8.** A

■ CHAPTER 4

1. **D.** This patient is demonstrating the Electra complex, which is part of the phallic stage of Freud's developmental stages.

2. **C.** Unsuccessful completion of the anal stage would lead to these behaviors and to more serious disorders, according to psychoanalytic theory. These people would be termed "anal retentive" in some social and professional circles today.

3. **D.** This option states that Y's behavior is not appropriate and lets Y tell you that the consequences have been discussed. Y is able to make a choice. Options A and B sound harsh and threatening and are not helpful forms of communicating. C is very close to letting the nurse "caretake" for Y. In behavior modification, Y would most likely be responsible for his or her own actions and choices.

4. **A.** Cell differentiation, the process whereby cells "specialize" into their particular type, is generally complete by the end of the first trimester (third lunar month).

5. **D.** Women are successfully having children at young ages; however, it is generally believed that a woman's body is not completely mature until the age of 18 years. Because the young woman's body is not completely mature, it is difficult to sustain her health and the life of the fetus; therefore, infant mortality as well as danger to the mother's health is greatest before this age. Older women are next in line as a risk group for infant mortality because of changing hormones that can jeopardize the woman's ability to support a fetus and carry it to term. Certainly, there are exceptions in both of these age groups regarding pregnancy and successful delivery. These are broad, general beliefs that are held among many in the medical and nursing community.

6. **B.** Option A describes "animus," the balance to the female, according to Jung.

7. **D.** According to Erikson, the stage or task for children in the 3- to 6-year-old group is the stage or task of "initiative." The stage or task of "industry" (the stage at which integration of life experiences or the confusion of those experiences develops) covers ages 16 to 20 years. "Intimacy" (the stage at which the main concern is developing intimate relationships with others) begins at approximately age 18 and continues through approximately age 25.

8. **C.** It is believed that infants develop in a very similar rate and pattern (physically, behaviorally, and cognitively) until the age of 10 months. Again, this is based on

generalizations; there are always exceptions (e.g., a child who is longer than most of his or her particular age group because of the gene pool from parents who are taller than the average).

9. **B.** Assimilation is the process of taking in and processing information. It is generally learned by experiencing through the senses. "Accommodation" is the process of working with the information that has been assimilated and making that information a working part of the toddler's daily life. "Autonomy" is the stage or task Erikson believes a toddler should be achieving. "Adjustment" is a general term related to change. It is not always a healthy response to change.

10. Matching

   1. Skinner, III, E
   2. Jung, IV, C
   3. Freud, VI, B
   4. Maslow, II, D
   5. Kohlberg, I, F

Note: V and A are not used. They are part of Carl Rogers' theory.

■ CHAPTER 5

1. **B.** Proxemics, or spatial distances vary among the cultures. What is comfortable and appropriate for some is not appropriate for others.

2. **C.** Prejudice means to "pre-judge." It is making a decision about a person, situation, etc. prior to having all necessary information.

3. **B.** Homelessness is not a mental illness but may be a condition of mental illness. It is difficult for this population of people to access the health-care and community services available.

4. **B.** Approximately one-third of the homeless in the United States are mentally ill.

5. **D.** Enlist the assistance of a religious representative to negotiate removal of the item(s) in question. Other safety actions may also be required, but right now, relating to this individual at his or her spiritual level is necessary not only for the patient's religious freedom of expression, but also to get him or her to be able to cooperate with additional nursing actions.

6. **D.** Actually all of the responses are correct. Nurses are mandatory reporters for suspected abuse/neglect/endangerment of children. Certainly, the child could ultimately die from uncontrolled diabetes. It is appropriate to call the RN and MD to the exam room, but a stat call would not be necessary. You are there: The best choice is to sit with the family for a time, gain their trust, and collect more information that could be used to modify the care plan or assist the MD in appropriate referrals for the best care of this child and family.

7. **B, C, D.** Many homeless fall into the "working poor" category and are actually working full-time jobs. Approximately one-third of the homeless also have a mental illness, quite often schizophrenia.

■ CHAPTER 6

1. **C.** Rationalization is the defense mechanism that sounds like "excuses."

2. **A.** Denial is the refusal to accept situations for what they really are. This is a classic example of denial.

3. **D.** This child is using compensation, which is finding some other strength that will make up for a real or imagined inadequacy.

4. **D.** He is "blaming" his wife for his actions rather than taking responsibility for his thoughts, feelings, and actions.

5. **A.** Rationalization. Certainly, eating a meal of burgers and fries does not depict mental illness! Even though the person may be joking, and there is an element of truth, this statement depicts an "excuse" for one's behavior and choice of menu selection.

6. **B.** Undoing. This is a tricky one. Many may have chosen C, Symbolization. The reason this would be more likely an example of "undoing" is because Tara is trying

to make up for a negative behavior that affected her daughter. While words have not been spoken, there is not really an "emotion" that is being represented, as would be the case in symbolization. Rather, Tara seems to be offering the tickets to "undo" the embarrassment she caused her daughter by her drunk and inappropriate public behavior.

7. Matching

1. G
2. I
3. D. To regress means to go backward.
4. E. Denial is failure to accept behaviors or situations as they truly are.
5. H. Conversion is anxiety that is converted from emotional symptoms to physical symptoms.
6. F. Pointing the blame at another takes the responsibility from the individual and projects it onto the other person.
7. A. Emotional pain that is too severe for the individual to endure is divorced or dissociated from the conscious memory.
8. C. As a defense mechanism, this is a form of escaping mental trauma. *Caution:* Fantasy can be used consciously in some forms of therapy.

■ CHAPTER 7

1. A. Nursing process is a systematic way of collecting data to have consistency in patient care. Options B and C are incorrect, even though nurses do document patient needs and RN and LPN/LVN roles are different in the nursing process. Patient needs are not usually documented as part of the nursing process per se. D is incorrect because the nurse needs to know the difference between medical and nursing care prior to writing the nursing process. Only nursing care is incorporated into the nursing process.

2. C. This is the best choice of those listed. It asks what you need to know, but it asks from the patient's perspective. It is less judgmental than the other choices.

3. B. Return demonstration (redemonstration) is the best method for evaluating the patient's learning. Option A is a method of teaching. C and D are steps in the nursing process and steps in developing a teaching plan.

4. A. Mental status examinations are made as part of the assessment or data collection part of the nursing process.

5. Matching

Nursing Process: A, M
NANDA: R
PES: H
NIC: D, O, P
NOC: C, I, L, Q
Data Collection: E, K
Nursing Diagnosis: N
Planning Care: G, S, T
Intervention/Implementation: B, F, J

■ CHAPTER 8

1. B. Options A, C, and D are commonly seen in the crisis (or third) phase of crisis; feeling of well-being is observed in the precrisis phase of crisis, when the patient thinks and states that everything is "fine."

2. D. The patient needs to know that he or she is away from the stress, even if it is only temporary. The person may not be able to think rationally, and to hear that safety and help are being offered can be the start of stress reduction and intervention. The following explain why the other options are not correct. A: "Why" needs to be avoided when possible to decrease the chance of the statement sounding judgmental and allowing the patient to feel defensive. B: Besides the fact that this is a closed-ended question, the person may not know the answer to this. It may, in fact, be one of the major causes of the stress that led to the crisis. C: This is an open-ended statement and will be valid to ask—later. As one of the first questions a person in crisis hears, it can lead to increased confusion and guilt. He or she might not have a clue as to what led to the attack or may be blaming himself or herself needlessly.

Because nobody deserves to be abused, asking the question of the person experiencing crisis can sound as though the nurse thinks the perpetrator had just cause to abuse.

3. C. Milieu is the therapeutic environment. It should be stress-free, or at least minimally stress-producing, and should make the patients feel comfortable to practice new, healthy behaviors. It might be locked, depending on the patients, but it is not required to be. The patients will not usually be hospitalized "for life" (however, some might be); a 72-hour-hold situation should have a milieu that corresponds to the needs of the patient being held.

4. D. Avoidance and denial are some targets for treatment with psychotherapy, not goals of psychotherapy. Options A, B, and C are all goals of psychotherapy.

5. B. ECT is not used to treat convulsive disorders. That is a mistake people make because of the name "electroconvulsive therapy." The treatment causes a light seizure but does not treat seizure disorders. Options A, C, and D are all true about ECT.

6. D. The use of psychoactive medications can change the person's ability to think and process information and help him or her to feel different about the situation, which may allow other therapies to work in adjunct to the medication, to help the person toward wellness. These medications do not cure mental illness. They are used for more than just violent behavior, and although they may have an effect on pain receptors, that is a side effect rather than a primary use for this group of medications.

7. A. Photosensitivity is a frequent side effect of this group of medications, especially thorazine. Patients need to understand that they can burn easily if out in the sun and should take precautions to stay shaded or keep their skin covered.

8. C. Patients treated with the MAOI group of medications should avoid certain foods and beverages that contain tyramine to avoid hypertensive crisis.

9. B. One of the goals of crisis intervention is to decrease anxiety. The person may feel a temporary increase in anxiety (e.g., at the time of being arrested or taken to the "detox" center), but that should resolve fairly quickly with effective intervention.

10. A. Repression is a defense mechanism and is therefore counterproductive in therapy. All other choices are correct.

11. B. Mental health nursing is a holistic practice. We take care of the whole person, not just the mind or the body. Treatment in many cases will not be achieved quickly and may involve lifelong work on the part of the patient. Evaluating the plan is another part of the nursing process.

12. A. It is your responsibility as a nurse to notify the supervisor and to call the physician, according to your scope of practice. Other choices are not independent nursing functions.

13. B. These are symptoms of the EPSEs of parkinsonism.

14. A. Anticholinergics are the usual drugs of choice for decreasing the effects of EPSEs.

15. B. The antianxiety drugs are potentially addictive. Patients with addictive tendencies may become addicted to these medications more easily than they would to drugs from other categories.

16. C. The newest research shows this classification of medications may produce an increase of suicidal ideation and attempts for children and adolescents. They can be very effective medications, but nurses must watch for and instruct patients and family members regarding the possibility of increased chance for suicide attempts while taking the medication.

17.   Matching

1.	H	**5.**	C
2.	G	**6.**	B
3.	F	**7.**	D
4.	A		

Option E defines the action of the medication classification monoamine oxidase inhibitors but does not correspond with any of the listed TREATMENTS.

■ CHAPTER 9

1. **C.** The definition of an alternative therapy is one that is used in place of conventional medicine. Option A suggests that such therapy has no value, which is very dependent upon the patient's beliefs. Option B is the definition of complementary therapies. Option D is incorrect; many cultures and people use alternative modalities as first-line treatment for all types of illness.

2. **D.** Complementary therapies are used with conventional medicine. Option A is vague; medical treatment is not defined simply by Western standards. Option B is incorrect because a model refers to a picture or idea. Option C infers that conventional medicine is holistic, when in fact it is disease-oriented.

3. **A.** *Integrative* refers to the use of conventional and less traditional methods in harmony. Option B is incorrect because such combinations are not exclusive to any one belief system. Option C would leave the decision-making to a physician without patient input, which is not holistic. Biofeedback, option D, is a complementary therapy.

4. **D.** The mind-body connection correctly describes why belief and expectation have an effect on health and disease. Option A is an incorrect definition; complementary therapies are used with conventional medicine. Option B is an opinion based on the notion that the mind and body operate independently of one another. Option C describes a treatment modality rather than a mechanism.

5. **B.** Regardless of the nurse's own feelings, remaining open and supportive encourages communication and rapport. Option A would have the effect of destroying rapport by making Mrs. Lucas wrong for her beliefs. Option C might be an observation better reported to the physician for his decision. Option

D would have the LPN/LVN performing well outside of his or her scope of practice in most states.

6. **D.** Aromatherapy, biofeedback, and massage are either alternative or complementary. In options A, B, and C, ECT (electroconvulsive therapy), antianxiety medications, and psychotherapy are considered conventional.

7. **A.** Reiki is a therapy involving energy manipulation and unblocking energy flow. Options B, C, and D are all forms of massage therapy.

8. **A.** Trance *is* an altered state of consciousness, but it is assuredly *not* sleep. Much of the therapeutic value of the work done in trance is lost if the client falls asleep. Options B, C, and D are all correct statements about trance.

9. **C.** This statement uses "see" and "clearly" to communicate that the speaker prefers a visual channel. Through the predicates "feels good" and "gut feeling" in option A, the speaker reveals a kinesthetic channel preference. In option B, the speaker demonstrates an auditory preference through the predicates "sounds good" and "paying attention to." Option D reflects the rarely-used *olfactory* preference; many practitioners treat these predicates as kinesthetic for therapeutic purposes.

10. **B.** Presupposing, or assuming, that the patient will not improve will directly and indirectly negatively affect the thoughts, feelings, and actions of the nurse as well as the patient. Often mentally ill patients are more sensitive to unspoken assumption, especially when it is communicated nonverbally. Options A, C, and D will positively impact unspoken communication and improve chances for better rapport.

■ CHAPTER 10

1. **B.** Watching the patient's behavior in specific situations gives the nurse insight into the patient's ability to think, be flexible, and maintain balance in stressful situations, among other things. Option A, intelligence, can be part of this assess-

ment, but it is not the only variable; C is not correct because the patient is entitled to an opinion, and we do not know from this response how the opinion is being expressed. D is also incorrect because the family itself is not a reliable predictor of behaviors of the individual members of that family.

2. A. A patient who is always happy and smiling may not be responding to the continuum or balance of fluctuations in daily life, so this is not always a healthy response. Options B, C, and D are all conditions of a person who is maintaining positive mental health.

3. D. Mental illnesses have etiologies that are based in physical, emotional, and environmental theories. They are complex; proof of any of the theories has yet to be provided.

4. Answers:
   A. Inorganic or functional rationales for mental illnesses
   B. Implies that poor relationships with the significant people in a young person's life set the stage for a life of compensating
   C. Postulates or suggests that the person with altered mental functioning endured a situation, often unknown, that happened early in life, over which the person had no control and that he or she can't be held responsible for subsequent behaviors

5. Answers (all of the following four are correct):
   A. Organic, altered mental status
   B. Result of genetic malfunction of the brain
   C. Result of physical malfunction of the brain
   D. Result of neurochemical malfunction of the brain

■ CHAPTER 11

1. B. The vividness of the description suggests that the person is having a flashback. Auditory hallucinations would most likely involve "voices" or "hearing" the guns. Delusions of grandeur might cause the person to go after the people with guns, while being unarmed himself or herself. Free-floating anxiety would be less descriptive. The person would not know the cause of the anxiety.

2. C. The behaviors indicate the probability of PTSD.

3. D. Repetitive behavior that interferes with daily functioning is indicative of OCD.

4. D. This is the best of the four choices because you are simply stating for the patient to relax. You are helping him reoxygenate and refocus and you are calming him by offering to stay with him. It also buys you some time to make a visual assessment. Option A would be appropriate nursing actions, but not as the first priority. Your first action needs to be calming the patient and continuing to assess. B and C are nontherapeutic responses.

5. C. Multiple personality disorder, or dissociative identity disorder, is considered to be a dissociative disorder rather than an anxiety disorder. Some theorists believe that the dissociative disorders are also anxiety disorders, but most are now differentiating the two types of disorders.

6. B. The feeling of impending doom is characteristic of free-floating anxiety. Signal anxiety is an anxiety response to an expected event, such as a test.

7. D. Rigid and inflexible behaviors are characteristic of OCD. These persons would like to be able to control those behaviors, but without treatment it is very difficult for them. They are not usually hostile, unless they are prevented from performing the obsession or compulsion, because that decreases the anxiety.

8. D. Phobia is an irrational fear that cannot be changed by reason or logic. The patient usually understands it is irrational, but the fear remains.

9. C. Withholding information that the nurse thinks might cause stress is not a helpful action for the patient. If the physician has not already informed the patient, or if the nurse states his or her discomfort about discussing the information, that is another consideration, but arbitrarily deciding to withhold information may actually increase the patient's anxiety.

10. **B.** A compulsion is a repetitive act; an obsession is a repetitive thought.

11. **B.** FEAR would be the most appropriate choice for NANDA diagnosis among these choices. There is no indication that the patient has anything to be compliant or noncompliant with. Low self-esteem and risk for self-directed violence may become issues later, if the anxiety goes untreated, is misdiagnosed, or becomes part of a dual-diagnosis.

12. **C.** Luvox (fluvoxemine) is the current drug of choice for OCD. Effexor (venlaxofine) is a close second. Be careful! These drugs are all used in treating mental illnesses. All sound similar and are spelled similarly.

13. Agoraphobia

14. **A, E,** and **F** are NOT appropriate nursing interventions. Stimuli should be diminished to decrease the stressors present. All changes in behavior and responses to treatment should be documented. Activities should be encouraged, but only those that are enjoyable and do not produce additional stress. People need to acknowledge the stressors and deal with them. Avoiding or creating "diversion" is not the best nursing care. Creating an environment where individuals feel comfortable and want to participate in activities is more therapeutic.

■ CHAPTER 12

1. **D.** Men as well as women can suffer from this type of "empty nest syndrome." This patient's symptoms are not consistent with those of the other depressive disorders, and the fact that his medication is not helping him may be a clue that this is a harder form of depression to treat, although it has been only a short treatment time.

2. **A.** This is selective reflecting. You have repeated the patient's exact words in a way that encourages her to either explain herself or rephrase her response in some way. Options B, C, and D are all blocks to therapeutic communication. B

is challenging her, C uses the word "why," and D is giving advice.

3. **B.** Play therapy is the most common and most effective form of therapy for children. Work (or occupational) kinds of therapy, behavior modification, and rational-emotive therapy are a little advanced for a child of this age.

4. **B.** Lithium is an electrolyte. Dehydration could increase the chances of severe side effects from the lithium.

5. **D.** Affect is the outward or physical display of an emotion.

6. **C.** Communicating in a judgmental manner is always a block to therapeutic, helping relationships.

7. **A.** These are the best nursing actions to take at this time. Omitting part of the conversation is not appropriate because all data relating to the patient's care and condition are relevant. Maintaining patient confidentiality is required.

8. **D.** From the patient's comments about feeling responsible for the plight of his family, guilt would be the best choice. Manipulation sounds plausible, but people in this condition are generally not trying deliberately to manipulate others.

9. **C.** Major depression usually manifests itself with symptoms of extreme sadness that is the prevalent mood for a period of 2 years. Euphoria would be more indicative of bipolar depression.

10. **D.** This is the block of false reassurance, which is never appropriate in therapeutic relationships. The other choices are all appropriate nursing interventions for a person who is depressed.

11. **D.** One of the main side effects of lithium is dehydration and fluid and electrolyte imbalance. Her dry lips, staggering gait, and statement of feeling confused are all symptoms of dehydration and sodium depletion. She may also be taking an incorrect dose. We do not have enough information with this situation to make that determination.

12. **B.** Showing empathy for this woman and her family is the best nursing action you

can take now. Asking more questions would certainly be helpful but may be too overwhelming at this time. Sharing information in this manner is not helpful and may trigger anger at the situation. Changing the subject may lighten the mood temporarily but would not show support at this time.

13. A. This may be a form of the involutional/empty nest-type of depression. This woman just had the majority of her family go away. She has not been in the situation long enough to meet the 2-year criteria for dysthymic disorder and she has not exhibited any mania to give her the bipolar diagnosis.

14. Serotonin, norepinephrine; lower

■ CHAPTER 13

1. D. Consequences should always be stated at the time the limits are set, to increase consistency. The problems with options A through C are as follows. A: When the behavior occurs, the patient may be testing, but if the consequences are not known, the patient has not been given enough information to make an appropriate choice. B: Anticipating a behavior is presuming, and you may be presuming incorrectly. This sets up negative expectations from the patient. C: The limits should not be set for the convenience of the staff or family or anyone but the patient. Family should be involved in the care plan if the patient is agreeable.

2. C. David is most likely displaying signs of antisocial personality disorder. He is not exhibiting signs of suspiciousness or paranoia, nor is he behaving in a dependent manner.

3. A. Manipulation is used by patients with personality disorders. It is not, however, commonly used by patients who have other threats to their mental health.

4. D. Interpersonal relationships are among the most difficult activities for a person with a personality disorder to develop. They can participate in group activities because they can excel and bring attention and gratification to themselves, but developing a close personal relationship is very difficult.

5. C. Antisocial (psychopathic) personality is usually the type of disorder in which a person would be in trouble with the law.

6. D. Erratic behavior is most characteristic of borderline personality.

7. A. Suspicion and mistrust, especially of other people, are characteristics of paranoid personality disorder. They are not as serious as they appear when part of paranoid schizophrenia.

8. C. This patient is displaying behaviors consistent with passive-aggressive personality disorder.

9. D. Vague communication is not acceptable. Honesty and clarity in communication are always necessary. The patient may feel inferior, which may be part of the manipulation. The nurse needs to confront the feelings of inferiority or any others that the patient might state.

10. B. Borderline personality. This group tends to engage in self-mutilating behaviors.

11. D. People with borderline personality disorder have a tendency toward sexual promiscuity and do run the risk for sexually transmitted diseases. CDC Infection Control policies should be carefully followed.

12. Matching

1. D	**5.** B
2. F	**6.** C
3. G	**7.** E
4. A	

Option H is not true for any of the personality disorders.

■ CHAPTER 14

1. C. The main symptom of paranoid schizophrenia is suspiciousness. Options A and D are symptoms of catatonic schizophrenia. B is a general symptom of schizophrenia. It is one of Bleuler's "4 As."

2. D. Inviting the patient to the party brings him into the present and allows him to make the choice for himself. This will help increase self-esteem and diminish other symptoms. Option A begins to reinforce the hallucinations, which is never appropriate for nurses. B and C are forms of demands, which may cause the patient to revert to negative and possibly aggressive behaviors.

3. A. Shawna's symptoms are consistent with patients who have catatonic schizophrenia. Option D, schizotypal, is a type of personality disorder but not actually a form of schizophrenia.

4. A. This is an example of a hallucination. The patient is seeing something that is not there. There is nothing actually visible that could be misinterpreted as a snake; if there were, this would be an illusion.

5. C. This is the honest response and it focuses on returning the patient to reality. The other responses play into the hallucination or border on belittling the patient.

6. C. Patients with schizophrenia do not function well in society without treatment. Even with treatment, some patients have a difficult time. The "reality" of schizophrenic people is their *own* reality and not the reality of the rest of society.

7. B. It is important always to deal with reality and the present when dealing with people with schizophrenia. Never reinforcing hallucinations and directing people away from situations that are stressful or competitive are also important. ECT is not a nursing function.

8. B. This time you are dealing with an illusion. There is something on the ceiling, and the patient is misinterpreting what is there.

9. C. Once again, maintaining honesty and reality is the best response.

10. D. These symptoms are characteristic of catatonic schizophrenia.

11. A. Ecolalia is the behavior or symptom of catatonic schizophrenia involving the patient repeating a word or part of word or phrase over and over. Ecopraxia is repetitive movement or actions.

12. D. Pha is of a cultural group that may require a lower than normal dose of the medication. In addition, nurses must always err on the side of patient safety and ask the physician to clarify an order they are not certain of.

13. Illusion

14. Delusion or delusion of grandeur

■ CHAPTER 15

1. B. Delirium is probably the best choice, since the patient presented as alert and oriented before surgery. Nothing indicates dementia at this point. She is not delusional; she is having a hallucination. The dilemma may be in what the nurse chooses to do next!

2. A. Your best action is to call your charge nurse and/or physician immediately. Your state Nurse Practice Act will dictate whom you should call first. Turning on the light may be helpful, but asking about the spiders plays into the hallucination, which is not therapeutic. Stopping the patient's pain medications is not an independent nursing function; you need to make that call to the physician first. Checking her medical record should have been done earlier, and it will not be helpful to her right now.

3. D. You have restated what the physician has already told Mrs. H, you have reinforced reality, and you have been honest. You offered to help the patient, which shows concern for her needs. The other choices are all blocks to therapeutic or helping communication.

4. B. Aricept can cause bradycardia.

5. D. Although Alzheimer's-type dementia is not a result of aging or arteriosclerosis, these conditions may be present in addition to the dementia.

6. C. You would expect to see memory and other cognitive processes impaired in someone with an organic mental disorder. The person will probably not be oriented to at least one of the three spheres of person, place, or time.

7. B. These symptoms are consistent with a person's having delirium. The admission of alcohol use adds to this conclusion. Time or decompensation of memory and behavior might change this initial diagnosis to a form of dementia.

8. C. This is the best option. You are showing concern for the patient, the family, and their situation. You have stated the implied message and offered to get the physician, who must be the one to give the initial information. You have maintained dignity for all, while behaving professionally.

9. D. Vascular or multi-infarct dementia is usually the result of several smaller strokes. The patient has usually had conditions such as high blood pressure for quite some time. The condition displays many of the same behaviors as other types of dementia but is also usually irreversible.

10. **1, 3, 5, 6, 8, 9** Incorrect Answers:

> **2.** Dementia patients may not remember what they were just asked to do. In a room with others, this could be an embarrassing, demeaning situation. If the nurse feels compelled to remind the patient, it should be done in private for that patient's dignity.
>
> **4.** Radios and televisions on at all times or on too loudly may provide too much stimulation and may cause increased agitation in some patients.
>
> **7.** Restraints, physical and chemical, are a legal issue. Safety is certainly an issue, but in some states, physical restraints are actually illegal or allowed only in certain situations. Nurses need to be aware of their state requirements, obtain the proper physician order to cover either physical or chemical restraints, and will need to find creative alternatives of diversion for the "wandering" patient or resident.

11. Reality orientation may be appropriate for some patients with early stages of dementia or with delirium; however, it is not appropriate for all and can cause increased anxiety for both the patient and the nurse.

■ CHAPTER 16

1. A. "Soma," from medical terminology, means "body." Somatoform disorders manifest themselves with body-related symptoms.

2. D. In somatoform disorders patients have physical symptoms but with no organic findings to support these symptoms.

3. B. These are symptoms of a person with a conversion disorder. They would not fit the definition of catatonia because only one limb is rigid and the person is not exhibiting negativism.

4. C. The best choice is to incorporate Mr. Icantdoit into activities that focus on neither arm but automatically require both arms to function. The thinking here is similar to the idea of not focusing on hallucinations. Take a very matter-of-fact approach, avoid focusing on the affected arm, and keep the patient oriented to the present. Positive reinforcement is appropriate when the right arm functions.

5. D. This apparent lack of concern for the blindness is called "la belle indifference."

6. A. The reason for the blindness is to alleviate the underlying anxiety. Alleviating the anxiety is called primary gain. Secondary gain would be sympathy, support, financial gain, or any other "perk" the patient may receive as a result of her blindness.

7. B. Belief of having an illness that cannot be treated or belief that one is getting an unidentified illness are symptoms of hypochondriasis.

8. A. The most appropriate nursing action is to be supportive. Assisting the patient to focus on strengths gives you and the patient a place to start with a care plan as well as showing the patient she or he in fact has strengths.

9. Somatoform pain disorder

10. Somatization disorder

■ CHAPTER 17

1. A. The desired effects of Antabuse, when the patient uses alcohol, are to produce nausea, vomiting, and heart palpitations. All other choices are possible side effects.

2. C. Denial is the most common defense mechanism used by people who are chemically dependent. Rationalization is also used by some patients.

3. D. Maintaining safety is very important during DTs or withdrawal. Nurses should never encourage hallucinations. This is not the time for trying to assess the situation or educate the patient. He or she will probably not want to listen, let alone be *able* to listen while withdrawing from the chemical.

4. A. Alcohol is a CNS depressant. The "high" that people feel is temporary and very misleading.

5. B. Delirium tremens is associated with frequency of visual hallucinations.

6. D. Sally may very well be codependent in her sister's alcohol abuse. Sally is taking responsibility for Susie's behavior instead of having Susie take care of herself.

7. B. This response addresses both sisters and tells them they both need help. It is honest, caring, and puts the responsibility on them to help themselves through this situation.

8. A. Susie should be encouraged to attend weekly AA meetings and Sally to attend weekly Al-Anon meetings. We do not know from the information if they are adult children of alcoholics; therefore, that would not be the best choice at this time. There is no need to check into the unit weekly, but they can be told that it is acceptable to call or check in if they choose to. The psychologist will tell them the meeting schedule; this would not be a nursing function for discharge planning.

9. C. The person who is dependent on a substance will display all these behaviors.

10. A. Honest communication is necessary for the person and family to heal.

11. B. Codependent. In an effort to be caring, you are inadvertently making excuses and encouraging the drinking behavior.

12. D. Let's hope they are planning a camping trip or even getting sick! In today's world, astute nurses and parents need to be alert to the fact that with these materials, children could be well on the way to making methamphetamine.

13. Matching

1. F		6. G	
2. D		7. K	
3. E		8. J	
4. H		9. C	
5. A		10. B	

Not Used: I. This option refers to Alcoholics Anonymous

■ CHAPTER 18

1. C. Anorexia nervosa is the fear of food. Bulimia nervosa is termed "binge eating." Pica is an eating disorder seen in young children.

2. D. Current statistics point to the African-American group as having a higher percentage of obesity than the national average as a whole.

3. B. Patients who have anorexia have an intense fear of being fat. They have an inaccurate sense of their size and body image and will not develop normal eating patterns without much help and behavior modification.

4. A. A nutritional deficit, and probably a fluid imbalance, exists in patients who are anorectic. The fluid imbalance is caused by the lack of intake and perhaps vomiting. There is also a body image disturbance, but it is a negative self-perception rather than a positive one.

5. D. Unlocking the feelings surrounding an eating disorder can be very helpful to the patient and treatment team. Focusing on the food and the destructive behaviors associated with the food puts the emphasis on the wrong area.

6. C. Patients with bulimia nervosa cannot control their eating. They binge and purge, and they are overly concerned and preoccupied with body shape and size.

7. D. This statement conveys your desire to help with ANY concern this patient may have postoperatively. The other options do show a concern and interest in this patient, but focusing on food and weight may limit the patient's willingness to offer other needs. The patient may also not be ready to talk about weight yet. This is a hopeful, yet a traumatic step for many.

8. B. This response is a combination of the therapeutic techniques of parroting and open-ended question. It uses the patient's words and leaves the question open for Donald to elaborate. The other choices are nontherapeutic and do not allow for patient expression.

9. Bulimia or bulimia nervosa

■ CHAPTER 19

1. D. Teaching skills to help the patient deal with the problems of day-to-day life will be helpful in the long run. Option B is a mistake made by people who believe the myth that some suicide attempts are not serious. C is a block to therapeutic communication (disagreeing) and may give false hope. The patient does not see that there is much to live for, or the suicide would probably not have been attempted. A is also incorrect because reporting the patient to the police is not required in most communities and could be a threat to the patient.

2. B. People are more likely to carry out the suicide when they appear to feel better. This is when they have the energy to create a plan and carry it out. When they are deeply depressed or confused, they often are not able to think clearly enough to do these things. When people feel loved and appreciated, they are less likely to think about suicide. This may be a temporary feeling on their part, however.

3. C. If a person is talking about suicide, the possibility for carrying it out is very real and must be taken seriously. In very few situations is suicidal ideation a manipulative behavior.

4. D. This man has definite potential for self-harm. He is not attempting to manipulate his wife's feelings, although she may feel that he is.

5. B. Your first action is to place the patient on one-on-one observation. Some facilities accomplish this by having staff perform rounds at a minimum of every 15 minutes; most facilities assign a staff person to stay with the patient. There is no need to place the patient in a locked unit at this time, nor is it appropriate to publicize the precautions to the whole facility. It would not be appropriate to give him his razor, as this could be an implement he could use to perform the suicide.

6. C. Document the discussion but explain that the precautions remain in effect. It is for his safety and the safety of others that the precautions are policy, generally. You may thank him for sharing his beliefs, and depending on where he is in his treatment, it may become appropriate for him to share his belief system with others. Not just yet, though!

7. D. All of these are true. Religious and cultural beliefs are strongly engrained in people and will dictate behavior. In some cases such as this or suicide bombings, notes are not left. They are not seen as necessary. People with a strong plan, regardless of the nature of the suicide, will usually find a way to be successful.

8. Possible answers:

1. Religion: Suicide may be an act of honor; repeating the religious phrase may be an indication of his intention to kill himself for his beliefs.
2. Ethnicity: May see America and its citizens as "evil," may have been raised to hate certain people.
3. Age: Is in a risk group for depression and drug use and may be under the influence of some chemical.
4. Injuries: May have had head injury, may be in shock, may have been

exposed to some toxins that affect his mental status.

5. **Lack of Information:** We do not know at this time if this man is a perpetrator or if he is a worker and an innocent victim of the accident.

▪ CHAPTER 20

1. **B.** MPD is thought to be an unconscious maladaptive response to a psychological trauma. It is not done consciously.

2. **B.** This gives exact, nonjudgmental documentation of what is happening to the patient at this particular time. By being factual and nonjudgmental, this response implies understanding of the condition of MPD.

3. **A.** The treatment goal for this patient is to integrate the personalities into one personality or into as few as possible. Treatment is difficult and will take a long time, but it is not hopeless.

4. **C.** Obsessive-compulsive disorder is an anxiety disorder. Dissociative disorders are probably anxiety-related but have their own classification.

5. **A.** Sudden inability to recall personal information is the main symptom. Forgetfulness, confusion, and disorientation may also be present. It is not "selective" and the person does not exhibit separate personalities.

▪ CHAPTER 21

1. **B.** Safety for children with conduct disorder is primary in importance. Chances are that the child will not settle quickly, and asking the parent to leave with the child is not a supportive action for either the parent or child.

2. **B.** Offering empathy and providing privacy will help calm the mother. Options A and C might take place later at the mother's discretion. D is not an appropriate choice because it is a block to therapeutic communication. The nurse does not know "just how they feel," and it is belittling to state so.

3. **D.** Children often act out or draw pictures about what is troubling them. Offering toys or drawing materials and observing the child discreetly can tell you much about what he or she has experienced. It may also serve as a diversion, but offering toys or drawing materials is meant to encourage self-expression rather than as a diversion from the situation.

4. **B.** Gender of the parent is not a strong indicator for the potential for abusing a child. Stress, parenting skills, and the experience of being abused him or herself as a child are strong indicators for the potential of abusing children. Cultural beliefs and behaviors, while accepted in one's native country and not interpreted by the parent as "abuse" may, however, not be acceptable here, and certain behaviors may be interpreted and reported as abusive.

5. **D.** The person committing the abusive behavior is also a "patient" and deserves empathy and nonjudgmental care. Not all child abusers will be required to go to jail and not all are dangerous to society as a whole. Child Protection or the agency responding to the report of suspected abuse will assist in determining if the child should stay in the abusive home, depending on many variables.

6. **D.** Being impulsive and inattentive are two main characteristics of ADD/ADHD. While the child may not work up to his or her potential, they are usually of average or even above average intelligence.

7. **B.** The most common symptom of autism is impaired social functioning. The patient does not make strong friendships. Emotions may be completely opposite of what would be appropriate, and the patient may achieve an appropriate developmental task and then regress, or may not achieve appropriate developmental tasks at all.

8. **C.** This is the best choice of the options listed, because it implies the nurse heard the parents' concerns and recognized the need to get them appropriate help right away. The other options are either nontherapeutic or provide false hope to the parents. They may sound polite but are

not helpful for the parents, who are concerned they did something wrong and want to know how they can help their child.

9. A. In most situations, the chain of reporting is from first-line staff (nurses and intake staff) to the immediate supervisor or manager. In part, this is to protect the "reporter" from the suspected abuser. In some smaller clinics, you may need to make a call to the reporting agency directly. You may also express empathy with the person bringing in the child, but your primary objective is to report the suspected abuse. At this time, it is still "suspected," as the uncle has not told us he actually "shook" the baby, only that he tried to get her to stop crying.

■ CHAPTER 22

1. B. Reinforce the word by showing or handling the object. Trying to guess the word or finishing the patient's sentence can be frustrating and insulting and can discourage the patient from attempting to communicate. Asking the patient to think about the word while you do something else is distracting.

2. D. Federal regulations require that the assessment be conducted by an RN for purposes of consistency. All other people on the health-care team supply input and documentation to assist with the assessment.

3. C. Medication side effect would be the most obvious possibility, as the medication is a recent change in routine, and normal vital signs should help rule out the possibility of a recent stroke. Depression is a more distant possibility.

4. C. You have been assertive and told the patient what you wanted in a way that encouraged the patient to participate in a specific activity. This also supports the person's self-esteem.

5. B. The losses experienced as people age are frequent causes of depression.

6. D. Dementia is not a part of normal aging. Other possibilities for unusual behavior

should be ruled out before diagnosing a person with dementia.

7. B. Aphasia is the speech complication that often results from stroke. Affect can also change after a stroke, but that is not a speech difficulty.

8. B. Drugs are metabolized more slowly in older people, which results in a cumulative effect that leads to toxicity.

9. C. These could be symptoms of elder abuse. The location of the bruises is consistent with shaking or beating. The lack of eye contact or verbal response indicates that the patient fears that the beatings might get worse.

10. D. The Omnibus Budget Reconciliation Act (OBRA) is the law that attempts to provide consistency in assessment and care of the aging.

11. B. Memory loss is NOT a normal part of aging.

12. A. This response corrects the name of the illness while still addressing the emotional response of the housekeeper. Option B is factually correct. It is important to call the disorder by its correct name, but the statement does not go on to help the staff member. Options C and D show some interest, but neither serve to educate or be helpful to the staff member.

13. Complementary (modality used in conjunction with traditional treatments).

14. Alternative (nontraditional modality used independent of traditional treatment).

■ CHAPTER 23

1. D. Showing empathy for the patient, offering to provide further assistance, and reassuring safety will help the patient to trust you and probably to be more comfortable and compliant with examinations.

2. B. Getting a statement in the patient's own words and documenting it in the medical record are required. Option A is information that the patient may not know. The word "why" is counterproductive in therapeutic communication. C is not recommended for reasons of liability for both the nurse and the patient. It is most likely a violation of your agency policy as well as a violation of professional ethics.

3. **C.** You need to be helpful to both people. You will need to take care of the physical and emotional health of both patients, and you will do it according to the degree of immediacy called for. A physician must be called if one is not in the area, but until he or she arrives, your nursing care, observation, and documentation will help ensure the best possible care for the patients.

4. **C.** You let Mrs. X know that you hear her concern and need for help. You are offering the best help you can at the moment, while allowing her to make the decision about speaking to the social worker.

5. **C.** While some patients may express displeasure at someone going ahead, most will realize something is terribly wrong. Apologize for their inconvenience and have someone assist them as soon as possible. Attending to this woman, her immediate needs, and those of her children is the best nursing choice. You may also let her know that someone will be in who can help her with safety issues, but it is important to get her in a quiet, safe room. After all, the perpetrator may be right behind her. She knows that!

6. **A.** You are showing empathy, being nonjudgmental, and offering the patient assistance. Offering to her that she needs to leave sounds helpful and may be true, but she has to make that decision on her own. The organization you offered her in option A may assist with that as well. "Why" is a nontherapeutic response. Asking if he's done that before does make an attempt at gathering information and showing concern, but the more immediate need now is to support her and offer her some options for assistance.

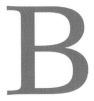
Agencies That Help People Who Have Threats to Their Mental Health

1. **National Institute of Mental Health (NIMH)**
   6001 Executive Boulevard, Room 8184, MSC 9663
   Bethesda, MD 20892-9663
   (301) 443-4513 (local) 1-866-615-6464 (toll-free) 301-443-8431 (TTY)
   Fax: (301) 443-4279
   www.nimh.nih.gov

2. **Depression and Bipolar Support Alliance**
   730 Franklin Street, Suite 501
   Chicago, IL 60610-7224
   1 (800) 826-3632 Fax: (312) 642-7243
   www.dbsalliance.org

3. **National Alliance for the Mentally Ill***
   Colonial Place Three
   2107 Wilson Blvd., Suite 300
   Arlington, VA 22201-3042
   Main: (703) 524-7600 Fax: (703) 524-9094
   TDD: (703) 516-7227
   www.nami.org
   *Your state probably has a chapter of Alliance for the Mentally Ill (AMI) as well.

4. **National Foundation for Depressive Illness**
   P.O. Box 2257
   New York, NY 10116
   (212) 268-4260 Fax (212) 268-4434 1 (800) 248-4344
   www.healthfinder.gov/orgs

5. **National Mental Health Association**
   2001 N. Beauregard Street, 12th Floor
   Alexandria, VA 22311
   Phone: (703) 684-7722 Fax: (703) 684-5968
   Mental Health Resource Center 800/969-NMHA
   TTY Line (800) 433-5959
   www.nmha.org

6. **American Association of Retired Persons (AARP)**
   Widowed Persons Services
   Social Outreach and Support
   1909 K Street NW
   Washington, DC 20049
   (202) 728-4370
   www.aarp.org

7. **National Hospice & Palliative Care Organization (NHPCO)**
   1700 Diagonal Road, Suite 625
   Alexandria, VA 22314
   Phone: (703) 837-1500 Fax: (703) 837-1233
   www.nhpco.org

8. **Child Abuse Prevention Association**
   503 E. 23rd Street,
   Independence, MO 64055
   (816) 252-8388
   www.childabuseprevention.org

Organizations That Support the Licensed Practical/Vocational Nurse

The following is a partial list of organizations that support and foster the role of the licensed practical/vocational nurse in the United States.

1. **National Association for Practical Nurse Education and Services (NAPNES)**
   8607 2nd Avenue, #404A
   Silver Spring, MD 20910
   (301) 588-2491 Fax: (301) 588-2839
   www.napnes.org
   Founded in 1941. Aims: promotion and consultation of setup of Practical Nursing programs, CEU offerings, etc. Publications: *Journal of Practical Nursing, NAPNES Forum,* pamphlets, brochures, and reports.

2. **National Federation of Licensed Practical Nurses (NFLPN)**
   605 Poole Drive
   Garner, NC 27529-4547
   (919) 779-0046 Fax: (919) 779-5642
   www.nflpn.org
   Founded in 1949. Aims: preserve and foster the ideal of comprehensive nursing care for the ill and the aging; improve the standards of practice for the LPN; gain recognition for the LPN; define effective utilization of LPNs; suggest further improvement in the education of practical nurses. Publications: *Licensed Practical Nurse,* journal published quarterly.

3. **American Psychiatric Nurses Association (APNA)**
   1555 Wilson Boulevard, Suite 515
   Arlington, VA 22209
   703-243-2443 Fax: 703-243-3390
   www.apna.org/membership
   Offers affiliate memberships for LPN/LVNs

4. **American Association for Men in Nursing (AAMN)**
   AAMN % NYSNA
   11 Cornell Road
   Latham, NY 12110-1499
   (518) 782-9400 Ext. 346
   aamn@aamn.org
   www.aamn.org
   Founded in 1973. Aims: advance new concepts in nursing and health care; identify and explore issues in health. Affiliated with the American Nurses Association (ANA).

5. **National Coalition of Ethnic Minority Nurse Associations Inc. (NCEMNA)**
   Dr. Betty Smith Williams, President
   6100 West Centinela Avenue, Suite 378
   Culver City, CA 90230
   (310) 258-9515 Fax: (310) 258-9513
   betwilliams@sbcglobal.net
   www.ncemna.org

6. **National Alaska Native American Indian Nurses Association, Inc. (NANAINA)**
   Multiple contacts.
   www.nanaina.com

7. **National Association of Hispanic Nurses, Inc. (NAHN)**
   1501 Sixteenth Street, NW
   Washington, DC 20036
   (202) 387-2477 Fax: (202) 483-7183
   info@thehispanicnurses.org

8. **National Black Nurses Association, Inc. (NBNA)**
   8630 Fenton Street, Suite 330
   Silver Spring, MD 20910-3803
   301-589-3200 or 1-800-575-6298
      Fax: 301-589-3223
   NBNA@erols.com
   www.nbna.org

9. **Philippine Nurses Association of America, Inc. (PNAA)**
   Philippine Nurses Association Hawaii
   P.O. Box 19085
   Honolulu, HI 96817
   (808) 341-2014
   pna_hawaii@yahoo.com
   www.geocities.com/pna

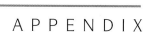
DSM-IV-TR Classification

NOS = Not Otherwise Specified.

An x appearing in a diagnostic code indicates that a specific code number is required.

An ellipsis (...) is used in the names of certain disorders to indicate that the name of a specific mental disorder or general medical condition should be inserted when recording the name (e.g., 293.0 Delirium Due to Hypothyroidism).

Numbers in parentheses are page numbers.

If criteria are currently met, one of the following severity specifiers may be noted after the diagnosis:

> Mild
> Moderate
> Severe

If criteria are no longer met, one of the following specifiers may be noted:

> In Partial Remission
> In Full Remission
> Prior History

■ DISORDERS USUALLY FIRST DIAGNOSED IN INFANCY, CHILDHOOD, OR ADOLESCENCE (39)

Mental Retardation (41)

Note: ***These are coded on Axis II.***

317	Mild Mental Retardation (43)
318.0	Moderate Mental Retardation (43)
318.1	Severe Mental Retardation (43)
318.2	Profound Mental Retardation (44)
319	Mental Retardation, Severity Unspecified (44)

Learning Disorders (49)

315.00	Reading Disorder (51)
315.1	Mathematics Disorder (53)
315.2	Disorder of Written Expression (54)
315.9	Learning Disorder NOS (56)

Motor Skills Disorder (56)

315.4	Developmental Coordination Disorder (56)

Communication Disorders (58)

315.31	Expressive Language Disorder (58)
315.32	Mixed Receptive-Expressive Language Disorder (62)
315.39	Phonological Disorder (65)
307.0	Stuttering (67)
307.9	Communication Disorder NOS (69)

Pervasive Developmental Disorders (69)

299.00	Autistic Disorder (70)
299.80	Rett's Disorder (76)
299.10	Childhood Disintegrative Disorder (77)
299.80	Asperger's Disorder (80)

299.80   Pervasive Developmental Disorder
          NOS (84)

Attention-Deficit and Disruptive Behavior Disorders (85)

314.xx   Attention-Deficit/Hyperactivity Disor-
          der (85)
   .01   Combined Type
   .00   Predominantly Inattentive Type
   .01   Predominantly Hyperactive-
             Impulsive Type
314.9   Attention-Deficit/Hyperactivity Disor-
          der NOS (93)
312.xx   Conduct Disorder (93)
   .81   Childhood-Onset Type
   .82   Adolescent-Onset Type
   .89   Unspecified Onset
313.81   Oppositional Defiant Disorder
          (100)
312.9   Disruptive Behavior Disorder NOS
          (103)

Feeding and Eating Disorders of Infancy or Early Childhood (103)

307.52   Pica (103)
307.53   Rumination Disorder (105)
307.59   Feeding Disorder of Infancy or Early
          Childhood (107)

TIC Disorders (108)

307.23   Tourette's Disorder (111)
307.22   Chronic Motor or Vocal Tic Disorder
          (114)
307.21   Transient Tic Disorder (115)
          Specify if: Single Episode/Recurrent
307.20   Tic Disorder NOS (116)

Elimination Disorders (116)

—.—   Encopresis (116)
787.6   With Constipation and Overflow
             Incontinence
307.7   Without Constipation and Overflow
             Incontinence
307.6   Enuresis (Not Due to a General Med-
          ical Condition) (118)
          Specify type: Nocturnal Only/ Diurnal
          Only/ Nocturnal and Diurnal

Other Disorders of Infancy, Childhood, or Adolescence (121)

309.21   Separation Anxiety Disorder (121)
          Specify if: Early Onset

313.23   Selective Mutism (125)
313.89   Reactive Attachment Disorder
          of Infancy or Early Childhood (127)
          Specify type: Inhibited Type/
          Disinhibited Type
307.3   Stereotypic Movement Disorder (131)
          Specify if: With Self-Injurious Behavior
313.9   Disorder of Infancy, Childhood, or
          Adolescence NOS (134)

■ DELIRIUM, DEMENTIA, AND AMNESTIC AND OTHER COGNITIVE DISORDERS (135)

Delirium (136)

293.0   Delirium Due to … *[Indicate the Gen-
          eral Medical Condition]* (141)
—.—   Substance Intoxication Delirium *(refer
          to Substance-Related Disorders for
          substance-specific codes)* (143)
—.—   Substance Withdrawal Delirium *(refer
          to Substance-Related Disorders for
          substance-specific codes)* (143)
—.—   Delirium Due to Multiple Etiologies
          (code each of the specific etiologies)
          (146)
780.09   Delirium NOS (147)

Dementia (147)

294.xx*   Dementia of the Alzheimer's Type,
          With Early Onset *(also code 331.0
          Alzheimer's disease on Axis III)*
          (154)
   .10   Without Behavioral Disturbance
   .11   With Behavioral Disturbance
294.xx*   Dementia of the Alzheimer's Type,
          With Late Onset *(also code 331.0
          Alzheimer's disease on Axis III)* (154)
   .10   Without Behavioral Disturbance
   .11   With Behavioral Disturbance
290.xx   Vascular Dementia (158)
   .40   Uncomplicated
   .41   With Delirium
   .42   With Delusions
   .43   With Depressed Mood
          Specify if: With Behavioral Distur-
          bance

*Code presence or absence of a behavioral dis-
turbance in the fifth digit for* **Dementia Due to
a General Medical Condition:**

0 = Without Behavioral Disturbance
1 = With Behavioral Disturbance

294.1x* Dementia Due to HIV Disease (*also code 042 HIV on Axis III*) (163)

294.1x* Dementia Due to Head Trauma (*also code 854.00 head injury on Axis III*) (164)

294.1x* Dementia Due to Parkinson's Disease (*also code 332.0 Parkinson's disease on Axis III*) (164)

294.1x* Dementia Due to Huntington's Disease (*also code 333.4 Huntington's disease on Axis III*) (165)

294.1x* Dementia Due to Pick's Disease (*also code 331.1 Pick's disease on Axis III*) (165)

294.1x* Dementia Due to Creutzfeldt-Jakob Disease (*also code 046.1 Creutzfeldt-Jakob disease on Axis III*) (166)

294.1x* Dementia Due to ... [*Indicate the General Medical Condition not listed above*] (*also code the general medical condition on Axis III*) (167)

—.— Substance-Induced Persisting Dementia (*refer to Substance-Related Disorders for substance-specific codes*) (168)

—.— Dementia Due to Multiple Etiologies (*code each of the specific etiologies*) (170)

294.8 Dementia NOS (171)

Amnestic Disorders (172)

294.0 Amnestic Disorder Due to ... [*Indicate the General Medical Condition*] (175)
Specify if: Transient/Chronic

—.— Substance-Induced Persisting Amnestic Disorder (*refer to Substance-Related Disorders for substance-specific codes*) (177)

294.8 Amnestic Disorder NOS (179)

Other Cognitive Disorders (179)

294.9 Cognitive Disorder NOS (179)

■ MENTAL DISORDERS DUE TO A GENERAL MEDICAL CONDITION NOT ELSEWHERE CLASSIFIED (181)

293.89 Catatonic Disorder Due to ... [*Indicate the General Medical Condition*] (185)

310.1 Personality Change Due to ... [*Indicate the General Medical Condition*] (187)
Specify type: Labile Type/Disinhibited

Type/Aggressive Type/Apathetic Type/Paranoid Type/Other Type/ Combined Type/Unspecified Type

293.9 Mental Disorder NOS Due to ... [*Indicate the General Medical Condition*] (190)

■ SUBSTANCE-RELATED DISORDERS (191)

The following specifiers apply to Substance Dependence as noted:

[a]With Physiological Dependence/Without Physiological Dependence

[b]Early Full Remission/Early Partial Remission/Sustained Full Remission/Sustained Partial Remission

[c]In a Controlled Environment

[d]On Agonist Therapy

The following specifiers apply to Substance-Induced Disorders as noted:

[I]With Onset During Intoxication/[W]With Onset During Withdrawal

Alcohol-Related Disorders (212)

Alcohol Use Disorders (213)

303.90 Alcohol Dependence[a,b,c] (213)

305.00 Alcohol Abuse (214)

Alcohol-Induced Disorders (214)

303.00 Alcohol Intoxication (214)

291.81 Alcohol Withdrawal (215)
Specify if: With Perceptual Disturbances

291.0 Alcohol Intoxication Delirium (143)

291.0 Alcohol Withdrawal Delirium (143)

291.2 Alcohol-Induced Persisting Dementia (168)

291.1 Alcohol-Induced Persisting Amnestic Disorder (177)

291.x Alcohol-Induced Psychotic Disorder (338)

.5 With Delusions[I,W]

.3 With Hallucinations[I,W]

291.89 Alcohol-Induced Mood Disorder[I,W] (405)

291.89 Alcohol-Induced Anxiety Disorder[I,W] (479)

291.89 Alcohol-Induced Sexual Dysfunction[I] (562)

291.89 Alcohol-Induced Sleep Disorder[I,W] (655)

291.9 Alcohol-Related Disorder NOS (223)

---

*ICD-9-CM code valid after October 1, 2000.

Amphetamine (or Amphetamine-Like)–Related Disorders (223)

Amphetamine Use Disorders (224)

304.40   Amphetamine Dependence[a,b,c] (224)
305.70   Amphetamine Abuse (225)

Amphetamine-Induced Disorders (226)

292.89   Amphetamine Intoxication (226)
          Specify if: With Perceptual Distur-
          bances
292.0   Amphetamine Withdrawal (227)
292.81   Amphetamine Intoxication Delirium
          (143)
292.xx   Amphetamine-Induced Psychotic
          Disorder (338)
   .11   With Delusions[I]
   .12   With Hallucinations[I]
292.84   Amphetamine-Induced Mood
          Disorder[I,W] (405)
292.89   Amphetamine-Induced Anxiety
          Disorder[I] (479)
292.89   Amphetamine-Induced Sexual
          Dysfunction[I] (562)
292.89   Amphetamine-Induced Sleep
          Disorder[I,W] (655)
292.9   Amphetamine-Related Disorder NOS
          (231)

Caffeine-Related Disorders (231)

Caffeine-Induced Disorders (232)

305.90   Caffeine Intoxication (232)
292.89   Caffeine-Induced Anxiety Disorder[I]
          (479)
292.89   Caffeine-Induced Sleep Disorder[I] (655)
292.9   Caffeine-Related Disorder NOS (234)

Cannabis-Related Disorders (234)

Cannabis Use Disorders (236)

304.30   Cannabis Dependence[a,b,c] (236)
305.20   Cannabis Abuse (236)

Cannabis-Induced Disorders (237)

292.89   Cannabis Intoxication (237)
          Specify if: With Perceptual Distur-
          bances
292.81   Cannabis Intoxication Delirium (143)
292.xx   Cannabis-Induced Psychotic Disorder
          (338)
   .11   With Delusions[I]
   .12   With Hallucinations[I]
292.89   Cannabis-Induced Anxiety Disorder[I]
          (479)
292.9   Cannabis-Related Disorder NOS (241)

Cocaine-Related Disorders (241)

Cocaine Use Disorders (242)

304.20   Cocaine Dependence[a,b,c] (242)
305.60   Cocaine Abuse (243)

Cocaine-Induced Disorders (244)

292.89   Cocaine Intoxication (244)
          Specify if: With Perceptual Distur-
          bances
292.0   Cocaine Withdrawal (245)
292.81   Cocaine Intoxication Delirium
          (143)
292.xx   Cocaine-Induced Psychotic
          Disorder (338)
   .11   With Delusions[I]
   .12   With Hallucinations[I]
292.84   Cocaine-Induced Mood Disorder[I,W]
          (405)
292.89   Cocaine-Induced Anxiety Disorder[I,W]
          (479)
292.89   Cocaine-Induced Sexual Dysfunction[I]
          (562)
292.89   Cocaine-Induced Sleep Disorder[I,W]
          (655)
292.9   Cocaine-Related Disorder NOS (250)

Hallucinogen-Related Disorders (250)

Hallucinogen Use Disorders (251)

304.50   Hallucinogen Dependence[b,c] (251)
305.30   Hallucinogen Abuse (252)

Hallucinogen-Induced Disorders (252)

292.89   Hallucinogen Intoxication (252)
292.89   Hallucinogen Persisting Perception
          Disorder (Flashbacks) (253)
292.81   Hallucinogen Intoxication Delirium
          (143)
292.xx   Hallucinogen-Induced Psychotic
          Disorder (338)
   .11   With Delusions[I]
   .12   With Hallucinations[I]
292.84   Hallucinogen-Induced Mood Disorder[I]
          (405)
292.89   Hallucinogen-Induced Anxiety Disor-
          der[I] (479)
292.9   Hallucinogen-Related Disorder NOS
          (256)

Inhalant-Related Disorders (257)

Inhalant Use Disorders (258)

304.60   Inhalant Dependence[b,c] (258)
305.90   Inhalant Abuse (259)

Inhalant-Induced Disorders (259)

292.89	Inhalant Intoxication (259)
292.81	Inhalant Intoxication Delirium (143)
292.82	Inhalant-Induced Persisting Dementia (168)
292.xx	Inhalant-Induced Psychotic Disorder (338)
.11	With Delusions[I]
.12	With Hallucinations[I]
292.84	Inhalant-Induced Mood Disorder[I] (405)
292.89	Inhalant-Induced Anxiety Disorder[I] (479)
292.9	Inhalant-Related Disorder NOS (263)

Nicotine-Related Disorders (264)

Nicotine Use Disorder (264)

305.1   Nicotine Dependence[a,b] (264)

Nicotine-Induced Disorder (265)

292.0   Nicotine Withdrawal (265)
292.9   Nicotine-Related Disorder NOS (269)

Opioid-Related Disorders (269)

Opioid Use Disorders (270)

304.00   Opioid Dependence[a,b,c,d] (270)
305.50   Opioid Abuse (271)

Opioid-Induced Disorders (271)

292.89	Opioid Intoxication (271) *Specify if:* With Perceptual Disturbances
292.0	Opioid Withdrawal (272)
292.81	Opioid Intoxication Delirium (143)
292.xx	Opioid-Induced Psychotic Disorder (338)
.11	With Delusions[I]
.12	With Hallucinations[I]
292.84	Opioid-Induced Mood Disorder[I] (405)
292.89	Opioid-Induced Sexual Dysfunction[I] (562)
292.89	Opioid-Induced Sleep Disorder[I,W] (655)
292.9	Opioid-Related Disorder NOS (277)

Phencyclidine (or Phencyclidine-Like)–Related Disorders (278)

Phencyclidine Use Disorders (279)

304.60   Phencyclidine Dependence[b,c] (279)
305.90   Phencyclidine Abuse (279)

Phencyclidine-Induced Disorders (280)

292.89	Phencyclidine Intoxication (280) *Specify if:* With Perceptual Disturbances
292.81	Phencyclidine Intoxication Delirium (143)
292.xx	Phencyclidine-Induced Psychotic Disorder (338)
.11	With Delusions[I]
.12	With Hallucinations[I]
292.84	Phencyclidine-Induced Mood Disorder[I] (405)
292.89	Phencyclidine-Induced Anxiety Disorder[I] (479)
292.9	Phencyclidine-Related Disorder NOS (283)

Sedative-, Hypnotic-, or Anxiolytic-Related Disorders (284)

Sedative, Hypnotic, or Anxiolytic Use Disorders (285)

304.10   Sedative, Hypnotic, or Anxiolytic Dependence[a,b,c] (285)
305.40   Sedative, Hypnotic, or Anxiolytic Abuse (286)

Sedative-, Hypnotic-, or Anxiolytic-Induced Disorders (286)

292.89	Sedative, Hypnotic, or Anxiolytic Intoxication (286)
292.0	Sedative, Hypnotic, or Anxiolytic Withdrawal (287) *Specify if:* With Perceptual Disturbances
292.81	Sedative, Hypnotic, or Anxiolytic Intoxication Delirium (143)
292.81	Sedative, Hypnotic, or Anxiolytic Withdrawal Delirium (143)
292.82	Sedative-, Hypnotic-, or Anxiolytic-Induced Persisting Dementia (168)
292.83	Sedative-, Hypnotic-, or Anxiolytic-Induced Persisting Amnestic Disorder (177)
292.xx	Sedative-, Hypnotic-, or Anxiolytic-Induced Psychotic Disorder (338)
.11	With Delusions[I,W]
.12	With Hallucinations[I,W]
292.84	Sedative-, Hypnotic-, or Anxiolytic-Induced Mood Disorder[I,W] (405)
292.89	Sedative-, Hypnotic-, or Anxiolytic-Induced Anxiety Disorder[W] (479)
292.89	Sedative-, Hypnotic-, or Anxiolytic-Induced Sexual Dysfunction[I] (562)

292.89   Sedative-, Hypnotic-, or Anxiolytic-
          Induced Sleep Disorder[I,W] (655)
292.9   Sedative-, Hypnotic-, or Anxiolytic-
          Related Disorder NOS (293)

Polysubstance-Related Disorder (293)

304.80   Polysubstance Dependence[a,b,c,d] (293)

**Other (or Unknown) Substance–Related
Disorders (294)**

*Other (or Unknown) Substance Use Disorders
    (295)*

304.90   Other (or Unknown) Substance
          Dependence[a,b,c,d] (192)
305.90   Other (or Unknown) Substance Abuse
          (198)

*Other (or Unknown) Substance–Induced
    Disorders (295)*

292.89   Other (or Unknown) Substance Intoxi-
          cation (199)
          Specify if: With Perceptual Distur-
          bances
292.0   Other (or Unknown) Substance With-
          drawal (201)
          Specify if: With Perceptual Distur-
          bances
292.81   Other (or Unknown)
          Substance–Induced Delirium (143)
292.82   Other (or Unknown)
          Substance–Induced Persisting
          Dementia (168)
292.83   Other (or Unknown)
          Substance–Induced Persisting
          Amnestic Disorder (177)
292.xx   Other (or Unknown)
          Substance–Induced Psychotic Disor-
          der (338)
    .11   With Delusions[I,W]
    .12   With Hallucinations[I,W]
292.84   Other (or Unknown)
          Substance–Induced Mood Disorder[I,W]
          (405)
292.89   Other (or Unknown)
          Substance–Induced Anxiety Disor-
          der[I,W] (479)
292.89   Other (or Unknown)
          Substance–Induced Sexual Dysfunc-
          tion[I] (562)
292.89   Other (or Unknown)
          Substance–Induced Sleep Disorder[I, W]
          (655)
292.9   Other (or Unknown)
          Substance–Related Disorder NOS (295)

■ SCHIZOPHRENIA AND OTHER PSYCHOTIC DISORDERS (297)

295.xx   Schizophrenia (298)

*The following Classification of Longitudinal
Course applies to all subtypes of Schizophrenia:*

Episodic With Interepisode Residual Symp-
    toms (*Specify if:* With Prominent Negative
    Symptoms)/Episodic With No Interepisode
    Residual Symptoms
Continuous (*specify if:* With Prominent Nega-
    tive Symptoms)
Single Episode in Partial Remission (*specify
    if:* With Prominent Negative Symptoms)/
    Single Episode in Full Remission
Other or Unspecified Pattern
    .30   Paranoid Type (313)
    .10   Disorganized Type (314)
    .20   Catatonic Type (315)
    .90   Undifferentiated Type (316)
    .60   Residual Type (316)
295.40   Schizophreniform Disorder (317)
          Specify if: Without Good Prognostic
          Features/With Good Prognostic Fea-
          tures
295.70   Schizoaffective Disorder (319)
          Specify type: Bipolar Type/Depressive
          Type
297.1   Delusional Disorder (323)
          Specify type: Erotomanic
          Type/Grandiose Type/Jealous Type/
          Persecutory Type/Somatic Type/Mixed
          Type/Unspecified Type
298.8   Brief Psychotic Disorder (329)
          Specify if: With Marked
          Stressor(s)/Without Marked
          Stressor(s)/With Postpartum Onset
297.3   Shared Psychotic Disorder (332)
293.xx   Psychotic Disorder Due to … *[Indicate
          the General Medical Condition]* (334)
    .81   With Delusions
    .82   With Hallucinations
—.–   Substance-Induced Psychotic Disorder
          *(refer to Substance-Related Disorders
          for substance-specific codes)* (338)
          Specify if: With Onset During Intoxica-
          tion/With Onset During Withdrawal
298.9   Psychotic Disorder NOS (343)

■ MOOD DISORDERS (345)

*Code current state of Major Depressive Disor-
der or Bipolar I Disorder in fifth digit:*

1 = Mild
2 = Moderate
3 = Severe Without Psychotic Features
4 = Severe With Psychotic Features
    Specify: Mood-Congruent Psychotic
    Features/Mood-Incongruent Psychotic
    Features
5 = In Partial Remission
6 = In Full Remission
0 = Unspecified

The following specifiers apply (for current or most recent episode) to Mood Disorders as noted:

[a]Severity/Psychotic/Remission
Specifiers/[b]Chronic/[c]With Catatonic Features/[d]With Melancholic Features/[e]With Atypical Features/[f]With Postpartum Onset

The following specifiers apply to Mood Disorders as noted:

[g]With or Without Full Interepisode Recovery/[h]With Seasonal Pattern/[i]With Rapid Cycling

Depressive Disorders (369)

296.xx	Major Depressive Disorder (369)	
.2x	Single Episode[a,b,c,d,e,f]	
.3x	Recurrent[a,b,c,d,e,f,g,h]	
300.4	Dysthymic Disorder (376)	

Specify if: Early Onset/Late Onset
Specify: With Atypical Features

311   Depressive Disorder NOS (381)

Bipolar Disorders (382)

296.xx   Bipolar I Disorder (382)
.0x   Single Manic Episode[a,c,f]
Specify if: Mixed
.40   Most Recent Episode Hypomanic[g,h,i]
.4x   Most Recent Episode Manic[a,c,f,g,h,i]
.6x   Most Recent Episode Mixed[a,c,f,g,h,i]
.5x   Most Recent Episode Depressed[a,b,c,d,e,f,g,h,i]
.7   Most Recent Episode Unspecified[g,h,i]
296.89   Bipolar II Disorder[a,b,c,d,e,f,g,h,i] (392)
Specify (current or most recent episode): Hypomanic/Depressed
301.13   Cyclothymic Disorder (398)
296.80   Bipolar Disorder NOS (400)
293.83   Mood Disorder Due to...
[Indicate the General Medical Condition] (401)
Specify type: With Depressive Features/With Major Depressive–like Episode/With Manic Features/With Mixed Features

—.–   Substance-Induced Mood Disorder
(refer to Substance-Related Disorders for substance-specific codes) (405)
Specify type: With Depressive Features/With Manic Features/With Mixed Features
Specify if: With Onset During Intoxication/With Onset During Withdrawal
296.90   Mood Disorder NOS (410)

■ ANXIETY DISORDERS (429)

300.01   Panic Disorder Without Agoraphobia (433)
300.21   Panic Disorder With Agoraphobia (433)
300.22   Agoraphobia Without History of Panic Disorder (441)
300.29   Specific Phobia (443)
Specify type: Animal Type/Natural Environment Type/Blood-Injection-Injury Type/Situational Type/Other Type
300.23   Social Phobia (450)
Specify if: Generalized
300.3   Obsessive-Compulsive Disorder (456)
Specify if: With Poor Insight
309.81   Posttraumatic Stress Disorder (463)
Specify if: Acute/Chronic
Specify if: With Delayed Onset
308.3   Acute Stress Disorder (469)
300.02   Generalized Anxiety Disorder (472)
293.84   Anxiety Disorder Due to...
[Indicate the General Medical Condition] (476)
Specify if: With Generalized Anxiety/With Panic Attacks/With Obsessive-Compulsive Symptoms
—.–   Substance-Induced Anxiety Disorder
(refer to Substance-Related Disorders for substance-specific codes) (479)
Specify if: With Generalized Anxiety/With Panic Attacks/With Obsessive-Compulsive Symptoms/With Phobic Symptoms
Specify if: With Onset During Intoxication/With Onset During Withdrawal
300.00   Anxiety Disorder NOS (484)

■ SOMATOFORM DISORDERS (485)

300.81   Somatization Disorder (486)
300.82   Undifferentiated Somatoform Disorder (490)

300.11   Conversion Disorder (492)
          Specify type: With Motor Symptom or
          Deficit/With Sensory Symptom or
          Deficit/With Seizures or Convul-
          sions/With Mixed Presentation
307.xx   Pain Disorder (498)
  .80   Associated With Psychological
            Factors
  .89   Associated With Both Psychological
            Factors and a General Medical
            Condition
          Specify if: Acute/Chronic
300.7   Hypochondriasis (504)
          Specify if: With Poor Insight
300.7   Body Dysmorphic Disorder (507)
300.82   Somatoform Disorder NOS (511)

■ FACTITIOUS DISORDERS (513)

300.xx   Factitious Disorder (513)
  .16   With Predominantly Psychological
            Signs and Symptoms
  .19   With Predominantly Physical Signs
            and Symptoms
  .19   With Combined Psychological and
            Physical Signs and Symptoms
300.19   Factitious Disorder NOS (517)

■ DISSOCIATIVE DISORDERS (519)

300.12   Dissociative Amnesia (520)
300.13   Dissociative Fugue (523)
300.14   Dissociative Identity Disorder (526)
300.6   Depersonalization Disorder (530)
300.15   Dissociative Disorder NOS (532)

■ SEXUAL AND GENDER IDENTITY DISORDERS (535)

Sexual Dysfunctions (535)

The following specifiers apply to all primary Sexual Dysfunctions:

Lifelong Type/Acquired Type
Generalized Type/Situational Type
Due to Psychological Factors/Due to Com-
bined Factors

Sexual Desire Disorders (539)

302.71   Hypoactive Sexual Desire Disorder
          (539)
302.79   Sexual Aversion Disorder (541)

Sexual Arousal Disorders (543)

302.72   Female Sexual Arousal Disorder
          (543)
302.72   Male Erectile Disorder (545)

Orgasmic Disorders (547)

302.73   Female Orgasmic Disorder (547)
302.74   Male Orgasmic Disorder (550)
302.75   Premature Ejaculation (552)

Sexual Pain Disorders (554)

302.76   Dyspareunia (Not Due to a General
          Medical Condition) (554)
306.51   Vaginismus (Not Due to a General
          Medical Condition) (556)

*Sexual Dysfunction Due to a General Medical
Condition (558)*

625.8   Female Hypoactive Sexual Desire Dis-
          order Due to … *[Indicate the General
          Medical Condition]* (558)
608.89   Male Hypoactive Sexual Desire Disor-
          der Due to … *[Indicate the General
          Medical Condition]* (558)
607.84   Male Erectile Disorder Due to … *[Indi-
          cate the General Medical Condition]*
          (558)
625.0   Female Dyspareunia Due to … *[Indi-
          cate the General Medical Condition]*
          (558)
608.89   Male Dyspareunia Due to … *[Indicate
          the General Medical Condition]*
          (558)
625.8   Other Female Sexual Dysfunction
          Due to … *[Indicate the General Medical
          Condition]* (558)
608.89   Other Male Sexual Dysfunction Due
          to … *[Indicate the General Medical
          Condition]* (558)
—.–   Substance-Induced Sexual Dysfunction
          *(refer to Substance-Related Disorders
          for substance-specific codes)* (562)
          Specify if: With Impaired Desire/With
          Impaired Arousal/With Impaired
          Orgasm/With Sexual Pain
          Specify if: With Onset During
          Intoxication
302.70   Sexual Dysfunction NOS (565)

Paraphilias (566)

302.4   Exhibitionism (569)
302.81   Fetishism (569)
302.89   Frotteurism (570)

302.2   Pedophilia (571)
         Specify if: Sexually Attracted to Males/Sexually Attracted to Females/Sexually Attracted to Both
         Specify if: Limited to Incest
         Specify type: Exclusive Type/Nonexclusive Type
302.83   Sexual Masochism (572)
302.84   Sexual Sadism (573)
302.3   Transvestic Fetishism (574)
         Specify if: With Gender Dysphoria
302.82   Voyeurism (575)
302.9   Paraphilia NOS (576)

Gender Identity Disorders (576)

302.xx   Gender Identity Disorder (576)
  .6   in Children
  .85   in Adolescents or Adults
         Specify if: Sexually Attracted to Males/Sexually Attracted to Females/Sexually Attracted to Both/Sexually Attracted to Neither
302.6   Gender Identity Disorder NOS (582)
302.9   Sexual Disorder NOS (582)

■ EATING DISORDERS (583)

307.1   Anorexia Nervosa (583)
         Specify type: Restricting Type; Binge-Eating/Purging Type
307.51   Bulimia Nervosa (589)
         Specify type: Purging Type/Nonpurging Type
307.50   Eating Disorder NOS (594)

■ SLEEP DISORDERS (597)

Primary Sleep Disorders (598)

Dyssomnias (598)

307.42   Primary Insomnia (599)
307.44   Primary Hypersomnia (604)
         Specify if: Recurrent
347   Narcolepsy (609)
780.59   Breathing-Related Sleep Disorder (615)
307.45   Circadian Rhythm Sleep Disorder (622)
         Specify type: Delayed Sleep Phase Type/Jet Lag Type/Shift Work Type/Unspecified Type
307.47   Dyssomnia NOS (629)

■ PARASOMNIAS (630)

307.47   Nightmare Disorder (631)
307.46   Sleep Terror Disorder (634)
307.46   Sleepwalking Disorder (639)
307.47   Parasomnia NOS (644)

Sleep Disorders Related to Another Mental Disorder (645)

307.42   Insomnia Related to ... *[Indicate the Axis I or Axis II Disorder]* (645)
307.44   Hypersomnia Related to ... *[Indicate the Axis I or Axis II Disorder]* (645)

Other Sleep Disorders (651)

780.xx   Sleep Disorder Due to ... *[Indicate the General Medical Condition]* (651)
  .52   Insomnia Type
  .54   Hypersomnia Type
  .59   Parasomnia Type
  .59   Mixed Type
—.—   Substance-Induced Sleep Disorder *(refer to Substance-Related Disorders for substance-specific codes)* (655)
         Specify type: Insomnia Type/Hypersomnia Type/Parasomnia Type/Mixed Type
         Specify if: With Onset During Intoxication/With Onset During Withdrawal

■ IMPULSE-CONTROL DISORDERS NOT ELSEWHERE CLASSIFIED (663)

312.34   Intermittent Explosive Disorder (663)
312.32   Kleptomania (667)
312.33   Pyromania (669)
312.31   Pathological Gambling (671)
312.39   Trichotillomania (674)
312.30   Impulse-Control Disorder NOS (677)

■ ADJUSTMENT DISORDERS (679)

309.xx   Adjustment Disorder (679)
  .0   With Depressed Mood
  .24   With Anxiety
  .28   With Mixed Anxiety and Depressed Mood
  .3   With Disturbance of Conduct
  .4   With Mixed Disturbance of Emotions and Conduct
  .9   Unspecified
         Specify if: Acute/Chronic

■ PERSONALITY DISORDERS (685)

Note: *These are coded on Axis II.*

301.0   Paranoid Personality Disorder (690)
301.20   Schizoid Personality Disorder (694)
301.22   Schizotypal Personality Disorder (697)
301.7   Antisocial Personality Disorder (701)
301.83   Borderline Personality Disorder (706)
301.50   Histrionic Personality Disorder (711)
301.81   Narcissistic Personality Disorder (714)
301.82   Avoidant Personality Disorder (718)
301.6   Dependent Personality Disorder (721)
301.4   Obsessive-Compulsive Personality Disorder (725)
301.9   Personality Disorder NOS (729)

■ OTHER CONDITIONS THAT MAY BE A FOCUS OF CLINICAL ATTENTION (731)

Psychological Factors Affecting Medical Condition (731)

316   ... *[Specified Psychological Factor] Affecting ... [Indicate the General Medical Condition]* (731)
           Choose name based on nature of factors:
           Mental Disorder Affecting Medical Condition
           Psychological Symptoms Affecting Medical Condition
           Personality Traits or Coping Style Affecting Medical Condition
           Maladaptive Health Behaviors Affecting Medical Condition
           Stress-Related Physiological Response Affecting Medical Condition
           Other or Unspecified Psychological Factors Affecting Medical Condition

Medication-Induced Movement Disorders (734)

332.1   Neuroleptic-Induced Parkinsonism (735)
333.92   Neuroleptic Malignant Syndrome (735)
333.7   Neuroleptic-Induced Acute Dystonia (735)
333.99   Neuroleptic-Induced Acute Akathisia (735)
333.82   Neuroleptic-Induced Tardive Dyskinesia (736)
333.1   Medication-Induced Postural Tremor (736)

333.90   Medication-Induced Movement Disorder NOS (736)

Other Medication-Induced Disorder (736)

995.2   Adverse Effects of Medication NOS (736)

Relational Problems (736)

V61.9   Relational Problem Related to a Mental Disorder or General Medical Condition (737)
V61.20   Parent-Child Relational Problem (737)
V61.10   Partner Relational Problem (737)
V61.8   Sibling Relational Problem (737)
V62.81   Relational Problem NOS (737)

Problems Related to Abuse or Neglect (738)

V61.21   Physical Abuse of Child (738) *(code 995.54 if focus of attention is on victim)*
V61.21   Sexual Abuse of Child (738) *(code 995.53 if focus of attention is on victim)*
V61.21   Neglect of Child (738) *(code 995.52 if focus of attention is on victim)*
—.–   Physical Abuse of Adult (738)
V61.12   (if by partner)
V62.83   (if by person other than partner). *(code 995.81 if focus of attention is on victim)*
—.–   Sexual Abuse of Adult (738)
V61.12   (if by partner)
V62.83   (if by person other than partner) *(code 995.83 if focus of attention is on victim)*

Additional Conditions That May Be a Focus of Clinical Attention (739)

V15.81   Noncompliance With Treatment (739)
V65.2   Malingering (739)
V71.01   Adult Antisocial Behavior (740)
V71.02   Child or Adolescent Antisocial Behavior (740)
V62.89   Borderline Intellectual Functioning (740)
           Note: This is coded on Axis II.
780.9   Age-Related Cognitive Decline (740)
V62.82   Bereavement (740)
V62.3   Academic Problem (741)
V62.2   Occupational Problem (741)
313.82   Identity Problem (741)
V62.89   Religious or Spiritual Problem (741)
V62.4   Acculturation Problem (741)
V62.89   Phase of Life Problem (742)

■ ADDITIONAL CODES (743)

300.9	Unspecified Mental Disorder (nonpsychotic) (743)
V71.09	No Diagnosis or Condition on Axis I (743)
799.9	Diagnosis or Condition Deferred on Axis I (743)
V71.09	No Diagnosis on Axis II (743)
799.9	Diagnosis Deferred on Axis II (743)

■ MULTIAXIAL SYSTEM

Axis I	Clinical Disorders Other Conditions That May Be a Focus of Clinical Attention
Axis II	Personality Disorders Mental Retardation
Axis III	General Medical Conditions
Axis IV	Psychosocial and Environmental Problems
Axis V	Global Assessment of Functioning

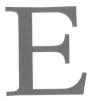

Standards of Nursing Practice for LPN/LVNs

■ NATIONAL FEDERATION OF LICENSED PRACTICAL NURSES (NFLPN) CODE FOR LICENSED PRACTICAL/VOCATIONAL NURSES

- Know the scope of maximum utilization of the LPN/LVN as specified by the nursing practice act and function within its scope.
- Safeguard the confidential information acquired from any source about the patient.
- Provide health care to all patients regardless of race, creed, cultural background, disease, or lifestyle.
- Refuse to give endorsement to the sale and promotion of commercial products or services.
- Uphold the highest standards in personal appearance, language, dress, and demeanor.
- Stay informed about issues affecting the practice of nursing and delivery of health care and, where appropriate, participate in government and policy decisions.
- Accept the responsibility for safe nursing practice by keeping oneself mentally and physically fit and educationally prepared to practice.
- Accept the responsibility for membership in NFLPN and participate in its efforts to maintain the established standards of nursing practice and employment policies that lead to quality patient care.

NFLPN Nursing Practice Standards

Introductory Statement

Definition: Practical/vocational nursing means the performance for compensation of authorized acts of nursing that utilize specialized knowledge and skills and that meet the health needs of people in a variety of settings under the direction of qualified health professionals.

Scope: Practical/vocational nursing comprises the common case of nursing, and, therefore, is a valid entry into the nursing profession.

Opportunities exist for practicing in a milieu where different professions unite their particular skills in a team effort for one common objective—to preserve or improve an individual patient's functioning.

Opportunities also exist for upward mobility within the profession through academic education and for lateral expansion of knowledge and expertise through both academic and continuing education.

Standards

Education

The licensed practical/vocational nurse

1. Shall complete a formal education program in practical nursing approved by the appropriate nursing authority in a state.

2. Shall successfully pass the National Council Licensure Examination for Practical Nurses.
3. Shall participate in initial orientation within the employing institution.

Legal/Ethical Status

The licensed practical/vocational nurse

1. Shall hold a current license to practice nursing as an LPN/LVN in accordance with the law of the state wherein employed.
2. Shall know the scope of nursing practice authorized by the Nursing Practice Act in the state wherein employed.
3. Shall have a personal commitment to fulfill the legal responsibilities inherent in good nursing practice.
4. Shall take responsible actions in situations wherein there is unprofessional conduct by a peer or other health care provider.
5. Shall recognize and have a commitment to meet the ethical and moral obligations of the practice of nursing.
6. Shall not accept or perform professional responsibilities which the individual knows (s)he is not competent to perform.

Practice

The licensed practical/vocational nurse

1. Shall accept assigned responsibilities as an accountable member of the health care team.
2. Shall function within the limits of educational preparation and experience as related to the assigned duties.
3. Shall function with other members of the health care team in promoting and maintaining health, preventing disease and disability, caring for and rehabilitating individuals who are experiencing an altered health state, and contributing to the ultimate quality of life until death.
4. Shall know and utilize the nursing process in planning (assessing [data gathering]), implementing, and evaluating health services and nursing care for the individual patient or group.
   - Planning (assessing [data gathering]): The planning of nursing includes

   - Assessment of health status of the individual patient, the family, and community groups
   - An analysis of the information gained from assessment
   - The identification of health goals
- Implementation: The plan for nursing care is put into practice to achieve the stated goals and includes
   - Observing, recording, and reporting significant changes which require intervention or different goals
   - Applying nursing knowledge and skills to promote and maintain health, to prevent disease and disability, and to optimize functional capabilities of an individual patient
   - Assisting the patient and family with activities of daily living and encouraging self-care as appropriate
   - Carrying out therapeutic regimens and protocols prescribed by an RN, physician, or other persons authorized by state law
- Evaluations: The plan for nursing care and its implementations are evaluated to measure the progress toward the stated goals and will include appropriate persons and/or groups to determine
   - The relevancy of current goals in relation to the progress of the individual patient
   - The involvement of the recipients of care in the evaluation process
   - The quality of the nursing action in the implementation of the plan
   - A reordering of priorities or new goal setting in the care plan
5. Shall participate in peer review and other evaluation processes.
6. Shall participate in the development of policies concerning the health and nursing needs of society and in the roles and functions of the LPN/LVN.

Continuing Education

The licensed practical/vocational nurse

1. Shall be responsible for maintaining the highest possible level of professional competence at all times.

2. Shall periodically reassess career goals and select continuing education activities which will help to achieve these goals.
3. Shall take advantage of continuing education opportunities which will lead to personal growth and professional development.
4. Shall seek and participate in continuing education activities which are approved for credit by appropriate organizations, such as the NFLPN.

NFLPN Specialized Nursing Practice Standards

The licensed practical/vocational nurse

1. Shall have had at least one year's experience in nursing at the staff level.
2. Shall present personal qualifications that are indicative of potential abilities for practice in the chosen specialized nursing area.
3. Shall present evidence of completion of a program or course that is approved by an appropriate agency to provide the knowledge and skills necessary for effective nursing services in the specialized field.
4. Shall meet all of the standards of practice as set forth in this document.

Bibliography

Aguilera, DC (1994). *Crisis Intervention Theory and Methodology*, 7th ed. St. Louis: Mosby-Year Book.

Aiken, LR (1991). *Psychological Testing and Assessment*, 8th ed. Needham Heights, MA: Allyn and Bacon (Simon and Schuster).

Aiken, TD, with Catalano, JT (1994). *Legal, Ethical, and Political Issues in Nursing*. Philadelphia: FA Davis.

Al-Anon Family Group Headquarters (1981). *Al-Anon's 12 Steps and 12 Traditions*. New York: Al-Anon Family Group Headquarters.

American Nurses Association (1988). *Standards of Psychiatric and Mental Health Nursing Practice*. Kansas City, MO: The Association.

American Psychiatric Association (2000). *Diagnostic and Statistical Manual of Mental Disorders-IV-TR*, 4th ed., Text revision. Washington, DC: American Psychiatric Association.

Anderson, C (1990). *Patient Teaching and Communicating in an Information Age*. Albany, NY: Delmar Publishers.

Anderson, RA (2001). *Clinician's Guide to Holistic Medicine, Hazelden Chronic Illness Series*. New York: McGraw-Hill.

Anderson, S, and Kaleeba, N (1994, July-August). The challenge of AIDS home care. *World Health Magazine (WHO), 47,* 20.

Baer, CL, and Williams, BR (1992). *Clinical Pharmacology and Nursing*, 2nd ed. Springhouse, PA: Springhouse Corp.

Bailey, DS, and Bailey, DR (1993). *Therapeutic Approaches to the Care of the Mentally Ill*, 3rd ed. Philadelphia: FA Davis.

Bandler, R, and Grinder, J (1979). *Frogs Into Princes: Neuro Linguistic Programming*, Ed. Andreas, S. Moab, UT: Real People Press.

Barry, PD (2004). *Mental Health and Mental Illness*, 7th ed. Philadelphia: JB Lippincott.

Bass, E, and Davis, L (1993). *Beginning to Heal—A First Book for Survivors of Child Sexual Abuse*. New York: Harper Perennial/Harper-Collins.

Bauer, BB, and Hill, SS (1986). *Essentials of Mental Health-Care Planning and Interventions*. Philadelphia: WB Saunders.

Beattie, M (1989). *Beyond Codependency and Getting Better All the Time*. New York: Harper/Hazelden–Harper and Row, the Hazelden Foundation.

Bete, CL, pamphlets (Channing L. Bete Co. Inc., South Deerfield, MA):

1. *A Christian Response to AIDS*, 1990
2. *About Adult Day Centers*, 1986
3. *About Employee Assistance Programs*, 1987
4. *About Home Health Care*, 1993
5. *About Patient Rights in Home Care*, 1998
6. *About Single Parenting*, 1983
7. *About Teens and Stress*, 1994
8. *About Widowhood*, 1998
9. *Are You a Single Parent?*, 1997
10. *Coping with the Stress of Parenting*, 1997
11. *Helping Your Child Grieve*, 1997
12. *Your Rights in Mental Health Care*, 1999

Bauer, B, and Hill, S (2000). *Mental Health Nursing—An Introductory Text*. Philadelphia: W.B. Saunders Company.

Bidi use among urban youth, Massachusetts, March–April, 1999. (1999, September 17). *Morbidity and Mortality Weekly, 48*(36), 796–799.

Bleuler, E (1911). *Dementia Praecox or the Group of Schizophrenias* (p. 26). New York: International Universities Press.

Boggs, W (2004). Brain-Penetrating ACE Inhibitors Slow Alzheimer's. *Neurology*, Online. (Any uses or copies of content from this journal in whole or in part must include the customary full bibliographic citation, including author attribution, date, article title, and the URL http://www.neurology.org/ and MUST include the copyright notice in the following format: Copyright 2004 by AAN Enterprises, Inc./Lippincott Williams & Wilkins, 351 West Camden Street, Baltimore, MD)

Bratman, S (1998). *The Alternative Medicine Ratings Guide*. Rocklin, CA: Prima Publishing.

Brickner, P, et al. (1990). *Under the Safety Net*. New York: WW Norton.

Bronston, B (2000, January 30). Some kids are worrying themselves sick. *Times-Picayune* (New Orleans).

Brumberg, JJ (1988). *Fasting Girls—The Emergence of Anorexia Nervosa as a Modern Disease.* Cambridge, MA: Harvard University Press.

Burnam, J (1995). *Mosby's Psychiatric Nursing Pocket Reference.* St. Louis: Mosby-Year Book.

Came, B (1994, October 31). The last trip: three teens die in a shocking suicide. *Macleans'* (Canada) 7, 14.

Carr, WHA (1995, September/October). A right to die. *The Saturday Evening Post.*

Carter, M, and Weber, T (1994). *Body Reflexology.* West Nyack, NY: Parker Publishing Company.

Cohn, R (1993, August 23). The troubled view from within—Whitehouse: not the ravings of a madman. *Newsweek,* p. 24.

Coleman, W (1990). *Understanding and Preventing Teen Suicide.* Chicago: Children's Press.

Community Health and Counseling Services (1999). Adult Mental Health Services, United Way of Eastern Maine. http://www.chcs-me.org.

Corsini, RJ (ed) (1994). *Encyclopedia of Psychology,* 2nd ed., Vol. 2. New York: John Wiley and Sons.

Culkin, J, and Perrotto, RS (1996). *Fundamentals of Psychology: Applications for Life and Work.* Cincinnati: South-Western Educational Publishing.

Deluca, J (1999, February). Preventing abuse and neglect. *Provider.*

Dennis, LB, and Hassol, J (1983). *Introduction to Human Development and Health Issues.* Philadelphia: WB Saunders.

DeWit, SC (1992). *Keane's Essentials of Medical-Surgical Nursing,* 3rd ed. Philadelphia: WB Saunders/Harcourt Brace Jovanovich.

Doenges, ME, Moorhouse, MF, and Burley, JT (1995). *Application of Nursing Process and Nursing Diagnosis—An Interactive Text for Diagnostic Reasoning,* 2nd ed. Philadelphia: FA Davis.

Donahue, MP (1985). *Nursing, The Finest Art.* St. Louis: CV Mosby.

Drickamer, MA, and Lachs, MS (1992, April 2). Should patients with Alzheimer's disease be told their diagnosis? *New England Journal of Medicine, 326,* 947–951.

Elias, TS, and Dykeman, PA (1990). *Edible Wild Plants—A North American Field Guide.* New York: Sterling Publishing Company.

Ellis, A (1988). A guide to rational living. Videocassette from the series *Thinking Allowed.* Oakland, CA: Thinking Allowed Productions.

Ellis, A (1994). *Reasons and Emotions in Psychotherapy.* Secaucus, NJ: Birch Lane Press.

Erikson, EH (1977). *Toys and Reasons—Stages in the Ritualization of Experience.* New York: WW Norton.

Eron LD, and Peterson, RA (1982). Abnormal behavior—social approaches. *Annual Review of Psychology, 33,* 231–264.

Fetrow, CW, and Avila, JR (1999). *A Professional's Handbook of Complementary and Alternative Medicines.* Springhouse, PA: Springhouse Corporation.

Finkel, SI (1993, November). The nursing home patient and prescribing psychotherapeutic drugs. *Nursing Home Medicine, 1*(6) 6–9.

Fischer, CA, and Schwart, CA (eds) (1996). *Encyclopedia of Associations,* 30th ed., Vols. 1 and 2. Detroit: Gale Research.

Foreman, J (1999, June 6). *Boston Globe.* Crisis intervention helps if it's used right. *Minneapolis Star Tribune.*

Foreman, J (1999, December 12). *Boston Globe.* Depressed? Help is just a click away (or is it?). *Minneapolis Star Tribune.*

Foreman, J (1999, April 11). *Boston Globe.* Finding the keys to alcohol abuse. *Minneapolis Star Tribune.*

Foreman, J (1999, May 30). *Boston Globe.* New treatment speeds up detox process. *Minneapolis Star Tribune.*

Foreman, J (1999, June 27). *Boston Globe.* Schizophrenia: incurable, but treatable. *Minneapolis Star Tribune.*

Foreman, J (1999, December 5). *Boston Globe.* Popular depression remedy gets mixed reviews. *Minneapolis Star Tribune.*

Foreman, J (2000, January 23). *Boston Globe.* St. Johnswort, antidepressants don't mix. *Minneapolis Star Tribune.*

Fossett, B, and Nader-Moodie, M (2004). *Psychiatric Principles and Applications for General Patient Care,* 4th ed. Brockton, MA: Western Schools.

Gardenswartz, L, and Rowe, A (1999). *Managing Diversity in Health Care Manual.* San Francisco: Jossey-Bass.

Gibson, D, and Aiken, MM (1994, June). When your patient is depressed. *JPN, 44,* 441.

Gilligan, C (1982). *In a Different Voice; Psychological Theory and Women's Development.* Cambridge, MA: Harvard University Press.

Gilligan, S (1987). *Therapeutic Trances: The Cooperation Principle in Ericksonian Hypnotherapy.* New York: Brunner/Mazel.

Goodnight, GT (1991). *Homelessness: A Social Dilemma.* Chicago: National Textbook Group.

Grainger, RD (1991, July). What does time mean to you? *AJN, 91,* 13.

Griffin, D (1998, November/December). Vocational rehabilitation. *Case Review.*

Griffin, KL (2000, February 6). *Milwaukee Journal Sentinel.* Drug appears to safely reduce craving for alcohol, study says. *Minneapolis Star Tribune.*

Griffith, HW (1995). *Complete Guide to Symptoms, Illness & Surgery,* 3rd ed. New York: The Body Press/Perigee.

Grinder, J, and Bandler, R (1981). *Trance-Formations: Neuro-Linguistic Programming and the Structure of Hypnosis,* Ed. Andreas, C. Moab, UT: Real People Press.

Gross, D (1999). *Good Endings—Caring for the Dying Resident.* Longmeadow, MA: Cinnabar Press.

Grossberg, G (1998). *Antipsychotic Treatment Options/Considerations in the Geriatric Population.* Distance Learning Network, Inc. http://distancelearninginc.com.

Hamilton, C (1999, May). Balancing life through the art of Feng Shui. *Stressfree Living,* pp. 20–21.

Hartmann, T (1998). *Healing ADD—Simple Exercises That Will Change Your Daily Life.* Grass Valley, CA: Underwood Books.

Hatton C, Valente S, and Rink A (1977). Assessment of suicide risk. In *Suicide Assessment and Intervention* (p. 56). New York: Appleton-Century Crofts.

Hazelden Foundation (2000, December 14). *National Survey Reveals Bias Against Recovering Alcoholics and Addicts.* Center City, MN: Hazelden Foundation.

Health News (1998). Mental illness in juvenile offenders. Empower Health Corporation. http://go.drkoop.com/healthnews.

Heinerman, J (1996). *Heinerman's Encyclopedia of Juices, Teas & Tonics.* Englewood Cliffs, NJ: Prentice-Hall.

Hill, SS, and Howlett, HA (1993). *Success in Practical Nursing,* 2nd ed. Philadelphia: WB Saunders.

Holton, B (1999, August 3). The healing power of creatures great and small. *Family Circle,* pp. 82–84.

House Select Committee on Aging (1991).

Congressional Quarterly Almanac, 102nd Congress, 1st Session, Washington, DC: CQ Inc.

Ireland, K (1992, April 21). Aiding the elderly. *Family Circle, 105,* 18.

Jellinek, EM (1952). Phases of alcohol addiction. *Quarterly Journal of Studies in Alcohol,* pp. 673–684.

Jellinek, EM (1960). *Disease Concept of Alcoholism.* New Haven, CT: College and Universities Press.

Johnson, DW (1993). *Reaching Out—Interpersonal Effectiveness and Self-Actualization,* 5th ed. Needham Heights, MA: Allyn and Bacon.

Josefson, D (2000, January 15). Pain relief in US emergency rooms is related to patients' race. *BMJ, 320,* 139.

Jordan, MR, and Danielsen, AV (1999). What is pastoral counseling? *Harvard Mental Health Letter,* MDX Health Digest, Thrive Partners.

Kalman, N, and Waughfield, CG (1993). *Mental Health Concepts,* 3rd ed. Albany, NY: Delmar Publishers.

Kaplan, HL, and Sadock, BJ (1985). *Modern Synopsis of Comprehensive Textbook of Psychiatry,* 4th ed (pp. 361–383). Baltimore: Williams and Wilkins.

Keller, V, and Baker, L (2000, January). Communicate with care. *RN,* (1), 32. www.rnweb.com.

Keltner, NL, Schweke, LH, and Bostrom, CE (2003). *Psychiatric Nursing,* 4th ed. St. Louis, MO: Mosby, Inc.

Kemper, DW (1997). *Medica Health Handbook,* 13th ed. Boise, ID: Healthwise Publications.

Keville, K (1996). *Herbs for Health and Healing.* New York: Berkley Publishing Group.

Kluft, RP (1987). First rank symptoms as a diagnostic due to multiple personality disorder. *Am J Psychiatry, 144,* 293–298.

Kluft, RP (1987). An update on multiple personality disorder. *Hospital Community Psychiatry 38,* 363.

Kneisl, CR (August 1990). Nursing the mind: tools that work combating anxiety. *RN,* p. 48.

Kroger, W (1963). *Clinical and Experimental Hypnosis in Medicine, Dentistry and Psychology.* Philadelphia: J. B. Lippincott Company.

Kübler-Ross, E (1969). *On Death and Dying.* New York: Macmillan.

Lachs, MS, and Pillemer, K (February 16, 1995). Current concepts—abuse and neglect of elderly persons. *New England Journal of Medicine, 332,* 437–443.

Late-life depression: Usually treatable, usually ignored. (1999, March). *Consumer Reports on Health 1998, 10*(3), 6-8mdx Health Digest, Medical Data Exchange, Thrive Partners.

Leuckenotte, AG (1990). *Pocket Guide to Gerontologic Assessment.* St. Louis: CV Mosby.

Levine, D (June 1995). Your aging parents: Choosing a nursing home. *American Health, 1,* 82.

Lidell, L, et al. (1984). *The Book of Massage.* New York: Simon & Schuster Inc.

Lipowski, ZJ (1987). Somatization: medicine's unsolved problem. *Psychosomatics, 28,* 294–297.

Living with Schizophrenia and Other Mental Illness. (1999). Arlington, VA: National Alliance for the Mentally Ill.

Maltby, N, et al. (1994, November 16). Efficacy of tacrine and lecithin in mild to moderate Alzheimer's disease: double blind trial. *JAMA, 272,* 1476t (Reprint request to G. Anthony Broe, University of Sydney, Dept. of Geriatric Medicine, Repatriation General Hospital, Concord 2139, Australia).

McCarty, P (1995). *A Beginner's Guide to Shiatsu.* Garden City Park, NY: Avery Publishing Group.

McGue, M, and Gottesman, II (1989). Genetic linkage in schizophrenia: perspectives from a genetic epidemiology. *Schizophrenia Bulletin, 15,* 453–464.

Meisol, P (1999, January 10). *Baltimore Sun.* A kinder, gentler shock therapy returns. *Minneapolis Star Tribune.*

Merriam-Webster Dictionary (1994). Springfield, MA: Merriam-Webster, Inc.

Milliken, ME (1993). *Understanding Human Behavior,* 5th ed. Albany, NY: Delmar Publishers.

Moseley, B (1995, January/February). PT interview: "Still crazy after all these years." *Psychology Today, 28,* 30.

Murray, B (2004). *Psychiatric Nursing: Current Trends in Diagnosis and Treatment.* Brockton, MA: Western Schools.

Neeb, K (1994, October). The culture of nurses. *Nursingworld Journal, 20,* 1.

Nemeth, M (1994, October 31). An alarming trend—suicide among the young has quadrupled. *Macleans'* (Canada), *107,* 15.

O'Connor, NK (1995, April 12). Physician-assisted death. *JAMA, 273,* 1088–1089.

Ode, K (1999, October 17). Kids not immune from depression. *Minneapolis Star Tribune,* E4.

Omnibus Mental Illness Recovery Act (OMIRA) (1999). (brochure). National Alliance for the Mentally Ill.

Park, CC, with Shapiro, LN (1976). *You Are Not Alone.* Boston: Little, Brown.

Parker, BA (1992, May). When your medical/surgical patient is also mentally ill. *Nursing 92, 22,* 66.

Peplau, HE (1952). *Interpersonal Relations in Nursing.* New York: GP Putnam's Sons.

Peterson, D (1992, July 19). Hennepin's alcoholic treatment questioned. *Minneapolis Star Tribune.*

Prochaska, JO (1984). *Systems of Psychotherapy.* Pacific Grove, CA: Brooks-Cole Publishing.

Purtilo, R, and Haddad, A (2002). *Health Professional and Patient Interaction,* 6th ed. Philadelphia: W.B. Saunders Company.

Quill, TE (1993). *Death and Dignity—Making Choices and Taking Charge.* New York: WW Norton.

RCS Rizzoli Libri (1994). *A-Z of Alternative Therapy.* Stamford, CT: Longmeadow Press.

Reiss, BS, and Evans, ME (1996). *Pharmacological Aspects of Nursing Care,* 5th ed. Albany, NY: Delmar Publishers.

Researchers question long-standing care for patients in isolation. (1999, October 17). *(Washington Post) Minneapolis Star Tribune.*

Rodgers, JE (1994, September/October). Addiction—a whole new view. *Psychology Today, 27,* 32.

Ross, CA, Anderson, G, Heber, S, and Norton, GR (1990). Dissociation and abuse among multiple personality patients, prostitutes, and exotic dancers. *Hospital Community Psychiatry, 41,* 328.

Rossi, EL, and Cheek, DB (1988). *Mind-Body Therapy: Methods of Ideodynamic Healing in Hypnosis.* New York: W. W. Norton & Co.

Rossi, PH (1989). *Down and Out in America—The Origins of Homelessness.* Chicago: University of Chicago Press.

Rubin, Z, Peplau, L, and Salovey, P (1993). *Psychology.* Boston: Houghton Mifflin.

Sarason, IG, and Sarason, BR (1996). *Abnormal Psychology—The Problem of Maladaptive Behavior.* Englewood Cliffs, NJ: Prentice-Hall.

Scherer, JC (1991). *Introductory Medical-Surgical Nursing,* 5th ed. Philadelphia: JB Lippincott.

Shapiro, PG (1982). *Caring for the Mentally Ill.* New York: Franklin Watts.

Schwartz, Mark S, and Olsen, RP (1995). *Biofeedback: A Practitioner's Guide,* 2nd ed., Ed. Mark S. Schwartz and Associates. New York: The Guilford Press.

Shives, LR and Isaacs, A. (2002). *Basic Concepts of Mental Health Nursing,* 5th ed. Philadelphia: JB Lippincott.

Sierpina, VS (2001) *Integrative Health Care— Complementary and Alternative Therapies for the Whole Person.* Philadelphia: F.A. Davis Company.

Smith, R (2000, January 15). A good death. *BMJ, 320,* (12)9–130.

Smyth, MG, and Hoult, J (2000, January 29). The home treatment enigma. *BMJ 320,* 305–309.

Skinner, K (1993, December). The hazards of chemical dependency among nurses. *JPN, 43,* 4.

Social science and the citizen: counting homelessness. (1994, November/December). *Society Magazine, 32,* 2.

Stogsdill, GW (1995). *Delmar's LPN/LVN Review Series: Mental Health.* Albany, NY: Delmar Publishers.

Stone, S (1999, February). Good health through good humor. *Nursing Homes Long Term Care Management,* pp. 53–54.

Storlie, FJ (1994, July). An unfinished symphony—the mind heals at its own tempo. *Nursing94, 24,* 88.

Subramanian, S (1995, January 16). The story in our genes—a landmark global study flattens the bell curve, proving that racial differences are only skin deep. *Time,* p. 34.

Sullivan PF, Neale, MC, and Kendler, KS (2000). Genetic epidemiology of major depression: review and meta-analysis. *American Journal of Psychiatry 157,* 1552–1562.

Taylor, BC (2003, August 12). Lawsuit alleges civil rights violations in Cook County jail; Complaint says inmates with mental illnesses face discrimination, lack of services. Chicago: Ascribe Newswire, Inc.

Thompson, M, and Johnson, KA (1993). *Black Health Guide to Obesity.* New York: Henry Holt and Company.

Tobacco use among middle and high school students—United States, 1999. (2000, January 28). *Morbidity and Mortality Weekly, 49*(3), 49–53.

Valfre, MM (2001) *Foundations of Mental Health Care,* 2nd ed. St. Louis, MO. Mosby.

Waughfield, CG (2002). *Mental Health Concepts,* 5th ed. Clifton Park, NY: Delmar/Thompson Learning, Inc.

Wei, JY, and Sheehan, MN (1997). *Geriatric Medicine: A Case Based Manual.* New York: Oxford Medical Publications, Oxford University Press, Inc.

West Publishing Company (1984). *The Guide to American Law* (Vol. 5, p. 388 and Vol. 8, p. 6). St. Paul, MN: West Publishing.

Will, GF (1999, December 5). Alternative to "mental cosmetic" Ritalin might be school choice. *(Washington Post). Minneapolis Star Tribune.*

Wolf, M (1992, June). Abuse of the elderly—How to spot it! How to help! *Good Housekeeping,* p. 221.

Woodward, KL (1994, May 23). An identity of wisdom ideas: Erik H. Erikson (1902–1994). *Newsweek,* p. 56.

Zamichow, N (1999, July 11). *Los Angeles Times.* Therapists use movies to give patients a new perspective. *Minneapolis Star Tribune.*

Zinn, L (1999, August). Is managed care in your future? *Nursing Homes Long Term Care Management,* pp. 28–30.

PUBLIC DOMAIN SOURCES

Caring for People with Severe Mental Disorders: A National Plan of Research to Improve Services (1995). National Institute of Mental Health, DHHS Pub. No. (ADM) 91–1762. Washington, DC: US Government Printing Office.

DHHS (NIOSH) (1996, July) *Violence in the Workplace—Risk Factors and Prevention Strategies.* Washington, DC: DHHS Publication No. 96–100.

Hendrix, ML (1993). *Bipolar Disorder—Decade of the Brain.* NIH Pub. No. 93–3679 (Formerly DHHS Publication No. (ADM) 90–1609. Washington, DC: Alcohol, Drug Abuse and Mental Health Administration).

Internet (1995). *Alzheimer's Disease— Decade of the Brain.*

www.allina.com
rnweb.com

ombudmhmr.state.mn.us
bmj.com/cgi/content/full/320/7228/139/a
hazelden.org
dlnetwork.com (Antipsychotic/elderly)
cdc.gov/niosh/homepage.html
http://go.drkoop.com/healthnews

Office of the Ombudsman for Mental Health and Mental Retardation, Suite 420, Metro Square Bldg., St Paul, MN 55101–2107 1-800-657-3506 TTY/voice 1-800-627-3529

Glossary

Abuse: Physical, verbal, or emotional mistreatment of self or others; misuse of chemicals, food, or other substances.

Abuser: One who abuses.

Accommodate: Process of adjusting one's schema to fit changing situations (Piaget).

Addiction: Condition of being physically and/or emotionally dependent on a substance or situation (e.g., alcohol, drugs, gambling). Withdrawal symptoms are experienced when the substance is removed or the activity is stopped.

Advocacy: Act of ensuring that patients, especially those classified as "vulnerable," are being treated in a safe, legal manner.

Affect: The outward display or expression of a feeling or mood.

Ageism: Form of discrimination against people on the basis of age.

Aggressive communication: Form of communication that hurts another and is not self-responsible ("you" statements).

Alcohol abuse: Compulsive use of alcohol usually lasting 1 month or longer.

Alcohol dependence: Improper use of alcohol with impairment of social or occupational functioning, which leads to signs of tolerance or withdrawal.

Alternative medicine: Modalities that replace those of conventional medicine.

Alzheimer's disease: Organic brain disorder; primary dementia.

Anorexia: Serious aversion to food, which can lead to malnutrition and death.

Antidepressant: Classification of psychoactive medication used to treat depression.

Antimanic: Classification of psychoactive medication used to treat manic behavior, such as in bipolar disorder.

Antiparkinson agent: Classification of medication used to treat the symptoms of both drug-induced and non-drug-induced parkinsonism.

Antipsychotics: Classification of psychoactive medications used to treat psychotic behavior found in disorders such as schizophrenia and organic brain disorders.

Antisocial personality: Personality type that requires immediate gratification. People with this personality type are often in trouble with the law. Also called sociopathic or psychopathic personality.

Anxiety: Feelings of uneasiness or apprehension.

Aphasia: Inability to speak, or speech that is ineffective.

Aromatherapy: Related to herbal therapy; provides treatment by both direct pharmacologic effects of aromatic plant substances and indirect effects of certain smells on mood and affect.

Assertive communication: Self-responsible statements that begin with the word "I" and deal with thoughts, feelings, and honesty.

Assimilating: Taking in, processing, incorporating new information (Piaget).

Autonomy: Development of a sense of self and independence (Erikson).

Bariatric: study of medicine and nursing involving weight management, treatment, and surgeries for morbidly obese patients.

Behavior: Any action or activity that can be observed.

Behavior modification: Form of treatment in which variables are manipulated to encourage and reinforce desired behavioral changes.

Beliefs: Concepts, opinions, and ideas that are accepted as true and are usually not exactly the same for each individual.

Biofeedback: Method of teaching patients to recognize tension within the body and to respond with relaxation.

Bipolar: Form of depression in which the person usually experiences cycles of extreme elation and extreme depression.

Body image: Individual's perception of his or her body.

Borderline personality: Disorder in which there is disturbance of self-image, moods, and relationships. May begin in early adulthood.

Bulimia: Eating disorder in which a person experiences eating binges, purging, or uncontrollable intake of food.

Catatonia: Rigidity and inflexibility of muscles, resulting in immobility or extreme agitation.

Collaborative: Form of care in which nurses work together and with other disciplines for the betterment of patient care.

Cognitive: Pertaining to the thought process and the ability to think.

Commitment: The act of forced hospitalization, frequently against the patient's will, for a specific purpose.

Communication: Method of transmitting messages between a sender and a receiver. Can be verbal or nonverbal.

Communication block: Method of communication that impedes helpful interactions with patients.

Community Mental Health Centers Act of 1963: A result of President John F. Kennedy's concern for the treatment of the mentally ill.

Complementary medicine: Alternative methods used with traditional treatments.

Compulsion: Unwanted, repetitive urge to perform or actual performance of a behavior.

Confidentiality: The act of maintaining privacy of patient information.

Conversion: Transference of anxiety into physical symptoms.

Coping: The act of successfully adapting psychologically, physically, and behaviorally to problems or stressors.

Counseling: One of several forms of therapy.

Crisis: Extreme state of emotional turmoil.

Culture: Nonphysical traits, rituals, values, and traditions that are handed down to others from generation to generation.

Culture of nurses: Professional values, rituals, and traditions passed down from one generation of nurses to the next.

DSM-IV-TR: *Diagnostic and Statistical Manual of Mental Disorders, Text Revision,* 4th edition.

Data collection: Gathering of information about a patient; part of nursing process.

Date rape: Unwanted sexual intercourse between people who have been together and in which the party who pays for the date expects sex in return.

Defense mechanisms: Group of behaviors used to reduce or eliminate anxiety. Unconsciously falling into habits that give the illusion of coping but produce ineffective results.

Deinstitutionalization: Policy in which people who had formerly required long hospital stays became able to leave the institutions and return to their communities and homes.

Delirium: Acute brain syndrome; rapid onset of cognitive impairments such as loss of memory and disorientation.

Delirium tremens (DTs): Form of withdrawal from alcohol in which the person experiences, among other symptoms, tremors, hallucinations, delirium, and diaphoresis.

Delusion: Fixed, false belief relating usually to persecution or grandeur.

Dementia: Gradual, progressive, chronic deterioration of intellectual functioning, judgment, memory, and so forth.

Dependent: Relying on another person or substance.

Dissociate: To separate a strong emotional response from the consciousness.

Drug abuse: Compulsive use of a drug, usually lasting 1 month or longer.

Drug dependence: Same as alcohol dependence, but with other drugs.

Dysfunctional: Having abnormal or ineffective function in mental health pertaining to coping and relationships.

Dysmorphophobia: Preoccupation with an imagined defect in appearance.

Dysphasia: Difficulty in speaking.

Dysthymia: Depressive neurosis.

ECT: Electroconvulsive therapy, reserved for types of depression or schizophrenia not responding to other forms of treatment. A current is passed through the patient, resulting in mild seizure and temporary coma.

Echolalia: Repetition of phrases, words, or part of a word; often part of catatonia.

Echopraxia: Repetition of movements; often part of catatonia.

Ego: Second part of Freud's personality development, balancing the id; the ego meets and interacts with the outside world.

Elder abuse: Physical, emotional, or sexual abuse of older adults.

Elderly: Pertaining to older people, often described as people over 60 years old.

Empathy: Therapeutic communication technique of understanding another person's emotion without actually experiencing the emotion.

Emotional abuse: Willful use of words or actions that undermine another person's self-esteem.

Ethics: Professional expectations that focus on legal issues.

Ethnic: Pertaining to races; physical or linguistic characteristics of a group of people.

Ethnicity: The condition of identifying with an ethnic group.

Eustress: Type of stress that results from the "good" life (experiences such as raises, promotions, and so on).

Evaluation: Part of nursing process that summarizes nursing interventions.

Feeling: Emotion.

Feeling statement: Statement that must identify an emotion that one is experiencing or trying to explore (e.g., "I feel proud" or "I feel frightened").

Free-floating anxiety: Anxiety that has no identifiable cause; feeling of "impending doom."

Geriatrics: Branch of medicine that deals with the illnesses and treatment of elderly people.

Gerontology: The study of aging and old age.

Hallucination: False sensory perception; can affect any of the five senses.

Health-illness continuum: Theory that physical and mental health and illness fluctuate somewhat on a daily basis, while staying within a social norm of behavior.

Hill-Burton Act: The first major act or law to address mental illness. It provided money to build psychiatric units in hospitals.

Hypnotherapy: Means for entering an altered state of consciousness, and in this state, use visualization and suggestion to bring about desired changes in behavior and thinking.

Hypochondriasis: Condition of unrealistic or exaggerated concern over minor symptoms.

Hypomania: Hyperactive behavior that consists of a less active manic state than mania.

Id: First part of Freud's personality theory, which is preoccupied with self-gratification.

Illusion: Misinterpretation of a sensory perception.

Implementation: Part of the nursing process that identifies specific actions a nurse will do to help a patient meet a goal; nursing intervention.

Incest: Sexual activity between people who are so closely related that marriage is illegal.

Insidious: Referring to onset that is so gradual it is hardly noticed.

Integrative medicine: Combines conventional and less traditional treatment methods.

"La belle indifférence": Inappropriate lack of concern for symptoms.

Language barrier: Any situation that impedes communication.

Laryngectomee: Person who has had a laryngectomy.

Laryngectomy: Partial or total removal of the larynx ("voice box").

Lunar month: Twenty-eight-day cycle in prenatal development.

Malingering: Deliberate faking or exaggerating of symptoms.

Mania: Mood disorder in which a person displays extremely elated, agitated mood without signs of fatigue.

Memory: Mental function that enables a person to store and recall information.

Menarche: First menstrual period.

Mental health: State of being able to work, love, and resolve conflicts simultaneously.

Mental illness: Disturbance of emotional homeostasis.

Methamphetamine: Illegal, highly addictive and highly dangerous substance, usually smoked; able to be made from common household items.

Milieu: Environment for treating patients.

Models: pictures or ideas that we form in our minds to explain how things work; they help us understand and interact with other people and our environment and help to formulate beliefs.

Monoamine oxidase inhibitors: Group of antidepressant medications used for people who do not respond to the tricyclic antidepressants.

Mood: Feeling state.

Morbid Obesity: Condition of being abnormally overweight; weight that is 100 pounds or more above established norms.

Narcissistic personality: Disorder that displays exaggerated self-love and self-importance.

National Mental Health Act of 1946: Part of the result of the first Congress to be held after World War II, providing money for training and research in nursing care (and other patient care disciplines) to improve care for people with mental illnesses.

Neglect: Omission of providing for the needs of a dependent person.

Neurolinguistic Programming (NLP): Theory that language cues can be used to understand how an individual experiences his or her world, allowing a practitioner to help patients change their experience and respond to problems in a different way; uses visual, auditory, and kinesthetic channels.

Nursing Interventions Classifications (NIC): A comprehensive standardized language of intervention labels and possible nursing actions.

Nursing Outcome Classifications (NOC): A standardized language that provides outcome statements and a set of indicators describing specific patient, caregiver, family, or community states related to the outcome.

Nonverbal communication: Actions, tone of voice, body motions, facial expressions, and so forth; the subjective part of the process.

Nursing process: Established system of data collecting and care planning performed by nurses.

Nursing diagnosis: Nonmedical statement of an existing or potential problem.

Nurse Practice Act: Act that dictates the acceptable scope of nursing practice for the different levels of nursing.

Obsession: Repetitive thought that cannot be ignored by the patient.

Omnibus Budget Reconciliation Act (OBRA): Act that was activated in 1981 to allow federal money to be allocated differently.

Orientation: Measurement of knowledge of person, place, and time in the mental health assessment.

Panic disorder: Condition of having one or more panic attacks, followed by the fear of having others.

Paranoid: Referring to a state of extreme suspiciousness.

Parenting: Raising children; referring to styles of raising children.

Passive/aggressive personality: Most common of the personality disorders; typified by dependent behavior; "chip-on-the-shoulder" attitude.

Patient Bill of Rights: Federal and state guidelines to ensure the civil rights of people who are entrusted to the care of health-care providers in hospitals, nursing homes, and so on.

Personality: Sum of the behaviors and character traits of a person.

Personality disorder: Nonpsychotic, maladaptive behavior that is used to satisfy the self.

Person-centered: Humanistic theory of unconditional positive regard for the person, involving treatment of the whole person rather than just the illness.

P.E.S.: Newer format diagnostic statement for care planning. Model. "P" the problem or need, "E" the etiology or cause, and "S" the signs, symptoms, or risk factors.

Phobia: Irrational fear.

Physical abuse: Any actions by omission or commission that cause physical harm to another.

Placebo: A neutral, inactive agent given in place of medication that produces symptom relief or other desired effects based upon the patient's expectations and beliefs.

Plan of care: Nursing process and medical orders that dictate a patient's daily care.

Post-traumatic stress: Reaction to witnessing or experiencing severe trauma that was not expected (e.g., rape, war).

Prejudice: Prejudging people or situations before knowing all the facts.

Presupposition: Assumptions we make when forming communication.

Primary gain: Relief of anxiety by use of defense mechanisms or the act of remaining physically or mentally unhealthy.

Professional: Refers to performing a skill for pay.

Proxemics: Study of spatial relationships including space, time, and waiting, which are all influenced by one's culture.

Psychoanalysis: Method of psychotherapy based in Freudian theory; uses free association and dream interpretation as part of the treatment. Treatment in this style is usually long-term.

Psychopharmacology: Medications as they are used and prescribed for mental illness.

Psychosexual: Referring to Freud's theory of personality and development in which behavior is related to the sexual gratification or lack of it received in early development.

Puberty: Stage of development at which sexual organs mature and one is capable of reproducing.

Rapport: the matching of speech patterns using auditory, kinesthetic, and visual references that provide a starting point for meaningful communication.

Rape: Violent sexual act that is performed against one's will.

Rational-emotive: Form of therapy involving a rational balance between thinking and feeling.

Reflexology: Massage and manipulation of the feet that acts upon energy pathways in the body, unblocking and renewing the energy flow.

Reiki: form of energy work incorporating touch that manipulates the client's energy along body meridians, or pathways.

Religion: Set of beliefs about one's spirituality, rituals, and worship.

Respite care: Relief supplied to primary caregivers (e.g., hospice).

Responsibility: Accountability.

Safe house: Specified "secret" place for people who are being abused to go for shelter.

Schizoid personality: Personality disorder characterized by being a loner and desiring little or no social contact.

Schizophrenia: Serious mental health disorder characterized by impaired communication, alteration of reality, and deterioration of personal and vocational functioning.

Secondary gain: Response to illness that results in attention, monetary benefits, and the like.

Sexual abuse: Unwanted sexual contact.

Sexual harassment: Unwanted sexual innuendo, often inflicted by a workplace superior on an employee or subordinate.

Signal anxiety: Stress response to a known stressor.

Social communication: The day-to-day interaction with personal acquaintances. Slang or "street language" may be used. Less literal and purposeful in social interactions.

Sociopathic: See Antisocial personality.

Somatization: Emotional turmoil that is expressed by physical symptoms, often loss of functioning of a body part.

Somatoform pain disorder: Anxiety that results in severe pain that is far in excess of what would normally be expected.

Spouse abuse: Physical, emotional, or sexual mistreatment of one's husband or wife.

Stereotype: A general opinion or belief.

Stimulant: Classification of medication that directly stimulates the central nervous system.

Stress: Emotional strain or anxiety.

Stressor: Condition that produces stress in an individual.

Suicide: The act of purposefully taking one's own life.

Suicide contract: Contract between the patient and nurse (or significant other) in which the patient will call the designated person when the patient has thoughts of suicide.

Suicide pact: Agreement made among a group of people (often adolescents) to kill themselves together.

Survivor: One(s) remaining after the death of another.

Survivor guilt: Feeling of guilt at being a survivor; often seen in post-traumatic stress disorder.

Superego: Third part of Freud's personality theory; the conscience, which deals with morality.

Sympathy: Nontherapeutic technique of experiencing the emotion along with the patient.

Therapeutic communication: Also called active or purposeful communication; communication that attempts to determine a patient's needs.

Thought: An opinion, idea, or fact that one wishes to express.

Tolerance: Ability to endure the effects of a chemical or the need for more to achieve a "high."

Trance: A state of altered awareness of a client's surroundings that brings the individual's focus of attention to an internal experience, such as a memory or imagined event.

Unconscious: Refers to idea and behaviors that are concealed from awareness.

Verbal abuse: Method of harming another by using degrading or foul language.

Verbal communication: Process of exchanging information by the spoken or written word; the objective part of the process of communication.

Victim: A person who is harmed by another.

Withdrawal: Physical and psychological effects of decreasing or stopping intake of a drug (e.g., alcohol, cocaine, and the like).

Index

Page numbers followed by t indicates tables.